Implementing
Women's Sexual Health and
Reproductive Rights
in South Asia

Credits

Original painting: Ms. Rabia Yaseen, Final year medical student, Services Institute of Medical Sciences, Lahore, Pakistan

Photography: Mr. Asad Shahzad, Fourth year medical student, Services Institute of Medical Sciences, Lahore, Pakistan

Implementing
Women's Sexual Health and
Reproductive Rights
in South Asia

Editors

Rubina Sohail
MBBS, FCPS, DCPS-HPE, FRCOG

Professor, Department of Obstetrics and Gynecology
Services Institute of Medical Sciences
President, South Asian Federation of
Obstetrics and Gynaecology (SAFOG)
Chair, FIGO Committee on Violence against Women
125-B, Ahmad Block, New Garden Town, Lahore, Pakistan

Narendra Malhotra
MD, FICMCH, FICOG, FICS, FRCOG, FMAS, AFIAP

Professor, Sarajevo School of Science and Technology, Croatia
Vice President, World Association of Perinatal Medicine (WAPM)
Director, Ian Donald School of Ultrasound
President, Indian Society of Prenatal Diagnosis and Therapy (ISPAT), 2017–2019
Secretary General, SAFOG, 2015–2019
Vice President, SAFOG, 2019–2021
84, MG Road, Agra 282010, Uttar Pradesh, India

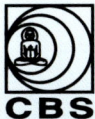

CBS Publishers & Distributors Pvt Ltd

New Delhi • Bengaluru • Chennai • Kochi • Kolkata • Mumbai
Hyderabad • Jharkhand • Nagpur • Patna • Pune • Uttarakhand

Implementing
Women's Sexual Health and
Reproductive Rights
in South Asia

ISBN: 978-93-89017-61-8

First Edition: 2021

Published by Satish Kumar Jain and produced by Varun Jain for

CBS Publishers & Distributors Pvt Ltd

4819/XI Prahlad Street, 24 Ansari Road, Daryaganj, New Delhi 110 002, India
Ph: 23289259, 23266861, 23266867 Website: www.cbspd.com
Fax: 011-23243014   e-mail: delhi@cbspd.com; cbspubs@airtelmail.in

Corporate Office: 204 FIE, Industrial Area, Patparganj, Delhi 110 092
Ph: 4934 4934   Fax: 4934 4935   e-mail: publishing@cbspd.com; publicity@cbspd.com

Branches

- **Bengaluru:** Seema House 2975, 17th Cross, K.R. Road, Banasankari 2nd Stage, Bengaluru 560 070, Karnataka
  Ph: +91-80-26771678/79   Fax: +91-80-26771680   e-mail: bangalore@cbspd.com
- **Chennai:** 7, Subbaraya Street, Shenoy Nagar, Chennai 600 030, Tamil Nadu
  Ph: +91-44-26680620/26681266   Fax: +91-44-42032115   e-mail: chennai@cbspd.com
- **Kochi:** 42/1325, 1326, Power House Road, Opp KSEB Power House, Ernakulam 682 018, Kochi, Kerala
  Ph: +91-484-4059061-67   Fax: +91-484-4059065   e-mail: kochi@cbspd.com
- **Kolkata:** 6/B, Ground Floor, Rameswar Shaw Road, Kolkata 700 014, West Bengal
  Ph: +91-33-22891126, 22891127, 22891128   e-mail: kolkata@cbspd.com
- **Mumbai:** 83-C, Dr E Moses Road, Worli, Mumbai 400018, Maharashtra
  Ph: +91-22-24902340/41   Fax: +91-22-24902342   e-mail: mumbai@cbspd.com

Representatives

- **Hyderabad**   0-9885175004   • **Jharkhand**   0-9811541605   • **Nagpur**   0-9421945513
- **Patna**   0-9334159340   • **Pune**   0-9623451994   • **Uttarakhand**   0-9716462459

Printed at: Goyal Offset Works (P) Ltd., India

"I fight for the dignity of all people, especially women, whose rights are trampled upon.
It is time that we all invest in the business of gender rights promotion"

—Amina Marie Grace Safi
Democratic Republic of Congo

Foreword

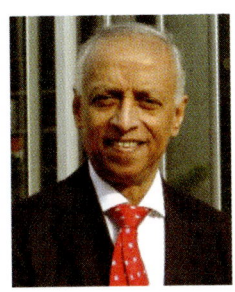

I am absolutely thrilled to see the South Asian Federation of Obstetricians and Gynaecologists (SAFOG) book *Implementing Women's Sexual Health and Reproductive Rights in South Asia*. In 1995 at the Women's Conference in Beijing, the world witnessed the declaration of 'Planet 50:50 by the year 2030'. Twenty years later in 2015, the UN made gender equality as SDG 5— a goal to be reached by 2030. These goals and declarations would not be achieved by 2030, unless every one of us work towards it individually and collectively. Mostly we hear of the problems and not the solutions that can be implemented. The book by SAFOG spearheaded by the dynamic President, Prof Rubina Sohail, addresses the issue of *strategy to action* steering SAFOG and its members to stand tall amongst the professional organisation and professionals to deliver solutions to empower women to exercise their sexual and reproductive health and rights. The contents of the book gives a clear message to its members and others to work hard and to assist the UN, Governments and Societies to achieve its SDG goals especially Goals 3 and 5. The globe cannot survive and thrive without gender equality and empowerment of women.

My sincere congratulations to the Editors, President of SAFOG, Prof Rubina Sohail and Prof Narendra Malhotra and the formidable authors from each of the countries which constitute the SAFOG. The book deserves credit for providing the situational analysis in each country in Part 1 followed by issues and solutions in Part 2 and progressing to description of practical steps for way forward in Part 3. Issues of contraception, safe abortion care, STD, HIV/AIDS, rape, gender violence, genital mutilation, other harmful practices and lack of empowerment are covered in detail.

As professionals we are good in providing the best medical care but in many instances we subconsciously forget the human rights issues of right for life, health, privacy, respectful care, confidentiality, information, decision making, reproductive choices, etc. These are well explained in Part 3 including the effect of religion and culture on sexual and reproductive health and rights of women.

This book should be in the hands of every health professional and the content taught to undergraduates, postgraduates and clinicians. Globally SAFOG has the biggest population of women and adolescents and witnesses a high burden of sexual and reproductive health and rights violation due to poverty, corruption, poor leadership, lack of political will exacerbated by natural and man-made disasters. I sincerely hope SAFOG will lead the way for other professional organisations to follow to establish 'Planet 50:50'.

With respect and kindest regards to members of SAFOG,

Yours sincerely,

Sir Sabaratnam Arulkumaran
Past President, RCOG, FIGO and BMA

Foreword

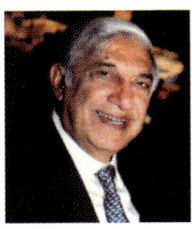

It gives me great pleasure in writing Foreword for the book written by multiple authors titled *Implementing Women's Sexual Health and Reproductive Rights in South Asia*. Being members of SAFOG we all understand the difficulties women face in our region, some difficulties are particularly our peculiar to this region due to our culture and traditions. To highlight these difficulties particularly related to sexual and reproductive rights in SAFOG countries is a great endeavor which I appreciate. The special feature of the book is that it is written by multiple authors from the SAFOG countries. I am sure it must have taken a lot of effort in organizing such a multiple authors' book.

I compliment Dr Rubina Sohail and Narendra Malhotra for undertaking this endeavor. I wish that this book is read by every practising gynecologist in SAARC countries. I hope it will achieve desired results or at least make a dent into the great mass of difficulties faced by women of this region and health care providers in our region.

Wishing you best of luck.

Rashid Latif Khan
Professor Emeritus
Past President, SAFOG

Message

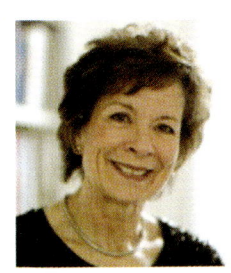

I n 2015, the world's nations came together to agree to end all forms of discrimination, violence and exploitation against women and girls, in total 193 nations signed. The General Secretary of the United Nations at the time, Ban Ki-moon, famously declared: "Let the 21st century be the century of women." To put this in context, to achieve this vision we must reach beyond the achievements made by our predecessors to ensure that for the first time in history the rights of women and girls are considered equal with the rest of society.

There is much to do. While we are continually making improvements and using our skills to advocate for safe, high quality and sustainable health care, we need to address both symptom and cause. For every instance of poor practice, inequality and harm done to women, there exists a system which actively supports or tacitly condones this violence. We must not forget that the health of women correlates to their educational achievement, which enriches and benefits all society and hugely reduces morbidity and mortality. It is time for all nations to prioritise education for girls and women and adopt a broader commitment to ending discrimination based on gender. By challenging the barriers women face when accessing health care, we must not forget to challenge the barriers to education which so often originate from the same source.

The Sustainable Development Goals set by the UN in 2015 provide us with a unique opportunity to address the inequality women and girls have experienced for millennia. We can join together, hold our governments and our societies accountable and create a healthier global population. Until this is achieved, we all must continue to advocate for the empowerment of women.

As obstetricians and gynaecologists we deal with many complex and difficult issues. However, safeguarding the dignity of women is neither complex nor difficult and should be at the centre of our practice and teaching. To deny access or to consider the rights of women and their choices as secondary issues in delivering health care is to misunderstand. Health care is not something given to a patient but a tool to empower them.

I would like to commend the editors who have gathered together so many colleagues dedicated to the advancement of women's rights in South Asia and beyond. I am especially pleased that we are not only shedding light on the current situation in many different nations, each with their own barriers and challenges, but collectively taking responsibility for the rights of women and girls and committing to driving change everywhere.

Lesley Regan
President, RCOG
Treasurer, FIGO

Message

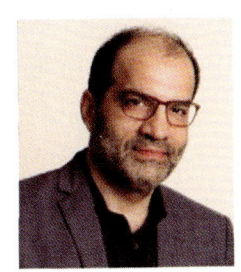

Sexual and reproductive health rights (SRHR) are essential for populations' health, economic development and survival. SRHR accounts for multiple components including sexual and reproductive health and well-being of humanity. Historically, two diverse movements achieved construction of reproductive rights as human rights: The population movement and the women's movement. Both movements traversed turbid paths and landmarks. From the first International Conference on Human Rights, held in Tehran, Iran in 1968, to the World Population Conference, 1974, in Bucharest, Romania, to Nederland, 1984, coining new ideologies linking population growth to reproductive rights. The term reproductive rights was later enshrined in the ground-breaking conference, the International Conference on Population and Development (ICPD) Cairo, 1994, and in Beijing, 1995. All countries around the globe have an obligation to fulfil, respect and protect women's sexual and reproductive health rights. As stated by the special rapporteur women must have access to reproductive good quality health care services (HCS) that are available, physically and economically accessible.

Despite, violation of woman's SRHR happens frequently, the Lancet Commission report of 2018, claims that around 4.3 billion people, mostly from developing and underdeveloped regions, have inadequate HCS that account for 200 millions of women who have no access to contraception and are unable to prevent unwanted pregnancy that result in yearly estimated 25 millions of unsafe abortions procedures. In addition, 30 million women have no access to safe childbirth under skilled attendance, and 45 million do not have access to antenatal care. Moreover, 350 million men and women are in need for STI treatment, where 2 millions are newly infected with HIV. WHO, UNFPA, FIGO, and other international organizations seriously addressed these SRHR violations. Sadly enough, and in many parts of the world, SRHR violations present in many forms and patterns including but not restricted to, poor access to HCS, forced sterilization, coercive sex/rape, virginity testing, selective feticide, female genital mutation, sexual orientation, and early marriage. Inadequate sexual and reproductive health adds to societal inequalities as well as contributes to poor social and economic development.

Looking at the SRHR status in the extended MENA and SEA regions, studies have shown that SRHR is particularly affected by the cultural sensitivies, politics, societal patriarchy, public space stigmatization, and most recently conflict and wars. Despite the presence of national strategies for youth, women and reproductive health in some of the countries, these strategies remain short of adopting the human rights approach and gender equality lens in implementation. Misrepresentation of human rights happens due to the multiple factors. Women are being deprived of their rights, especially in rural areas, due to the inherited patriarchal social and cultural traditions that disregard equality. Poor awareness about the importance of SRHR problem among local legal professionals, along with the lack of collaboration with health care workers led to the insufficient realization of SRHR. Another issue is the lack of awareness among women about their own health rights, which prevents them from the use of services.

Serious gaps were identified in SRHR among many countries in the region, gaps that will continue to deter the proper establishment and implementation of SRHR-based policies and programmes, and will keep the 2 regions lagging behind achieving SDG 2030. There are many entries to catch up with the global debate and pace regarding SRHR. This textbook represents a window of opportunity in that regard that will help raise awareness among both the professionals and the public helping steer SRHR implementation towards the right and appropriate direction.

Faysal El Kak
Vice President, FIGO
President, FAGOS

Message

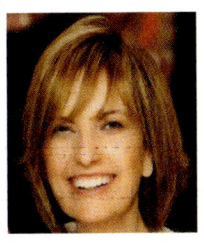

This book, fruit of contributions made by esteemed and knowledgeable colleagues, is a source of invaluable information on some of the greatest challenges in the field of women's health and well-being in the South Asian region. The layout chosen not only provides vital information on the current obstetrical and gynaecological situations in this area of the world, but also an overview of real-life situations and proposes solutions so as to apply a rights-based approach to health care.

It includes issues such as respectful maternity care, sexual health and reproductive rights, violence against women, child marriage, female genital mutilation, maternal mortality, women's empowerment, the control of STIs and much more, all of which are common to OB-GYN specialists, be they in more or less advantaged environments.

However, diversity, multiculturalism and customs on what women can, and are expected to do, often make for difficult trouble-shooting and solution finding.

This book provides those working in the field of obstetrics and gynaecology with a roadmap of how to improve women's health and rights and deserves to have a wide readership if we are to implement a rights-based approach to girls' and women's health and to meet the Sustainable Development Goals.

Chiara Benedetto
Chair, FIGO Committee for Women's Health
and Human Rights 2015–2018
Past President, EBCOG

Message

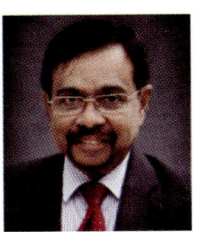

S exual and reproductive health and rights (SRHR), being the concept of human rights applied to sexuality and reproduction, is inevitably an important area of concern to practising obstetricians and gynecologists. This is more so, in the SAFOG region where countries differ widely in their socio-cultural dimensions in addition to their geography with wide-ranging hiatuses in the area of SRH rights enjoyed by women in respective countries especially in the poor, rural or migrant communities.

SAFOG has identified the glaring need of taking stock of the situation of SRHR within its member countries as the first initiative in addressing these issues which will underpin the efforts to follow to improve the reproductive health status of our sisters in the region.

The eminent professionals identified for the task were members of the national societies who had contributed much towards the well-being of women, especially in diverse areas related to SRHR and they as expected, have brought forth an excellent document which establishes clearly the current situation, future needs, as well as the challenges faced by individual countries together with specific suggestions towards overcoming them.

While congratulating Prof Rubina Sohail, President SAFOG, and Prof Narendra Malhotra, Secretary General, taking the initiative and the lead role in compiling this book, and thank them for producing a comprehensive book which will be of immense value not only for the practising obstetricians and gynaecologists, but also to all those involved with SRHR work. Let me also acknowledge the immense contribution made by the authors. I recommend everyone to carefully peruse the publication in order to expand their vistas on the subject of SRHR and move towards ensuring a better future for all women in our region.

Rohana Haththotuwa
Secretary General, AOFOG

Message

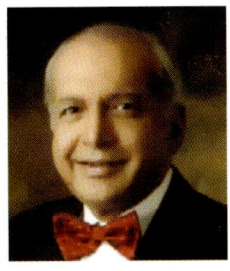

Human rights are the foremost and basic rights of all human beings, men as well as women. Sexual and reproductive rights in a way form essential components of various human rights pertaining to life, dignity, health and education. The practice of these rights can lead to improvement of the health and well-being of not only the women but also the society at large. Application of the principles enshrined in these rights ensures the well-being and empowerment of women that are so desirable in so many countries and regions of the world.

At present more than 200 million women in need lack access to effective contraception, unsafe abortion rates are unacceptably high, and preventable maternal and neonatal mortality though reduced considerably over the last three decades, requires significant efforts by many countries to be brought down to the levels enunciated in SDGs. All these are essentially interwoven with the sexual and reproductive rights of women.

South Asian countries, in particular, need to make progress in a number of areas pertaining to women's health and their rights situation. Social milieu of a male-dominated society is a major factor responsible for early marriages and repeated pregnancies with short intervals, many a times in quest for a male child. On the other hand, the woman is blamed for all that goes wrong, may that be infertility or abortion.

SAFOG's publication of *Implementing Women's Sexual Health and Reproductive Rights in South Asia* is a great step in highlighting the status of women's health as well as the rights situation in South Asia. The up-to-date data should be relevant to the policymakers to compare strategies adopted by various countries. The information given in the book makes it an essential read for health care professionals and all concerned with improvement of human rights. The attractive and uniform pattern of given information would help the reader putting things in perspective for these countries.

I would like to commend all the contributors and congratulate the members of the editorial board for their efforts in writing and compiling this very useful work.

CN Purandare
Past President, FIGO

Contributors

Aqeela Abbas
MBBS, FCPS
Coordinator, Maternal Nutrition and Lactation Management
Senior Registrar
Obstetrics and Gynaecology Services Hospital, Lahore, Pakistan

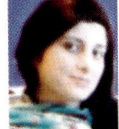

Asifa Naureen
MBBS, BSc, FCPS
Assistant Secretary General, SAFOG
Assistant Professor, Department of Obstetrics and Gynaecology
Services Institute of Medical Sciences, Lahore, Pakistan

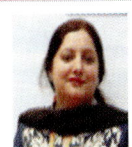

Athula Kaluarachchi
Professor, Department of Obstetrics and Gynaecology
University of Colombo, Sri Lanka

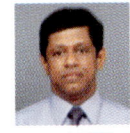

Asma Mushtaq
MBBS, FCPS
Assistant Professor, Department of Obstetrics and Gynaecology
Services Institute of Medical Sciences, Lahore, Pakistan

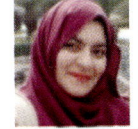

Augustus Keshala Probhodana Ranaweera
MBBS, MD, MRCOG
Senior Lecturer
Department of Obstetrics and Gynaecology
University of Colombo, Sri Lanka

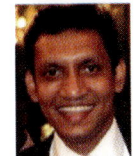
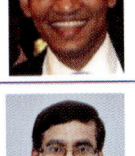

BB Rewari
MD, FRCP, FICP
Scientist HIV/STI Hepatitis
World Health Organization
Regional Office for South East Asia, New Delhi, India

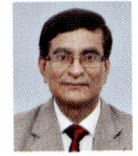

Bushra Haq
MBBS, MCPS, FCPS
Focal Person for PPIUCD
Assistant Professor, Department of Obstetrics and Gynaecology
Services Institute of Medical Sciences, Lahore, Pakistan

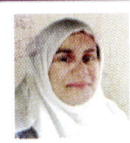

Chandana Jayasundara
MBBS, MD, MRCOG
Senior Lecturer
Department of Obstetrics and Gynaecology
University of Colombo, Sri Lanka

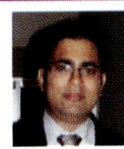

Fariha Nehreen Mirza
Final Year Medical Student
Ibrahim Medical College, Dhaka, Bangladesh

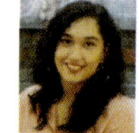

Ferdousi Begum
Professor, Department of Obstetrics and Gynaecology
Ibrahim Medical College and BIRDEM Hospital, Dhaka, Bangladesh

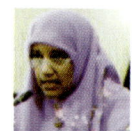

Hemantha Senanayake
President, Sri Lanka College of Obstetricians and Gynecologists
Professor, Department of Obstetrics and Gynaecology
University of Colombo, Sri Lanka

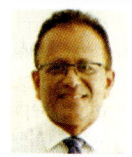

Humaira Saleem
MBBS, FCPS
Senior Registrar
Obstetrics and Gynaecology Services Hospital, Lahore, Pakistan

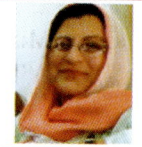

Kiren Khurshid
MBBS, FCPS, MHPE
Associate Professor, Department of Obstetrics and Gynaecology
Services Institute of Medical Sciences, Lahore, Pakistan

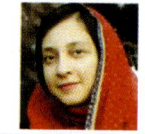

Kusum Thapa
Senior Maternal Health Advisor
Jhpiego, An Affiliate of Johns Hopkins University, US

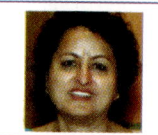

Laila Arjumand Banu
Immediate Past President OGSB
Secretary General FAOPS, Bangladesh

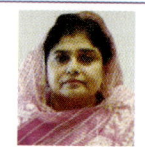

Madeeha Rashid
MBBS, MCPS, FCPS
Assistant Professor, Department of Obstetrics and Gynaecology
Services Institute of Medical Sciences, Lahore, Pakistan

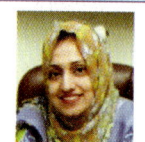

Malalai Jamshid Nejaby
MD, MPH
Board Member of Afghanistan Association of OB/GYN
Family Planning Maternal and Newborn Advisor Jhpiego, Afghanistan

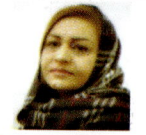

Mariam Iqbal
MBBS, FCPS, MHPE
Consultant, Department of Obstetrics and Gynaecology
Rashid Latif Medical College, Lahore, Pakistan

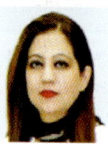

Mohammed Rishard
MBBS, MD, MRCOG, PG Cert Med
Senior Lecturer
Department of Obstetrics and Gynaecology
University of Colombo, Sri Lanka

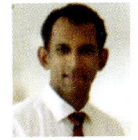

Mriganka Mouli Saha
MBBS, MS, DNB, MNAMS
Assistant Professor, Department of Obstetrics and Gynaecology
College of Medicine and JNM, WBUHS, Kalyani, West Bengal, India

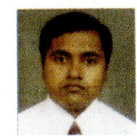

Narendra Malhotra
MD, FICMCH, FICOG, FICS, FRCOG, FMAS
Professor, Department of Obstetrics and Gynaecology
Dubrovnik International University

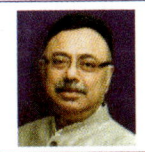

Neharika Malhotra Bora
MD, FICMCH, FMAS
Director Rainbow IVF, Agra
Consultant at Malhotra Nursing and Maternity Home, Agra, India

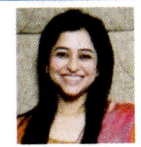

Noreen Rasul
MBBS, FCPS
Program Coordinator, Kangaroo Mother Care
Assistant Professor, Department of Obstetrics and Gynaecology
Services Institute of Medical Sciences, Lahore, Pakistan

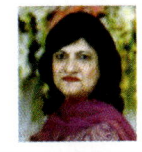

Noreen Zafar
MBBS, MRCOG, FRCOG
Consultant of Obstetrics and Gynaecology

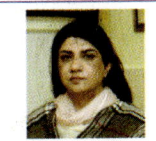

Nusrat Mahmud
MBBS, MS
Associate Professor, Department of Obstetrics and Gynaecology
BIRDEM General Hospital, Dhaka, Bangladesh

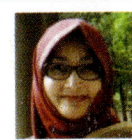

Parikshit Dahyalal Tank
Consultant Obstetrician and Gynaecologist
Ashwini Maternity and Surgical Hospital, Center for Endoscopy and
Assisted Reproduction, Ghatkopar, Mumbai, India

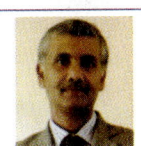

Rowshan Ara Khanom
Professor, Department of Obstetrics and Gynaecology
US Bangla Medical College, Rupganj, Narayanganj,
Dhaka, Bangladesh

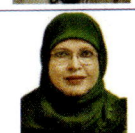

Rubina Sohail
MBBS, FCPS, DCPS-HPE, FRCOG
Professor, Department of Obstetrics and Gynecology
Services Institute of Medical Sciences, Lahore, Pakistan
President, South Asian Federation of Obstetrics and Gynaecology (SAFOG)

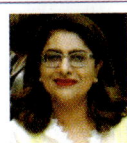

Ruchika Garg
MD, FICOG, FICMCH, MAMS, FMAS, CIMP, FIAOG
Associate Professor, Department of Obstetrics and Gynaecology
SN Medical College, Agra, India

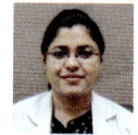

Sadia Ahsan Pal
MRCOG, FRCOG
Vice President, SOGP
Professor, Obstetrics and Gynaecology, OMI Hospital, Karachi, Pakistan

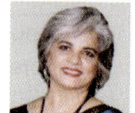

Sapna Amatya Vaidya
Senior Consultant, Obstetrics and Gynecologists, MOHP
Paropakaar Maternity and Women's Hospital, Kathmandu, Nepal

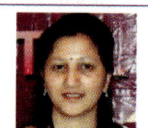

Saroja Pandey
Senior Consultant, Obstetrics and Gynecologists, MOHP
Paropakaar Maternity and Women's Hospital, Kathmandu, Nepal

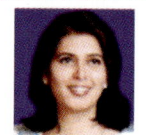

Shafiqa Breshna Babak
Associated Professor, Obstetrics and Gynaecology
President, Afghan Society of Obstetrics and Gynecologist

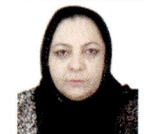

Shahla Kanwal
MBBS, FCPS
Research Coordinator
Senior Registrar
Obstetrics and Gynaecology Services Hospital, Lahore, Pakistan

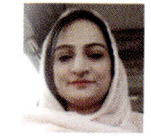

Sheikh Zinnat Ara Nasreen
MBBS, MPH, FCPS, MRCOG, FRCOG
Professor, Department of Obstetrics and Gynaecology
ZH Shikder Women's Medical College and Hospital, Bangladesh

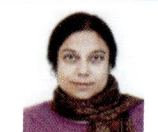

Shyam Desai
Professor, Department of Obstetrics and Gynaecology
Wadia Hospital, Mumbai
President, Mumbai Obs/Gyn Society
President, Indian Association of Gyn Endoscopy

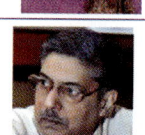

Syeda Batool Mazhar
MBBS, FRCOG, FCPS
Professor, Department of Obstetrics and Gynaecology
MCH Centre, PIMS, Islamabad, Pakistan

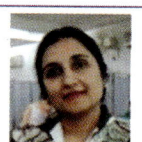

Udagamage Don Puspananda Ratnasiri
Consultant, Obstetrician and Gynaecologist
Castle Street Hospital for Women, Colombo 08, Sri Lanka

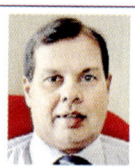

Uma Pandey
MD, FRCOG
Associate Professor, Department of Obstetrics and Gynecologists
Institute of Medical Sciences, Banaras Hindu University, Varanasi, India

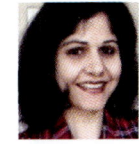

Yeasmin Jahan
Associate Professor, Department of Obstetrics and Gynaecology
Shaheed Suhrawardy Medical College, Dhaka
Govt. of the People's Republic of Bangladesh

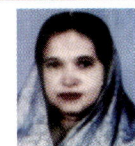

Preface

S outh Asia is home to one-sixth of the world's population, making it the most densely populated geographical region in the world. The region faces public health challenges on a demographic and geographic scale unmatched in the world. South Asia's low life expectancy, high rates of malnutrition, maternal mortality, infant mortality and incidence of tuberculosis are second only to those of sub-Saharan Africa. India, Pakistan and Bangladesh are burdened by the mammoth population load. The fact that the countries of the South Asian region are living on less than $1 a day makes the matters worse and solutions more difficult to find. The situation with sexual and reproductive rights is pretty much the same. There is preference for male child, lack of education, gender discrimination, and violence against women, lack of women empowerment, not enough laws on permissible age of marriage and lack of favorable family laws for women in areas such as inheritance, divorce and child custody.

As teachers in obstetrics and gynaecology and clinicians, we tend to focus on knowledge, clinical competencies and attitudes to ensure that our trainees become good doctors. During this time, we overlook many of our regional and country needs, thinking of them as only public health issues. Matters such as contraception, abortion, patient safety, neonatal mortality, maternal mortality, poverty, women empowerment, patient safety and quality of care are a few of such examples. Sexual and reproductive rights, is one such important area. It is high time that OB/GYN specialists take responsibility of working on these neglected areas and work towards improvement of women's health.

The objective of writing the book is to bring to light the situation of women sexual and reproductive rights in the region and to highlight the issues of gender-based violence. The book also aims at ensuring that the gynaecologists realize the situation and become partners in finding solutions to these important issues. The book comprises three parts—situation analysis of countries of South Asia, issues and solutions pertaining to gender-based violence and the way forward.

Hopefully, the book will serve as a tool to look at ways to advance women's health and improve sexual and reproductive rights of the women in the region.

Rubina Sohail

Narendra Malhotra

Acknowledgements

Writing an acknowledgement is the most difficult part of the book. The list of people I want to thank is long. I would like to start by thanking FIGO and Prof Rashid Latif Khan who introduced me to sexual and reproductive rights almost twenty years ago. Prof CN Purandare for having faith in me, Prof Chiara Benedetto for setting the stage by being an excellent Chair of Sexual Health and Human Rights Committee, where I was a member.

I have to thank each one of the authors of the book for agreeing to contribute to the book, for finding time out of their busy schedules and diligently working for completing their chapters. Special acknowledgement is due to some contributors who went out of the way to make the book possible and were only a call away. Thank you Dr Shyam Desai, Dr Kusum Thapa, Dr Sadia Ahsan Pal, Dr Ferdousi Begum, Dr Narendra Malhotra and Dr Hemantha Senanayke. The editorial team spent hours of their time, meticulously reading each word and going over the contents. Dr Asifa Naureen, you are my lifeline, this endeavor would not have been possible without you. I have to thank the young faculty Dr Kiren Sohail, Dr Madiha Rashid and the team of department of obstetrics and gynaecology at SIMS. I want to acknowledge the time given by the senior members of the faculty for going through the manuscript and giving their opinion. Prof Sabaratnum Arulkumaran and Prof Farrukh Zaman, you are my inspiration.

Mr Ghazanfar Ali and Mr Mohammad Afzal, thank you for your secretarial services and facilitating the entire process. Mr Ghazanfar Ali was the backbone in designing and shaping the book. Dr Mahad Khalid deserves mention for going over the script of the book. Thanks are due to the students of "Zephyr"—the art, photography and music society of Services Institute of Medical Sciences, Lahore, for helping in designing the cover of the book. They spent precious hours toiling over the design, finally reaching a consensus. I would like to thank the publishers for their valuable input in making this endeavor possible. Dr Narendra Malhotra is my coeditor—a big thank you.

Finally, thank you—team SAFOG for working together towards a common vision.

Rubina Sohail

Rubina Sohail

Contents

PART 3: THE WAY FORWARD

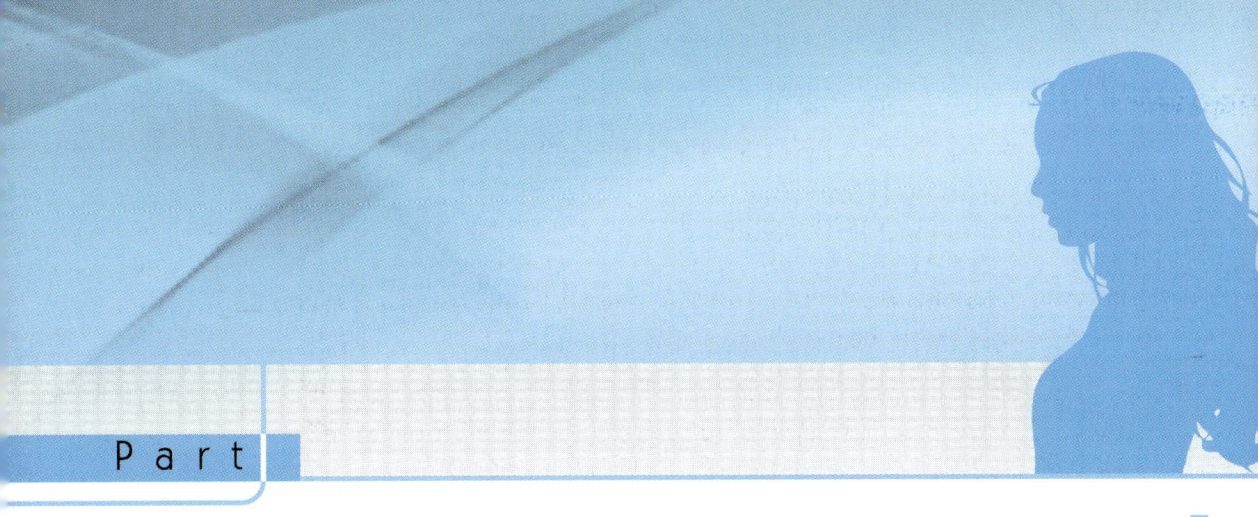

1

Situation Analysis
of Afghanistan

Shafiqa Breshna Babak, Malalai Jamshid Nejaby

INTRODUCTION

Afghanistan is a land-locked multiethnic country located in Southern Asia that borders China, Iran, Pakistan, Tajikistan, Turkmenistan, and Uzbekistan. The geography of Afghanistan is arid and mountainous, the Hindu Kush mountains run northeast to southwest and divide the northern provinces from the rest of the country. The government system is an Islamic Republic, the chief of state and head of government is the President. Afghanistan has a controlled economic system in which the central government directs the economy regarding the production and distribution of goods. Afghanistan is a member of the South Asian Association for Regional Cooperation (SAARC).

DEMOGRAPHICS

Afghanistan's population estimated at 34 million in 2018 (WHO country profile), with an annual growth of 2.03 percent is among the fastest growing in the world. Afghanistan also has one of the highest total fertility rates (TFR) in the world at 5.3 children per women (AfDHS, 2015). At that rate, the Afghan population is expected to double in 24 years. Because of relatively high fertility, nearly half of Afghanistan's population (47 percent) is under the age of 15 years, and 16 percent is under the age of 5 years.

Afghanistan's health sector made re-markable progress over the last decades,

which has translated into a decline in maternal mortality (616 deaths per 100,000 in 2015 compared to 1,600 deaths/100,000 in 2002). The promotion, delivery and utilization of family planning (FP) in Afghanistan improved between 2003 and 2010, with the use of modern contraceptive methods increasing from 10% to 20%. However, the AfDHS 2015 indicates that the modern contraceptive prevalence rate (mCPR) has since remained static at 20% over the last eight years. Overall, 25% of currently married women have an unmet need for family planning. Life expectancy was reported in 2015 at 60.5 years and only 0.04% of the population has HIV. It is assumed that roughly 600,000 to as high as 2 million Afghans may have been killed during the various 1979–2001 wars. These figures are highly questionable and no attempt has ever been made to verify them. The country's population is expected to reach 82 million by 2050.

Maternal mortality ratio (MMR)	661/100,000
Infant mortality rate (IMR)	165/1,000
Neonatal mortality rate (NMR)	22/1,000
Under-5 mortality rate	257/1,000
Pregnant women with at least one skilled ANC visit	59%
Births with a skilled attendant present	51%
Breastfeeding at age 2	54%
Couples using modern family planning method	20%
Total fertility rate	5.3

Sex ratio

At birth: 1.05 male(s)/female

Under 15 years: 1.05 male(s)/female

15–64 years: 1.05 male(s)/female

65 years and over: 0.93 male(s)/female

Afghanistan's population is young, which is typical of countries with high fertility rates. Forty-seven percent of the population is under age 15, while 3% of residents are age 65 or older. The average size of households in Afghanistan is 8.0 persons. Urban households are slightly smaller than rural households (7.7 persons versus 8.2 persons). Men head most of Afghan households (98%), with only 2% of households headed by women.

Male population: 52%

Female population: 24.2%

Literacy: In Afghanistan, both educational levels and literacy rates are low. The proportion of ever-married women with no education is higher than the proportion among men (84% versus 51%). Nine percent of women and 31% of men have completed at least some secondary education.

GDP: The Gross Domestic Product per capita in Afghanistan was last recorded at 1804 US dollars in 2017, when adjusted by purchasing power parity (PPP). The GDP per capita, in Afghanistan, when adjusted by purchasing power parity is equivalent to 10% of the world's average. GDP per capita PPP in Afghanistan averaged 1490.88 USD from 2002 until 2017, reaching an all-time high of 1848.70 USD in 2013 and a record low of 1062.20 USD in 2004.

Poverty is a prevalent issue as over one-third of the country's population lives below the national poverty line (less than USD 1/day). According to the 2015 Afghanistan Demographic Health Survey (AfDHS), 15% of women and 49% of men are literate, fertility rate is 5.3 children per woman, median birth interval is 28.4 months, median age at first birth among women is 20 years, and 89% of women reported having one or more problems in accessing health care for themselves.

The people and government of the Islamic Republic of Afghanistan, as well as international partners and stakeholders, still need to do a lot to reach the country's development goals.

Prevailing Cultural and Social Environment

Afghanistan is a multi-ethnic society, characterized by its diverse ethnic, linguistic and tribal groups. The government is an Islamic Republic and the guiding tenets of Islam dictate many social and behavioral norms in society. However, attitudes and values of Afghans have been significantly influenced by the invasions and wars they have been subjected to throughout the country's ancient and modern history. Modern aspirations of the younger generation have also changed with the arrival of the internet and mass media.

The recent relentless conflicts of the late 20th and 21st century have produced a generation of Afghans who have scarcely been afforded peace. Afghanistan has fiercely resisted the invasions from Great Britain and the Soviet Union, and continues to survive despite the ongoing insurgency by the Taliban and others. To this point, there is a definite feeling of self-pride amongst Afghans as survivors, and general public attitudes are strongly opposed to outside interference. This has translated into a prevailing national attitude that determinedly seeks independence from controlling bodies. However, interestingly, this assertion of the country's independence does not really manifest as national cohesiveness. In fact, Afghanistan has been late to embrace a national identity. Its people tend to feel a stronger sense of loyalty and belonging to their kin, tribe or ethnicity before sovereign state. Such loyalty to blood ties and ethnicity reflects the deep tribalism and collectivism of Afghan society. Dependence upon kin and community has long been so crucial to survival that there is a broad mistrust of government involvement in people's personal lives. This is exacerbated by the underfunded social services that are often unable to meet the basic needs due to corruption or lack of security. Therefore, if Afghans are in crisis and essential needs must be met, they are likely to turn to those of the same family, kinfolk, village/community, tribe or ethnicity for assistance (in that general order or preference).

Afghanistan is mostly an agricultural country with many people being produce or livestock farmers. The international community has tried to support the establishment of a modern democratic state in Afghanistan, however, most villages and rural regions tend to govern themselves. In small villages, there are frequently no schools, stores or government representation. There may be three authority figures: The village headman (*malik*), the master of water distribution (*mirab*) and the teacher of Islamic laws (*mullah*) whose role is to make judgments as to whether someone's behavior is observing the Qur'an. Often a village will have a large landowner (*khan*) who governs by assuming the role of both the malik and mirab. However, an assembly of men usually vote on the important decisions that affect the whole village or tribe.

Much social behavior is influenced by Afghans' awareness of their personal honor; 'honor' in this sense encompasses an individual's reputation, prestige and worth. Preservation of honor is often at the forefront of people's minds in Afghanistan. It influences people to behave in accordance with social expectations (following Islamic traditions) and maintain mostly conservative behaviors. People tend to avoid drawing attention to themselves or risk doing something perceived to be dishonorable.

PROBLEMS

Violence Against Women

Violence against women and girls is a grave violation of human rights. Its impact ranges from immediate to long-term multiple physical, sexual and mental consequences for women and girls, including death. It negatively affects women's general well-being and prevents women from fully participating in society. Violence not only has negative consequences for women but also their families, the community and the country at large. It has tremendous costs, from greater health care and legal expenses and losses in productivity, impacting national budgets and overall development. Decades of mobilizing by civil society and women's movements have put ending gender-based violence high on national and international agendas. An unprecedented number of countries have laws against domestic violence, sexual assault and other forms of violence. Challenges remain however in implementing these laws, limiting women and girls' access to safety and justice. Not enough is done to prevent violence, and when it does occur, it often goes unpunished.

According to 2010-2011 Afghanistan Multiple Indicator Cluster Survey, 15% of Afghan women (aged 15–49 years) were married before the age of 15, and 46% before the age of 18. Out of all women (aged 15–49 years), 92% believe that a husband is justified in beating his wife.

1. In March 2014, the government published its first report on the elimination of violence against women (VAW) in Afghanistan.
2. Overall 4,505 incidents of violence against women were registered in relevant Afghan ministries in 32 of Afghanistan's 34 provinces between 2012 and 2013. Available data show that violence against women is a pervasive problem in Afghanistan.

Almost 90% of women in Afghanistan have experienced at least one form of domestic violence. Percentage of ever-married women who have experienced any form of physical violence (by a spouse or anyone else) since age 15 and in the 12 months before the survey, 17% have experienced sexual violence and 52% have experienced physical violence.

In Afghanistan, women's experience of domestic violence cuts across all socioeconomic characteristics. 53% of ever-married women have experienced physical violence since age 15 with 46% experiencing violence in the 12 months before the survey. A larger percentage of women reported experiencing physical violence "often" in the past year (31%) than "sometimes" (15%) in the previous year.

Violence during pregnancy is also fairly common. Almost 1 of 5 (16%) ever-married women who have ever been pregnant has experienced physical violence during pregnancy.

Experience of physical violence since age 15 increases sharply with age and women's number of children. For example, 33% of women age 15–19 have experienced physical violence since age 15 compared with 60% of women age 40–49.

The likelihood of experiencing physical violence during pregnancy generally increases with number of living children. About one in five ever-married women with 5 or more children has experienced physical violence during pregnancy compared with 7% of women with no children. Women who are employed but are not paid in cash (63%) are more likely than unemployed women (52%) and those who are employed for cash (53%) to have experienced physical violence. Women's experience of physical violence varies greatly by province. Less than 1 in 10 women report experience of physical violence in Helmand (6%) and Badakhshan (7%), compared with more than 9 in 10 women.

Women who have no education are twice as likely (56%) as women who have secondary education (28%) to report the experience of violence. Fifty-six percent of ever-married women reported ever experiencing spousal violence (physical, sexual, or emotional) perpetrated by their husband and 52% reported experiencing such violence in the past 12 months, either often (36%) or some-times (16%). Women's experience of spousal (physical, sexual, or emotional) violence increases substantially with age and number of children. Thirty-one percent of ever-married women age 15–19 have ever experienced spousal violence compared with 61% of women age 40–49. Thirty-three percent of women with no living children have experienced spousal violence compared with 60% of women with 5 or more children. Eight in 10 women who seek help ask their own family for help and about one-third (34%) ask their husband's family for help. The next most common source of help is neighbors (18%). In Afghanistan women who seek help to stop the violence are unlikely to seek help from doctors, police, or any other civil or social organization.

Women and girls constitute nearly half of the country's population. However, the social structure in Afghanistan is still characterized by male dominance, leaving the status of women at the bottom of the social hierarchy. Gender inequality in Afghanistan is one of the highest in the world. The gender development index (GDI) in 2014 for Afghanistan at 0.310 was second lowest among all countries.

Moreover, there is a lack of gender sensitivity in data collection and analysis. Core development policies are guided more by security and military priorities rather than by concerns for sustainability and the fulfillment of human rights. Women's overall representation in decision-making positions in various government sectors is still low at 23%, in the health sector it is 24.1%.

Crisis Situations: Migrants and IDPs

The population of Afghanistan is around 34 million as of 2018 which includes roughly 3 million Afghan citizens living as refugees in both Pakistan and Iran. The nation is composed of a multi-ethnic and multilingual society, reflecting its location astride historic trade and invasion routes between Central Asia, Southern Asia, and Western Asia. Its largest ethnic group is the Pashtun, followed by Tajik, Hazara, Uzbek, Aimak, Turkmen, Baloch and a few others.

While Afghanistan is entering the 40th year of protracted displacement, UNHCR expects the humanitarian situation to remain complex, despite the encouraging efforts in peace negotiations and the strong political will in Afghanistan. Persistent socio-economic challenges compound protection risks and limit returnee reintegration prospects, which often results in negative coping mechanisms, such as child labour, early marriage, labour exploitation and debarment.

Under the Solutions Strategy for Afghan Refugees (SSAR) framework, the Government of Afghanistan will continue progress on development and sustainable reintegration through the implementation of the Displacement and Return Executive Committee (DiREC) policy framework and Action Plan, while challenges will likely persist in fully translating policy into implementation at the field level.

In July 2018, the Government of Afghanistan officially announced its decision to join and support the Comprehensive Refugee Response Framework (CRRF) as a country of origin. Government of Afghanistan developed a roadmap and decide upon the way forward in rolling out comprehensive responses in this specific context.

The planned Parliamentary and Presidential elections in Afghanistan during October 2018 and early 2019, respectively, may result in demonstrations and targeted attacks on election related premises.

Highly complex scenarios of internal displacement, compounded by insecurity and shrinking humanitarian space are expected to continue in 2019. Drought will create protection risks for IDPs, increasing their vulnerability and reliance on negative coping mechanisms.

Afghanistan suffers from one of the world's longest protracted complex emergencies due to conflict, natural disasters and mass population movements. In 2018, drought affected two-thirds of Afghanistan, leaving 3.6 million people in need of urgent humani-tarian assistance. In addition, increasing conflict in different regions resulted in higher numbers of internally displaced people and trauma cases. Nearly 800,000 displaced people have returned from Pakistan and Iran and the number is expected to increase in the coming years. Around 1.9 million people are now in need of humanitarian health services and additional emergency service support. Ongoing conflict results in the movement of more than 1 million people, increasing the need for humanitarian health services.

Ongoing food insecurity continues to exacerbate needs for health provision for populations on the move and around the country. Funding pledges are unpredictable due to extended emergencies in the region, reducing the response capacity. Insecurity and limited accessibility to emergency locations in high-risk provinces and damage to hospitals hamper the effort to provide essential emergency health services, capacity building and monitoring activities.

Abortion

Afghanistan is an Islamic country and according to the religious laws of Islam performing intended abortion is prohibited, addressing complications from unsafe abortion, whether spontaneous or induced, is an important step in reducing maternal mortality, and as outlined in the international guidance, post-abortion care (PAC) that includes family planning services and counseling is a key intervention in the path-way to maternal survival and the reduction of unplanned pregnancies.

In order to contribute to maternal death reduction, PAC services are included and reflected in the Ministry of Public Health's Reproductive Health Strategy of 2012–2016. PAC is aligned with other initiatives to further strengthen PAC services, both through improving the quality of services at the hospital level and through promoting the availability of PAC services at the health center level. By further expanding access for women, and improving the quality and reach of services, it will be possible to address unnecessary suffering and death due to complications of spontaneous and induced abortions.

One of the key innovations to support expansion of PAC services is the use of medical treatment for incomplete abortion with misoprostol, which is one of the two recommended treatment options, along with manual vacuum aspiration (MVA) (WHO, 2012a). For eligible clients, using a less invasive medical treatment will improve quality of service, while making it possible to offer these services at the primary and secondary levels. Furthermore, the training time of the providers and the cost of procedure to the patient and the health system will also be reduced through an integrated provision of services, to link the primary levels of care with the secondary and tertiary levels as needed. According to HMIS during first half of 2016, around 7,100 women have successfully received PAC services in four specialized hospitals, three regional hospitals, and two provincial hospitals (HMIS, 2016).

STI

The extent and nature of STIs in Afghanistan are largely unknown because no prevalence studies have been conducted. HIV is still predominantly a concentrated epidemic among injecting drug users (IDUs). Many of these IDUs have come from outside Afghanistan and are concentrated particularly in Herat, Kabul, and Balkh. The National AIDS Control Program has initiated provision of STI services as a prevention strategy for HIV because the presence of an STI greatly increases the risk of acquiring or transmitting HIV infection and according to AfDHS survey 2015 women were more likely than men to report having had an STI or having experienced STI symptoms in the 12 months before the survey, 2% of women reported that they had an STI; 13% had a bad smelling/abnormal genital discharge and 8% had a genital sore or ulcer. Among men, 2% reported

that they had an STI, 6% had a bad-smelling/abnormal discharge, and 4% had a genital sore or ulcer. Overall, 15% of women and 8% of men had either an STI or symptoms of an STI during the 12 months before the survey.

More than two in five women and one in four men who had an STI or STI symptoms sought advice or treatment from a clinic, hospital, private doctor, or other health professionals. Fifty-three percent of women and 45% of men did not seek any treatment when they had an STI or STI symptoms.

Contraceptives

Birth spacing and family planning are two of the most effective and cost-effective public health interventions for reducing maternal and infant mortality. A gap of less than two years between successive births is associated with higher maternal and infant mortality rates and higher rates of under nutrition and morbidity among children. Each additional pregnancy multiplies a woman's risk of dying from complications of pregnancy and childbirth. As the modern contraceptive prevalence rate (mCPR) increases, maternal mortality decreases, both because there are fewer pregnancies and because there are fewer high-parity, high-risk pregnancies. The current mCPR of 20% is preventing between 20% and 34% of potential maternal deaths (Figs 1.1a and b).

According to the AfDHS 2015, the median birth interval in Afghanistan is 28.4 months, and 32% of children are born less than 24 months after the previous one.

The population group at highest risk of short birth intervals is teenage mothers. Among women aged 15–19 years, 68% of second or subsequent births are within 24 months of the previous one. Eight percent of women in that age group have already had their first child and are at risk of another pregnancy.

A series of national surveys since 2003 have shown an increase in the mCPR from 10% in 2003 to 20% in 2010. Since then, the overall mCPR has remained unchanged (Fig. 1.2). The

Contraceptive knowledge and use in Afghanistan

Knowledge of contraceptive methods is high in Afghanistan, with 95% of currently married women and 92% of married men knowing at least one method of contraception. Pills, injectable, and male condoms are the most widely known methods among both women and men.

Percentage of currently married women and men age 15–49 who have heard of specific contraceptive methods

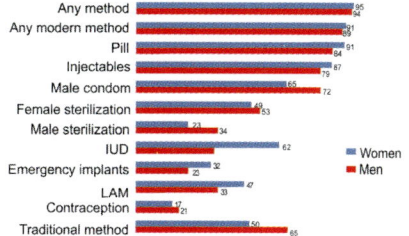

Contraceptive prevalence rate
Percentage who use any contraceptive method. Sample: Currently married women age 15–49

Fig. 1.1a: Knowledge of contraceptive methods

Overall 23% of currently married women use a method of family planning, with 20% using a modern method and 3% using a traditional method

Percentage of currently married women age 15–49 currently using a contraceptive method

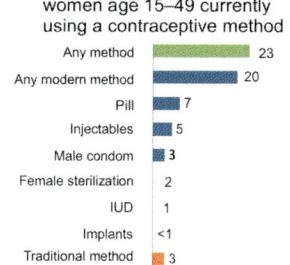

Fig. 1.1b: Contraceptive use

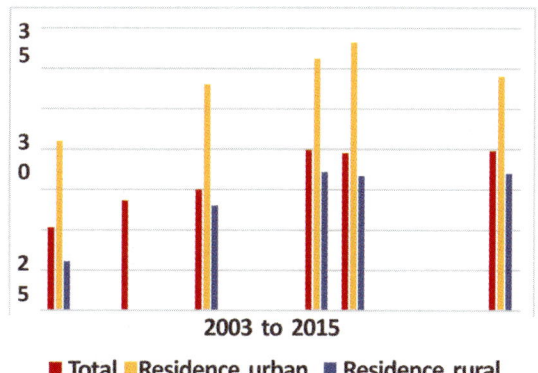

Total ■ **Residence urban** ■ **Residence rural**

Fig. 1.2: Modern contraceptive prevalence rate by residence

urban mCPR is 70% higher than the rural mCPR, and the mCPR of the wealthiest quintile is double that of the poorest quintile. Of the current mCPR of 20%, the main contributions by method are: Pills 6.8%, injectable 4.8%, condoms 3.3%, female sterilization 1.8%, IUDs 1.4%, and implants 0.2%. Contraceptives are obtained about equally from public and private health institutions, including 31% from pharmacies (pills and condoms) (AfDHS 2015).

The Afghanistan Demographic Health Survey (AfDHS) 2015 indicates that the modern contraceptive prevalence rate (mCPR) is 20% and the national family planning (FP) goal is 30% mCPR for married women by 2020.

Pills, injectable, and male condoms are the most commonly used methods.

The knowledge about at least one FP method is around 58% (2012 Afghanistan Health Survey), the estimated unmet need is 25%, and the total fertility rate (TFR) is 5.3 (AfDHS 2015).

According to 2016 National Maternal and Newborn Health QoC Assessment findings of the 246 facilities visited during the assessment, the majority of facilities had a mix of short- and long-term contraceptive methods available at the time of the assessment (91% facilities had male condoms, 94% had oral contraceptives, 92% had intrauterine devices [IUD] and 84% had injectable). Implants, which were only recently added to the Ministry of Public Health (MoPH) Essential Medicines list in 2016, were only available in 9% of the facilities. Based on service delivery observations, counseling on healthy timing and spacing of pregnancy was only provided in 20% of ANC consultations ($n = 467$ observations), 17% during the first hour after birth ($n = 714$ observations), and 29% for postnatal consultations before women were discharged after childbirth ($n = 436$ observations). Based on interviews with SBAs, health care providers' personal beliefs were found to be an important factor on both whether or not FP counseling is provided and on the content of information shared. More than one-third of SBAs interviewed (43%) reported believing that a woman should not choose a FP method until she consults with her husband, and 86% reported believing that a woman who has not had a boy child should not be encouraged to use FP.

The low levels of FP counseling observed in this assessment highlighted the significant gaps in provision of proper counselling and missed opportunities that needed to be promoted and strengthened at all levels of health facilities in Afghanistan. Because SBAs are instrumental in conveying information to families and communities, tackling the bias and preferences of service providers themselves was identified as another area to address effectively with limited resources in the context of Afghanistan. Multiple FP methods are available including implants and approved by MOPH but availability of implant was low and additional support is needed to increase the availability of implant. MOPH is keen to promote and strengthen FP counseling within the continuum of care of maternal and newborn health and designed interventions by the Reproductive Health Department of MOPH which prioritized client needs, values, and desires in the provision of quality FP services.

CONCLUSIONS

Afghanistan has been internationally recognized for the significant health gains made over the past 15 years, especially in maternal and child health outcomes, with the rebuilding of the health system. Yet much remains to be done, especially for the health and well-being of women, mothers, newborns, children, and adolescents, the Ministry of Public Health (MoPH) to make further gains to improve the health of Afghanistan's most vulnerable citizens in the coming years.

Afghanistan has made great progress in reducing maternal, infant, and child mortality since 2002 through implementation of the Basic Package of Health Services (BPHS) and the Essential Package of Hospital Services (EPHS). As a result, 60% of the population is within one hour of a health facility, and 88% within two hours' travelling time. Fifteen thousand rural communities have community health workers (CHWs) who are trained to treat childhood illnesses and provide condoms and contraceptive pills and injectable. By about 2010, 60% of pregnant women were using antenatal care (ANC), 50% were using a skilled birth attendant, and 20% of couples were using a modern contraceptive. However, since that time there has been no further progress in the use of these services.

BIBLIOGRAPHY

1. Afghanistan Economy 2018 https://theodora. com/wfbcurrent/afghanistan/afghanistan_ economy. html

2. Afghanistan National Maternal and Newborn Health Quality of Care Assessment 2016. Key Findings Report.

3. Central Statistics Organization (CSO) and UNICEF. Afghanistan Multiple Indicator Cluster Survey 2010-2011: Final Report. Kabul: Central Statistics Organization (CSO) and UNICEF, 2012. Available at: http://cso.gov.af/Content/files/AMICS.pdf

4. CSO, MoPH, and ICF. 2017. Afghanistan Demographic and Health Survey 2015. Kabul, Afghanistan: CSO.

5. Islamic Republic of Afghanistan, Ministry of Public Health, Gender Department. National Gender Strategy (2012–2016). Available: http://moph.gov.af/Content/Media/Documents/MoPH_National_Gender_Strategy_Final_English_201216420121212934246553325325.pdf

6. Islamic Republic of Afghanistan, Ministry of Public Health, National Family planning service Delivery guideline 2018.

7. Islamic Republic of Afghanistan. National Action Plan for the Women of Afghanistan (NAPWA). Available: http://www.svri.org/Afghanistan policy.pdf

8. Ministry of Public Health of the Islamic Republic of Afghanistan. Reproductive, Maternal, New-born, child and Adolescent strategy, 2016–22.

9. Ministry of Women's Affairs of the Islamic Republic of Afghanistan. First Report on the Implementa-tion of the Elimination of Violence against Women Law in Afghanistan, 2014. Available at: http://mowa.gov.af/Content/files/EVAW%20Law%20 Report_Final_English_17% 20%20March% 202014.pdf

10. Source: 2018 CIA World Factbook and other sources Afghan Public http://moph.gov.af/en/documents/category/bsc-reports.

11. UN Security Council Resolution 1325,2000. Available: http://www.un.org/en/ga/search/view_doc.asp?symbol=S/RES/1325

12. United Nations Assistance Mission in Afghanistan (UNAMA) and United Nations Office of the High Commissioner for Human Rights (OHCHR). Justice through the Eyes of Afghan Women: Cases of Violence against Women Addressed through Mediation and Court Adjudication. 2015. Available at https://unama.unmissions.org/Portals/UNAMA/UNAMA-OHCHR/UNAMA_OHCHR_Justice_through_eyes_of_Afghan_women_15_April_ 2015.pdf

13. WHO. WHO Guidelines on Integrated Management of Pregnancy and Childbirth. Available at: http://www.who.int/maternal_ child_adolescent/documents/impac/en/. https://www.mail-man.columbia.edu/research/averting-maternal-death-and-disability-amdd/toolkit.

Situation Analysis of Bangladesh

Fariha Nehreen Mirza, Nusrat Mahmud, Laila Arjumand Banu

INTRODUCTION

The People's Republic of Bangladesh, a country in South Asia, shares its borders with India and Myanmar and forms the largest and eastern-most part of the Bengal region. Its largest city is its capital Dhaka, followed by Chittagong, which is also the largest seaport in the world.

Bangladesh is the world's eighth most populous country (as of 2017, the population count is 164.7 million accommodated in 147,570 km² land).This also makes Bangladesh the 11th most densely populated country in the world. The population growth rate in Bangladesh was among the fastest in the world in 1960s and 1970s, which decelerated with the introduction of birth control in the 1980s. The current population growth rate is 1.0% with a fertility rate of 2.5.

The under-18 population of Bangladesh accounts for 40% of the population and this statistic is expected to continue till 2031. This warrants welcome growth in economy and is evidenced by increased of the gross national income from 1996 to 2014 by 3 times. Bangladesh is a lower middle income country and has been named one of the next eleven emerging markets, with the second highest foreign exchange reserves (after India). Its economy is ranked 43rd in nominal gross domestic product and 23rd in purchasing power parity.

PREVAILING CULTURAL AND SOCIAL ENVIRONMENT

Bangladesh has a rich cultural heritage. Modern Bangladesh has started its journey in

1971. The Bengal Sultanate and Mughal Bengal influenced this region to build Muslim domi-nance. The Bangladeshi culture is a mixture of Islam, Hinduism, Buddhism and Christianity. Music, dance and drama; art and distinct culinary tradition enriched Bengali culture. From the historic background, Bangladesh has appealing architecture influenced by Mughal and terracotta sculpture. Jamdani motifs and fine muslin are the cultural heritage of Bangladesh, recognized by UNESCO. White rice and fish are the staple food for Bangladeshis. "Pohela Boishakh", the Bengali New Year, is celebrated each Year on 14th April as major festival without any religious discrimination. The Bengali New Year's procession "Mongol Shovajatra" is the icon of Benagli art and cultural heritage, recognized by UNESCO. The Language Movement in 1952 established the identity of Bangla Nations. Every year on 21st February, people marked this day with respect for those who sacrificed their lives for their language. Bangla is the only language where people sacrificed their lives. The United Nation has declared this day as International Mother Language Day. Sports in Bangladesh are a popular form of entertainment. Cricket is the most popular sports. Bangladeshi people love to play football and kabaddi also.

IMPLICATIONS OF RELIGION FOR SEXUAL AND REPRODUCTIVE HEALTH

The major religion in Bangladesh is Islam (90%), but a significant percentage of the population adheres to Hinduism (9%). In rural Bangladesh due to lack of proper education, religion acts as a barrier for implementations of reproductive health in women. Early childbirth and teenage marriage acts as hindrance in reproductive needs of women in Bangladesh. Child marriage affects three out of five girls in Bangladesh. The adolescent pregnancy 113 per 1000 births, between the age group of 15 and 19 years and that is the highest in South Asia.

The Imams (religious leaders) in Muslim community and also the village head can be convinced to work together to improve the situations.

CURRENT SOCIAL ENVIRONMENT APROPOS WOMEN

Bangladesh's women have made progress in various aspects of health, education, and work, but still face sizable gender gaps. The vocational, and tertiary education, energy, transport, and urban development—these are major sectors where there are disparities in gender.

Sex selective health care and infanticide suggest a correlation between the number of females and males in Bangladesh and that ratio is 95:100. In terms of the population, that ratio accounts for approximately 5 million missing women. Women family members are less likely to receive modern medical care and are generally recipients of traditional remedies. The health situation for urban women is worse than that for rural women, especially those living in slums. The urban population living in the slum areas does not have adequate sanitation, water and health facilities which results in poor health.

Bangladeshi women face barriers and disadvantages in nearly every aspect of their lives, including access to health services, economic opportunity, political participation, and control of finances.

Bangladesh has been a role model in women's empowerment in the past decade, and the country is experiencing an appreciable change in society because of its efforts in this regard. The concept of women's empowerment and efforts in this area has helped the country attain a steady progress in gender equality, which helped Bangladesh to secure the first spot in gender equality (among South Asian countries) for the second consecutive year at the Gender Gap Index of 2017. The index, prepared by World Economic Forum, measures education, economic participation, health, and political empowerment to measure gender equality of any country.

Half of the population of Bangladesh is women and their economic participation has increased significantly. In fact, national and international policy strategies have also been reflected in the policy to ensure women's advancement so that they have control over their lives and play an influential role in society as decision makers. The number of working women increased to 18.6 million in 2016-17 from 16.2 million in 2010. Bangladesh secured the 47th position among 144 countries in 2017 as per The Global Gender Gap Report, whereas India, Sri Lanka, Nepal, Bhutan and Pakistan remain at 108, 109, 111, 124 and 143 positions respectively.

Situation is changing at present due to mobilization of rural women by NGOs in villages. They get services and use of women community level workers to provide doorstep services in health and family planning. This played an important role in improving infant, child and maternal health and income earning opportunities. Mobilization of women was important in strengthening their voice in demanding their rights and services. The last few years have been extremely positive for women working in different sectors—alongside a steady rise in female leadership. Given the country's current landscape where gender equity is not just a buzzword anymore, we can expect more visibility for working women in terms of availability and acceptability.

Participation of girls in primary schools is increasing as their overall enrollment rose from 57% in 2008 to 95.4% in 2017. Bangladesh has topped the Gender Gap Index in the primary and secondary education category, and to continue the efforts to this end, the government has extended its stipend program for female students, and undertaken initiatives to make women-friendly environment and infrastructures.

VIOLENCE AGAINST WOMEN

Bangladesh is one of the least developed countries in the world. The estimated prevalence rate of violence against women is extremely high. It acts as an obstacle for gender equality, development and peace. Definition of violence can be described as violation of human rights. This can be a major turning point in the struggle to end violence against women globally. Discrimination and inequalities of gender increase women's vulnerability to violence.

Violence against women has many forms including physical aggression or threats, sexual abuse, emotional abuse, controlling or domineering, intimidation, stalking, passive/covert abuse, and economic deprivations.

Violence can takes place in the home, on the streets, in schools, the workplace, in farm fields, refugee camps, during conflicts and crisis. Main reason behind Violence against Women was dowry (32.72%), familial conflict (32.54%), sexual assault (19.16%), extramarital relation (11.20%), others (3.06%) and domestic violence (1.31%). Marital rape is also quite prevalent. Alcohol consumption and mental illness can be co-morbid with abuse.

According to the UNFPA State of the World's Women Population Report, 47 percent of the women in Bangladesh testify to having ever been physically assaulted by a male partner. This report, and the fact that Bangladesh would thus rank second in a list of 12 countries with a high rate of violence against women.

Homicide, serious injuries, unwanted pregnancies are the consequences of violence against women. Sexually transmitted infections (STIs) and HIV/AIDS, and disease vulnerability. Violence may also be responsible for maternal mortality, especially among young, unwed, pregnant women. The gender-based violence may end up with the psychological consequences like suicide and mental health problems.

Gender-based violence also acts as barrier in socioeconomic development.

Improvement of economic status of women is a must, as well as women empowerment is essential to combat violence at community level. Strict enforcement of law and awareness about violence against women through mass media can improve the situation.

Rape

According to Section 375 of the penal code of Bangladesh, rape occurs when a man has sexual intercourse with a woman, against her will, without her consent or with consent if it has been acquired by threating death or hurt. Rape also occurs when the man gains consent, knowing that he is not the woman's husband but the woman thinks that he is another man that she is legally married to. Sexual intercourse with a girl below the age of sixteen years, also counts as rape. This statutory definition is far from gender neutral (excluding males as victims, and hermaphrodites and transgenders completely) and identifies only penovaginal intercourse as rape; oral and anal penetrations are excluded. The irony is that even though a woman cannot be convicted as the perpetrator, she can, under Section 30 of the Prevention of Oppression against Women and Children Act be punished for instigation with the same punishment as that for commission of rape. The law also fails to include marital rape, unless the wife is below the age of sixteen; a primitive contiguity when the laws were first established under colonial rule.

In Bangladesh, rape is a frequent and widely underreported incident. The reluctance in victims to report rape may be due to the societal stigmas that almost always place the burden of blame on the victim, fear of further harm to self and loved ones, a non-friendly and often sluggish justice system, which depends heavily on bribes, and demoralizing rates of conviction. From January 2014 to December 2017, there were 17,289 reported cases of rape against women and children. Only 3430 cases made it to court where 649 people were convicted. This may be due to the tendency in Bangladesh of settling cases by local council or "shalish".

The punishments range from monetary penalty to a verdict to marry the victim. A study by the United Nations in 2013, found that 82% rural men and 79% urban men in Bangladesh, thought they were entitled to rape, with 62.1% not feeling guilt or worry over consequences, and 95.1% not facing any legal consequences.

A recent order passed by the High Court of Bangladesh issued 18 directives for proper management of a rape complaint, failure of following which is to be regarded as punishable offense. These include mandatory DNA sampling and analysis within 48 hours of the reported incident, immediate opening of a server to register the complaint, the presence of a female officer not below rank of constable during examination of the victim, provision of a female social worker for mental support, strict safeguarding of the victim's identity, privacy and security at all times, amongst other things. Bangladesh has also recently done away with the "two-finger test" which has widely been criticized as a deterrent to reporting of rape. It is hoped that bringing more changes such as these, will streamline the judicial process and bring faster justice to victims.

SPECIAL SITUATIONS

Child Marriage

Bangladesh holds the fourth place in ranking of prevalence of child marriages in the world, along with the second highest number of child brides 4,451,000, according to Girls not Brides. This puts every three out of five girls at risk of early marriage (UNFPA). The legal age to wed in Bangladesh is 18 years for girls and 21 years for boys. However, the Child Marriage Act bill was passed in 2017 that allows girls to be married off at a younger age in "special cases", without specifying what those special cases are.

The reasons for high rate of early marriage are rooted in Banglasdeshi traditions and social codes of conduct. A major factor contributing to early marriage is poverty. In the poorest households, girls are married at the median age of 15, while in richer ones the age increases to 18. Getting a girl married off young, means lesser dowry to pay, one less mouth to feed and financial stability for the girl. A very patriarchal and gender-biased society exists in Bangladesh, so a fear of disgrace caused by sexual harassment or premarital sex, is taken care of by early marriage. There are also increased incidences of child marriage in the recent Rohingya refugee population, as a means to acquire more food rations and protect girls from abuse.

Early marriage brings its own sets of implications for the girl, mostly considerable health risks. According to UNICEF, girls are five times more likely to die during childbirth than if they had a child after twenty years. Also neonatal mortality is 60% greater when born to a mother under 18 years than to a mother over 19 years. Girls married early are also more likely to drop out of school, which reduced their productivity and eventual contribution to the economy.

Bangladesh has taken various steps to reduce the incidence of child marriage. One of the country's sustainable development goals is to eradicate child early marriage by 2030. It is compulsory to present birth certificate at the time of marriage. Local governments and Plan Bangladesh lead movements like Child Marriage Free Unions to enforce existing laws. The Ministry of Women and Children Affairs in partnership with UNICEF Bangladesh has developed the National Plan of Action (NPA). The goal is to reduce the rate of marriage for girls of 18 years in 2021, and to completely eliminate child marriages by 2041.

Contraception

As mentioned earlier, Bangladesh ranks as the 11th most densely populated country with 164.7 million accommodated in 147,570 km^2 land. The country has made intense efforts in controlling the population growth rate, and the total fertility rate has fallen significantly over the past four decades. The fertility rate has fallen from 6.3 births per woman in 1975 to 2.3 in 2011. A large contribution here is made by the increasing availability and use of contraceptives by Bangladeshi couples.

The current contraceptive prevalence rate in Bangladesh is 62% with modern methods of contraception adopted by 52% urban women as compared to 46% rural women. The most preferred method is the pill with 29% users, followed by injectable with 7% users, and only 5% women opting for tubal ligation. Condoms were the only method, that found a few users amongst males (5%).

In Bangladesh, contraception can be purchased without prescription. Also, social workers have been supplying contraceptives to people's doors since 1970s. The Guttmacher Institute reported that "The main reasons pill users gave for choosing their method (cited by 35-41%) were that it is easy to use, a field-worker had delivered it to their home and they had concerns about other methods' side effects." There are more than 10 contraceptive

pill brands in Bangladesh including Shukhi, Nordette, Minnicon, Marvelon, etc. Condom brands include Ovacon, Marvelon, Novacon. There is Norplant in the form of subdermal implants and injectables include Depo-Provera SAS 150 mg/ml, Megestron and Noristerat.

Multiple international organizations such as UNFPA, UNDP, UNICEF and NGOs such as NDSP, PSTC, BRAC, Engender Health, Marie Stopes Clinic Society have been working in Bangladesh to promote family planning. The Bangladesh government itself is running a program called the Health Population and Nutrition Sector Development Program (HPNSDP) which aims reduce morbidity and mortality in the country and improve the nutritional status of the population, along with reduction of the population growth rate. A local daily listed social stigma, religious taboo, side-effect of contraceptives and lack of manpower in the healthcare field as major obstacles in family planning schemes of the country. Cohesive teamwork between the government and non-government along with method-mix cafeteria approach and commitment of the on-field workers can help further our progress and overcome all hurdles in achieving our targets in family planning.

Abortion

Abortion in Bangladesh, except when done to protect the life of the mother, is illegal. According to the penal code of Bangladesh Sections 312–316, severe punishment is reserved for causing miscarriage, causing miscarriage without women's consent and death caused by the act done with the intention to cause miscarriage. Exceptions are not made for the mental and physical health status of the mother, any impairments of the child or even for rape. Following the Liberation War, this ban had been lifted for sometime in 1972, for the women who had been raped during the war. In 1976, an attempt was made by the Bangladesh National Population Policy to legalize abortion in the first trimester, however that was unsuccessful. Menstrual regulation was introduced in 1979, and has since been the go to legal procedure for termination of pregnancy, but only in the first trimester.

According to the Guttmacher Institute, the rate of abortion in 2014 was 29 per 1000 women between the ages of 15–49. 430,000 had undergone MR procedures while 1,194,000 underwent induced abortions in most likely, unsafe conditions. An estimated 384,000 women had suffered from post-abortal complications such as hemorrhage, shock, sepsis, etc., and 91% of clinics capable of providing treatment for such complications, had done so. Urban women are approximately 1.8 times more likely to receive treatment for complications following abortion than rural women. This begets the question of whether menstrual regulation is sufficient for the country. In 2014, a National Demographic and Health Survey showed that half of married women had never heard of MR before. Only 53% of public sector facilities and 20% of private sector facilities, that were registered to provide MR services, actually did so. The reasons for this may be a lack of trained staff or proper equipment or both. Only one-third of the private facilities, having both trained personnel and proper equipment provided MR services in 2014, citing social reasons such as lack of husband's consent, marital status of the girl, age of the girl, etc. behind their decision. Even though most facilities provided the necessary counseling to post-abortal patients, very few provided contraceptive methods.

Multiple organizations are now working to provide their services in the field. A Bangladesh NGO, Marie Stopes, runs 132 clinics in the country, and provides family planning counselling and contraceptive methods, MR services and post-abortion care, antenatal and postnatal services as well as aids in management of STDs. Naribhandhob, an organization in collaboration with the Dutch organization Women on Waves,

Women on Web, Asia Safe Abortion Partnership, runs a free hotline that gives women access to information regarding drugs, procedures and post-abortal complications and care. The Federation of Gynaecology and Obstetrics (FIGO) has been running the initiative for unsafe abortion and its consequences in Bangladesh since 2008. They have contributed to the increased usage of manual vacuum aspiration in place of sharp curettage and have also legalized the use of a combination of Misoprostol and Mife pristone in 2012.

Crisis Situations: Refugees

In the 73rd United Nations General Assembly, Prime Minister Sheikh Hasina said that as of September 2018, there are 1.1 million Rohingya refugees in Bangladesh. The Muslim minority from Myanmar, have been slowly making their way across the border into Bangladesh since 1970s, however, the number has risen exponentially following the escalation of tensions in August 2017. The world's "most persecuted minority" have found shelter in the Kutapalong and Nayapara areas of Cox's Bazaar district in Bangladesh, where they now outnumber the locals by a 2:1 ratio. The majority are woman and children with 40% children under the age of 12 and 16% women single mother. According to a report by the Washington post, these children are suffering from severe mental trauma, malnutrition, diarrhea, while a majority of women are pregnant by sexual assault and are themselves in dire need of treatment and counseling.

According to a UNHCR report in 2017, 3422 cases of skin disease, 10846 cases of respiratory disease among the refugee population (United Nations Children's Fund. Bangladesh Humanitarian Situation report-10 (Rohingya Influx) New York: UNICEF, 2017). Another UNICEF report found 419 cases of measles in the same year (United Nations Children's Fund. Bangladesh Humanitarian Situation report-10 (Rohingya Influx) New York: UNICEF, 2017). As of February 2018, there were 5800 reported cases of diphtheria with 38 deaths. (World Health Organization. Weekly Situation Report. Bangladesh: WHO, 2018). The Ministry of Health and Family Welfare, in collaboration with organizations like WHO, UNICEF have been prompt in bringing out vaccines for diseases like measles, rubella, polio, tetanus and diphtheria. About 136,000 and 72,000 children up to the age of five were given vaccines for measles and polio (along with a dose of vitamin A) respectively.

In addition, antibiotics, ORS salines, 3.2 million water purification tablets as well and 18000 hygiene kits have been distributed. About 9 million liters of safe water are needed everyday, but only 30% of this is reaching the refugees. This is why despite a successful cholera vaccination campaign, many people are still falling ill due to unhygienic practices.

Pregnant women and lactating mothers have been named two of the most vulnerable groups among the Rohingya refugee population. About 12,000 pregnant and lactating women are said to be in need of treatment of malnutrition. There have been multiple reports of refugees having anxiety and panic attacks, difficulty sleeping and even eating disorders, as they recount the horrors they escaped. Social workers and psycho-therapists have been sent for counseling while children are undergoing therapy by being encouraged to draw pictures describing their ordeal.

The government of Bangladesh has been more than generous, and opened its arms to the influx of refugees. Locals have made every effort to rehabilitate the Rohingyas despite limited resources of their own. The local hospitals and local NGOs are working around the clock to provide healthcare to the people. World Food Program has been supplying rice rations, but is in need of more funds with the growing number of mouths to feed. Booths have been set up to unite loved ones. Lessons in English and Burmese are also being provided to them. To combat monsoon seasons, 63 km of retaining walls, 91 km of drainage pipes have been installed with the aid of UNHCR.

Despite its best efforts it is important to keep in mind that Bangladesh herself is a low middle-income country and also one of the most densely populated. The constant inflow of people will soon overwhelm, if it has not already, a country that is still trying to stand on her own feet. Multiple children have been reported to be missing and suspected to be trafficked to neighboring countries.

Accommodation of over one million people, means significant area has to be cleared by deforestation. For a country that is already dealing with rising sea levels, frequent landslides and floods, these do not bode well. Also the air is becoming polluted due to burning of firewood by the refugees, as well as the depletion of groundwater and contamination of streams. As the Rohingyas leave designated camps, and venture more inland, there is increased chances of conflict over resources, land and employment opportunities.

The world needs to take an active role in helping Rohingyas, rather than simply sympa-thizing. So far deals for repatriation with Myanmar have been unfruitful. Neighboring countries, while having condemned the actions against Rohingyas, have failed to mediate a solution.

Sexually Transmitted Diseases

Sexually transmitted diseases may affect people in all classes irrespective of gender and economic status in Bangladesh. The pre-valence of sexually transmitted disease is the major challenge in health sector in Bangladesh. A large number of migrant workers contribute the transmission of STDs in Bangladesh. Gonorrhea (29.5%), syphilis (12.6%), non-gonococcal urethritis (41.5%), genital herpes (8.4%) and HIV (0.7%) are the major infective organism for STDs.

HIV prevalence is very low in general population. In severe cases it is as high as 2.7% in casual sex workers. It is estimated that about 11000 people living with HIV are migrant workers. Other potential risk factors could be injectable drug users, female sex workers, male sex workers and transgenders.

Genital infections by Chlamydia are now recognized as highly prevalent sexually transmitted disease. Due to unprotected coitus, lack of sex education and migrant workers, STDs are becoming the burden in health sectors in Bangladesh. Mass education regarding sexual and reproductive health in primary and secondary school levels will help to reduce the STDs in Bangladesh. Injudicious use of antibiotics in the treatment of STDs causes antibiotic resistance in Bangladesh. There will be time, we will leave with no drugs for the treatment of STDs. Careful monitoring, mass education, proper guideline for the management of STDs are dare importance. Mass media can play a pivotal role for the elimination of STDs in Bangladesh.

CONCLUSIONS

Scenario for women in Bangladesh has improved in last 20 years. Maternal and child mortality is decreasing yet poor nutrition is a critical health problem in Bangladesh. Non-communicable diseases—chronic diseases, cancer, diabetes, cardiovascular diseases, and chronic respiratory disease are in increase trend.

Overpopulation, poverty, unemployment, crime, corruptions are the major problems which put health services of Bangladesh in back steps. Government has taken initiative to improve the situation by good governance, strengthened national policy in health sector by delivering mid-wife led continuous care and emergency obstetrics care.

The Government has set up a national committee for the adaptation and operationalization of the Sustainable Development Goals in the country. In near future Bangladesh will be a role model in women's health in this region.

BIBLIOGRAPHY

1. Adolescents in Bangladesh: A situation analysis of Pragmatic Approaches to Sexual and Reproductive Health Education Services. Sigma Ainul, Ashish Bajracharya.USADI.Jan 2017.
2. Bangladesh Wikipedia/gender equality.
3. Bangladesh.unfpa.org/en/topics/family-planing-4.
4. Bdnews24.com/Bangladesh/2018/02/19.
5. Bostonglobe.com/news/world/2017/01/31/rohingya-refuges-bangladesh-relocatedremote
6. Dhaka Tribune: 4/12/2018.
7. Dhakatribune.com/Bangladesh/2017/10/2 3/rohingya-influx-refuges-outnumber-ukhiya-teknaf-locals
8. Dhakatribune.com/health/201/1/04/chal-lenges-bangladesh-face-family-planing
9. Faxnews.com/world/Bangladesh-point-finger-at-myanmar-for-rohingya-genocide
10. Genital Infections by Chlamydia—An Overview: Hoque SM, Hossain MA, Paul SK. KYMAC Journal, Vol. 3, No. 1, June 2012.
11. Girlnotbrides.org/child-marriage/Bangladesh
12. Girlsnot.brides.org/child-marriage/Bangladesh/2017.
13. Guttamacher.org/fact-shed/menstrual regulation-unsafe-abortion-bangladesh
14. Guttamacher.org/fact-sheet/menstrual regulation-unsafe-abortion-bangladesh
15. Guttmacher.org/journal/iprsh/20013/03/Bangladesh-women-weigh-vriety-future-when-choosing-contraceptive
16. Independent.co.uk/news/world/rohingya muslim-crisis-burma-children-hungermal nutrition.
17. International Organization for Migration. Needs and Population Monitoring Round 6 Assessment Report-Cox's Bazar, Bangladesh. Geneva: International Organization for Migration; 2017.
18. Pattern of sexually transmitted diseases (STDs) among patients attending outpatient department of dermatology of Dhaka Medical College Hospital, Dhaka. AliCM, SikdarTK, Sultana N. J Dhak Med Coll.2010;1991:7–10.

19. Searo.who.int/entity/childadloscent/topics/child_health/fp-ban.pdf

20. Searo.who.int/mediacentre/releases/2017/1671/en.

21. Undp.org/content/dan/rbap/doc/womens empowerment/RBP-Gender/2013.

22. Unhcr.org/ph/campings/rohingyaemergency

23. Unhcr.org/ph/campings/rohingya-emergency

24. Unicef.org/sowc09/docs-country example-Mli-pdf

25. United Nations Children's Fund. Bangladesh Humanitarian Situation report-8 (Rohingya Influx). New York: UNICEF; 2017.

26. United Nations Children's Fund. Outcast and Desperate: Rohingya refugee children face a perilous Future. New York: UNICEF; 2017

27. Unwomen.org/en/news/stories/2018/feature-rohingya-humantarian -update.

28. Violence against women in Bangladesh. Nashid Tabassum Khan, Asma Begum. Delta Medical College Journal 5(1),25–29, 2017.

29. Washingtonpost.com/news/monkey-café/wp/2017/10/12/ there is a massivehumanatarian-crisis-in-bangladeshrohingya-refuge

Situation Analysis of Bhutan

Kiren Khurshid, Humaira Saleem, Shahla Kanwal

Bhutan

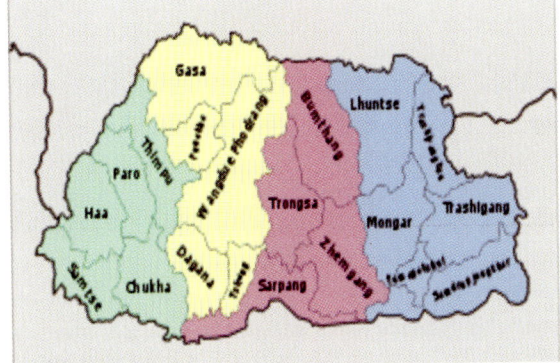

DEMOGRAPHICS

In South Asia Bhutan is a landlocked country located at the end of Himalayas between China and India.

Land area is 38,394 km². Its capital city is Thimphu. Country is divided in 20 Dzongkhags (districts), which are further subdivided in Dungkhags (subdistricts).

POPULATION AND POPULATION DENSITY

It is 164th most populous country of the world with one of the lowest population densities of the world. Official census was conducted in 2005–2006. The population in 2015 was 787356 which translates in 20.5 people/km², in 2018 population was 817054 (21.28 person/km²), in 2019 the estimate of population is 826229. Out of which 52% are males and 47% are females. Male to female ratio is 1.098. Currently projected

population is 900,000 by 2030. 30.5 percent of population is younger than 15 years, 62.7 percent between 15–64 years and the median age is 24 years. The average household size in Bhutan is 4.4 persons. Total fertility rate is estimated at 2.3 per 1000 live births and the population growth rate is estimated at 1.3 percent.

In 2019 annual growth rate is reported as 1.12 in different reports, previously in 2005 census it was 2% annually. There is one birth every 37 minutes that translates in 39 births per day and 17.3 births/1000 population. Reported death is one death every 103 minutes.

Life Expectancy

Life expectancy at birth in 1960 was 32.4 and it has improved enormously and in 2014 is reported to be 69.5. From 1950 to 2010, life expectancy at birth has nearly doubled and the values show, from 36.1 years to 66.8 years for females in 2010. This may be due to improved water, sanitation and health facilities.

Total Fertility Rate

Total fertility rate is 2 children per woman and in 2017 was reported 2.3 children.

CULTURAL AND ADMINISTRATIVE SETUP

Dzongkhag (Dzongkha: dzong khak) is an administrative and judicial district. The twenty dzongkhags are subdivided into 205 *gewogs*.

Some larger dzongkhags have one or more of an intermediate judicial division, known as *dungkhags* (subdistricts), which themselves comprise two or more *gewogs*. Legislation in 2002 was passed by The Parliament of Bhutan and in 2007 new legislation was for the status, structure, and leadership of local governments including dzongkhags. Its most recent legislation regarding dzongkhags is the Local Government Act of 2009.

An official who is elected head of a dzongkhag known as (district administrator or mayor) **dzongdag**. The Dzongkhag Tshogdus District Councils have the powers to enforce rules on health and public safety; advertising in regard to environmental aesthetics; to regulate environmental pollution, media in accordance with the Information, Communications, and Media Act; and to regulate gambling. These entities also generate their own finances and have an oversight on royal appointees and Dzongdags (governors).

Languages include Dzongkha which is national language and Nepali with other various regional dialects. The medium of instruction in schools is English. The primary basis of economy rests on agriculture, hydropower, forest industry and tourism. Bhutan's major trading partner is India, some other trading partners are Bangladesh, Thailand, Japan, Germany, UK and the USA. Main religion is Buddhists 75%, 22% are Hindus and 0.2% is Muslims.

WOMAN STATUS IN BHUTAN

Economic Participation

The Kingdom of Bhutan remains in isolation for many years, in cultural and economical terms, has gone through reforms politically with a government which is democratically elected and growing encounter due to influences from outside in the fields of trade, migration, education and tourism. These automatically influence all aspects of life in Bhutan. The mid-term report on the level of achievement of the Millennium Development Goals (MDG) has shown the development gains made by the country in recent years, and also highlighted some important challenges in future, especially in terms of equity of access to health and various socioeconomic benefits. Economic development in the country has led to increasing opportunities for men and women. Women in Bhutan have a major contribution towards economic development as their part in generation of economy is not less than men.

Literacy Rate

Current woman status in Bhutan is represented by many different indicators. Overall literacy rate is 60–64.9%. In woman literacy rate is 48.5% and this automatically translates into extent of economic and financial independence. By 1989 the percentage of women employees in government sector was only 10%, but the women were dominant labour force in agriculture. The government founded an association named the National Women's Association of Bhutan in 1981, with main intention to improve the socioeconomic status of women, with special attention to those living in rural areas. The total female workforce that was unemployed is less than 4%, compared with men out of which 10% possess no occupation.

There are many pro-women or women supporting organizations in the country which encourage women to raise their earnings by different ways as weaving, food business. One such organization is SABAH Bhutan. Women in labour force are 65.8% which is quite high.

Gender Gap

Global Gender Gap Index was 0.6651 (2013) which is 93rd out of 149 in the world in 2013. According to the Global Gender Gap Index 2016, Bhutan is at 21st position out of 144 countries. This clearly depicts a drop of almost 29 countries from 2013 when rank of Bhutan was at 93 out of 136 countries. The report found reasonable disparity against females in education and other sectors as health economy and politics in the Kingdom of Bhutan.

Women in parliament constitute 13.9% of the total. First woman minister was elected in 2013. In 2016, out of 26,954 civil servants, 35.5 percent were women which translate in a rise of 77 percent in the last decade. Although adult literacy rates are still lower than many other countries (particularly for women), primary school enrollment rates show a rise from 45% in 1990 to 84% in 2005. Health expenditure is 3.6% of GDP.

Health Indicators

Maternal mortality rate is reported as 148/ 100,000 live births by CIA world fact book and infant mortality rate is 32/1000 live births. According to Annual Health Bulletin 2017, maternal mortality has decreased from 255 in 2000 to 86/100000 live births in 2016. According to government statistics Bhutan has achieved Millennium Development Goal 5. Total fertility rate is 2 children/woman. This depicts a declining trend from 3.8 in 2000 to 2.6 in 2009 and now just 1.9–2. This is a clear indicator that country is focusing in woman health and population dynamics. The National Commission for Women and Children (NCWC) was established in 2004 and responsibility was assigned to take the lead in promoting and protecting the rights of women and children. Adolescent fertility rate which means births per 1000 women aged 15–19 years is 28.4.

Reproductive Health (RH) Indicators

Antenatal care coverage: It means at least one visit (ANC 1+) in Bhutan is 97.9%. Antenatal care coverage at least four visits (ANC 4+) is 81.7%. Antenatal care coverage at least 8 visits 26.1%. Percentage of women aged 15–49 years who received postnatal care for their most recent birth in the past 2 years before the survey 74.6%. The proportion of the births attended by skilled health personnel has rose from 23.7 percent in 2000 to over 89 percent in 2016. There were 10948 deliveries with 10781 deliveries conducted in the health centers while 230 deliveries had occurred at home, 13 both attended by trained birth attendants in 2016.

Percentage of women aged 15–49 years who were informed about the danger signs of pregnancy during antenatal visits for their most recent birth in the past 2 years were 46.2%. Women aged 15–49 years who knew at least one contraceptive method that could prevent or delay pregnancy were 96.3%. According to survey prevalence of colostrums feeding among women aged 15–49 years who received post-natal care for their most recent birth in the past 2 years preceding the survey was 87.5%. Percentage of women aged 20–59 years who are aware of breast cancer was 66.0.

74.6% women aged 20–59 years are aware of Pap smear test. HPV vaccination—girls who turned 13 years till 1st Jan 2013. In this group crude HPV vaccination coverage (card + history) was 73.3% and only Crude HPV vaccination coverage (by card only) was 90.5%. In a study in 2013 in Bhutan the prevalence of Anemia was reported as 54.8% in mothers of child bearing age.

Marriage

Child marriage was once widespread but now is a rare event in Bhutan. Marriage Law passed in 1980, age for girls was sixteen years for marriage. Polyandry is rare but Brokpas of Merak-Sakten still practice in Bhutan. Marriages with foreigners are discouraged by government. Polygamy is allowed in law, allowing up to three wives to a man with the permission of first wife.

ADOLESCENT SEXUAL AND REPRODUCTIVE HEALTH

Though child marriage is a rare event in Bhutan now but teenage pregnancies contribute a significant number in total births. According to Ministry of Health in 2008, 11% of total births were of mothers at a younger age and risks identified were there was lack of awareness among this age group about reproductive and sexual health. This area has not shown any progress in its indicators as adolescent fertility rate has rose up to 28% in 2012.

Contraceptive Prevalence Rate

Contraceptive prevalence rate (CPR) is 65.6% which is better than many other countries in this region.

Under Five Mortality Rate

In 2000 under five mortality rate was 84 /1000 live births and in 2016 reported as 37.3/1000 live births with a major chunk due to deaths of newborns, i.e. 21/1000 live births.

HEALTH FACILITIES FOR MATERNAL AND CHILD HEALTH

With the cooperation of UNICEF 1005 health workers are trained in early essential newborn care (EENBC) and Kangroo Mother Care (KMC) among ten high load delivery hospitals. This will result in decrease in perinatal mortality rate in upcoming years. Maternal and child health staff is trained in 20 districts for infant and young feeding, lactation management and nutrition counseling. Health assistants in rural areas are appointed at basic health units and this is major step towards reduction in unattended births. Moreover, initially emergency obstetric care (EmOC) was available in referral centers but now this essential service is available across the country and basic health units. This step has resulted in a significant fall in maternal mortality over the years. For the children health, the healthcare providers or healthcare assistants assess weight, height of a child and provide vitamin A and deworming tablets till a child reaches five years of age.

Violence

According to National Health Survey of Bhutan in 2012, in currently married women aged 15–75 years, 6.1% experienced physical violence by their intimate partner and 2.1% of currently married women aged 15–75 years experienced sexual violence by their intimate partner, in the same group of women aged 15–75 years, psychological violence by their intimate partner was 3.2%.

The knowledge and skills about how to protect oneself from violence was given to 3000 adolescents, 300 young monks and nuns, these trainings were supported by UNICEF as reported by UNICEF in 2017. Research on violence against children in Bhutan conducted by UNICEF reveals that commercial sexual exploitation has emerged as a serious issue in southern and south-eastern dzongkhags and girls experience sexual violence and harassment.

The emergence of drayangs, where women dance in bars to entertain men has been criticized as institutionalized prostitution. In National Assembly this issue has been raised. According to the Bhutan Infocomm and Media Authority (BICMA) records, there are 42 drayangs in the country today providing employment mostly for women. While the drayang owners deny the practice of commercial sex, people who visit the drayangs report that commercial sex is being practiced there.

In the year 2017, there was implementation of many recommendations from the 2016 Violence against Children research, with the Government initiating a review of the National Plan of Action for Child Protection (2013–2018). National Strategy and a Plan of Action for Protection of Children in Monastic Institutions (2017–2022) have been made. Major policymakers and eminent stakeholders are directly engaged with more than 3,000 adolescents and young people all over the country to offer suggestions and devise solutions on addressing challenges. While the strategic shift towards more upstream policy and UNICEF cooperation results are now showing up. In 2004, NGO Respect, Educate, Nurture, Empower Women (RENEW) was established. RENEW deals with domestic violence cases and its community-based support system extends to district level where domestic violence and sexual and gender-based violence survivors are identified and supported.

Abortion

The National Assembly's women, children and youth committees reported that in 2015, 1,556 women had undergone abortion in Bhutan. The mothers or health centers report the cases of abortion. The actual burden of abortions is believed to be much more. Medical termination of pregnancy was legalized in 1999 in cases of risk to maternal health.

Other Key Indicators

GDP per capita is around 3438 US dollars, and 3.6% of GDP is expenditure on health. Obesity prevalence is 6.4% and poverty rate is 8.2%. In general, improved water access is 98.6%. The percentage of pre-school education gross enrolment is 22 percent and transition rates for primary to secondary education is 97 per cent and these figures have surpassed the targets set for 2018 which were set as 20 per cent for preschool enrolment and 95 per cent for transition with the cooperation of UNICEF. All over Bhutan free medical services are provided through a network of district hospitals, connected with Regional Referral hospitals located in Gelephu, Phuentsholing and Mongar. The National Referral Hospital is in Thimphu, the capital city, and a network of

District Hospitals and Basic Health Units is present in the districts (2,3). According to the information given in Annual Health Bulletin 2013, 48.7% of the babies are exclusively breast fed in first six months of life.

General Medical Issues

Government has endorsed different plans as Bhutan's Every Newborn Action Plan 2016–2023, the National Sanitation, Hygiene Policy and the Accelerated Nutrition Plan 2016–2018 with UNICEF support to provide a strong framework for rapid progress in the areas of health, nutrition and water, sanitation and hygiene (WASH). UNICEF supported a temperature monitoring study for the immunization cold chain, a stillbirth estimate study, a determinant analysis of undernutrition and a menstrual hygiene management needs assessment to increase evidence-based policy making, UNICEF annual report 2017 revealed that a good indicator for general health especially of children is reported by decrease in stunting. In 1998 stunting in Bhutan was 61% which has decreased to 21% in 2015. This indicates an improvement in nutritional status of the country.

Immunization

Immunization coverage has been maintained above 95 per cent for 11 basic antigens, covering adolescent girls and pregnant women along with children. Bhutan is certified with measles elimination status. UNICEF and WHO provided critical support for the certification as reported in Annual Report 2017.

Special Situations

There is a rapid growth in household incomes and has gone to double digit. Poverty rates has gone down significantly, even then there are areas and population groups that lag behind. These include those residing in remote areas, immigrants and the urban poor. Urban population was just 25% in 2001 which has increased rapidly to 36% in 2009. Girls should be protected from harmful cultural practices such as **night hunting,** and from teenage pregnancies, and abortions and all other forms of violence. The establishment of a Women and Children bench at the Thimphu district court should be seen as a step forward to gender-friendly policies.

UNICEF is actively supporting six inter-agency theme teams in Bhutan to work at different sectors:

1. Disability
2. Data
3. SDGs
4. Emergency preparedness and response
5. Gender-based violence.
6. Nutrition.

Refugees

The Marriage Act and the Citizenship Law, 1985 have not accepted several thousand Lhotshampas as their nationals. As a result of the foreign wives of Lhotshampa husbands are not granted citizenship, so more than 60,000 children were not given Bhutanese citizenship. This is more than 20 percent of the total children population of Bhutan. Refugee children constitute a significant portion of the country's total population. More than 10,000 Lhotshampa wives are not nationals according to prevailing Marriage Act as stated by BWCO.

HIV and Tuberculosis

597 cases are reported from 1993 to 2018, out of which 309 are males and 288 are females. 452 are living now. 93% acquired infection through unprotected heterosexual relationship and 6% is mother to child transmission and 1% through injections. 29% are detected by contact tracing, 22% on voluntary testing and 9% on antenatal screening as reported by UNAIDS 2018. Tuberculosis mostly is affecting the productive age group between 15 and 44 years. The success of treatment is around 90 percent.

Multi-Drugs Resistance Tuberculosis (MDR-TB) is a public health concern, and of a total 1145 TB cases, 43 cases were MDR-TB in 2016 were reported. Poor compliance by patients during the course of treatment has resulted in emergence of MDR-TB.

Noncommunicable Diseases and Cancers

Noncommunicable diseases (NCDs) are on a rise as in other parts of South Asia. The prevalence of diabetes is 6.4 and proportion of hypertension is 37. This in turn leads to increase in cardiovascular diseases, stroke and cerebrovascular events. In 2014, from health centers 639 cases of cancers were reported in the country. By gender, the males had a higher incidence (61%) as compared to females (39%). The top ten cancers include stomach, cervix, colo-rectaectum, head and neck, oesophageal, ovary, breast, hepatobiliary and skin.

The head and neck cancer, hematological and cervical cancers are in the highest numbers in terms of the referrals and annually, about Nu. 160 million on an average is spent just for cancer referrals outside the country.

Various five year plans are functional in Bhutan to achieve different targets of above mentioned indicators as 11th Five Year Plan of Royal Government of Bhutan, WHO Country Cooperation Strategy and United Nations Development Assistance Framework 2014–2018 for Bhutan. All of them set up six different but interlinked strategic priorities. These focus on equal access to health, reduction in NCDs, morbidity and mortality and enhancing public health leadership.

CONCLUSION

In the context of development going on in the country at a larger level, the change and transformation to democracy in past few years has been a trendsetter towards decentrali-zation, and also with the formation of civil society agencies though in developmental stages collaboration of different sectors at various levels has started. This ongoing development has directed towards an increase in rural to urban migration, which in turn has led to changes in lifestyles and livelihoods being followed traditionally.

Overall, the rapidly enhancing effects of administrative reform (decentralization), globalization and economic development with a result of population movement will mean a peak shift for all sectors especially health sector in the context of planning and strategic development over the coming years in Bhutan. Hence, health reforms will require keeping up the pace with this social transition, and support from all is needed especially in the form of resource mobilization.

Although Bhutan is making progress in different parameters set internationally for a country development but still there is a lot of requirement of improvements in national health system. Bhutan has to reach targets set for maternal, adolescent and child health. Though maternal mortality is low as reported by government at 80/100,000 live births still has to reach up to 70 for sustainable development goals. The improvement in this indicator over the years can be attributed to improvement in women literacy rate and higher percentage in jobs and politics, leading to women empowerment. Moreover, decrease in total fertility rate and a rise in contraceptive prevalence rate translates in better women health and hence a decrease in maternal mortality rate. Government and other supporting agencies efforts in the form of extension of EmOC services up to basic health unit and training of health assistants has played a major role. Still hemorrhage is the leading cause of maternal death in Bhutan and targets can be achieved if qualification, management and information system of health sector is strengthened further.

To meet the challenges for sustainable development goals in Bhutan, the country needs to emphasize on early marriages and gender equality. This can be achieved by strengthening the institutions and community at large especially women and girls partici-pation. Increase in awareness about adolescent sexual and reproductive rights and protection from STIs are the major areas which need improvement and attention.

Gender-based violence reported by Government of Bhutan is around 2–3% that is low as compared to rest of the countries of the region. As reported in 2012 by WHO, it is 37.3% in South East Asia. The major determinants of low rate in Bhutan may be attributed to higher enrollment of girls at primary and secondary school education and acting of woman as majority in labour force work leading to financial independence and women empowerment. Even then further work has to be done with poor, unemployed less educated sectors of the population.

To conclude, for further improvement in women reproductive and sexual rights in Bhutan, academic institutions, health sector, training centers and capacity building of female community itself is the need of the day.

BIBLIOGRAPHY

1. "All in the Family", Kuensel 27 August 2007.
2. Annual Health Bulletin Bhutan 2017 MOH (Ministry of Health).
3. Annual Health Survey 2016: Ministry of Health 2016.
4. Bhutan women and child organization bulletin 2016.
5. Census report Bhutan 2005–2006.
6. CIA World Fact Book 2015
7. Data Bank: World Development Indicators. The World Bank 2017.
8. Department of Public Health. Maternal and Neonatal Deaths Review (Draft). Thimphu 2016.
9. "Dzongkhag YargayTshogdu Chathrim 2002" (PDF). Government of Bhutan. 23 July 2002. Retrieved 3 March 2016.
10. "Final Delimitation". Election Commission, Government of Bhutan. 2011. Retrieved 3 March 2013.
11. "Freedom in the World 2011 - Bhutan". UNHCR Refworld online. Freedom House. 2011-05-12. Retrieved 2011-05-20.

12. Health Management Information System Unit. Monthly activity report 2016.

13. Ministry of Health. Bhutan Cancer Report 2015.

14. Ministry of Health. National Child Health Strategy (2014–2018). In: Health DoP, editor. Thimphu 2014.

15. Ministry of Health. National Health Survey In: Thimphu, editor. 2012.

16. National Health Survey Bhutan 2012, Feature.

17. National Statistical Bureau, "Statistical Yearbook of Bhutan", 2016.

18. National TB Control Program, MoH 2016.

19. NCWC, "Bhutan Gender Policy Note", 2013.

20. Priyadarshini Verma. "Women in Bhutan: Exploring their Socio Cultural Status in the late 20th Century." Proceedings of the Indian History Congress 75 (2014):920–27.

21. The Global Gender Gap Report 2013 (PDF). World Economic Forum. pp. 12–13.

22. "The Local Government Act of Bhutan, 2009" (PDF). Government of Bhutan. 11 September 2009. Retrieved 3 March 2016.

23. "The Local Governments' Act of Bhutan 2007" (PDF). Government of Bhutan. 31 July 2007. Retrieved 3 March 2016.

24. This article incorporates public domain material from the Library of Congress document: Robert L. Worden (Sept. 1991). Andrea Matles Savada, editor. "Bhutan: A country study". Federal Research Division. Role of Women.

25. UNAIDS 2018.

26. UNICEF, 2016, A research on violence against children in Bhutan.

27. World Bank. Data Bank: Development Indicators 2017.

28. "World Health Organization, Kingdom of Bhutan". www.searo.who.int. ab Law, Gwillim (18 Dec. 2010). "Districts of Bhutan". Administrative Divisions of Countries ("Statoids"). Retrieved 31 December 2010.

4

Situation Analysis of India

Shyam Desai, Parikshit Dahyalal Tank

INDIA—DEMOGRAPHICS

Population and Population Density

India is the second most populous country in the world, after China. India s population in 2018 stands at 1.3 billion people. One in 6 people who are in the world are in India. By land area, India is the seventh largest country. Needless to say, there is a high population density of 412 people per square kilometer. This ranks 31st in the world. In some cities, such as Mumbai, the population density is very high and is believed to be about 21000 people per square kilometer.

Growth Rate

Over the last decade, India s population has been growing at 1.1% per year. India has doubled its population in the last 40 years. This rapid growth rate has been termed a population explosion. It led to various measures to curb population and family welfare became an integral part of every government s health policy. Even though the fertility rate has declined and total fertility rate (TFR) is approaching replacement levels (2.3 in 2016), it is estimated that India will overtake China as the most populous country in the next 20 years.

Urban–Rural Mix

There is an often quoted refrain that India lives in its villages. This does hold true even today.

However, the scenario is changing fast. In the year 1947 when India became independent, less than 5% of India lived in cities. By 2011, census data showed that over a third of Indians lived in cities. However, satellite imagery studies have shown that this figure may be higher. Current estimates of urban population have crossed the halfway mark, even though definitions and estimates differ. This is important from the point of view of allocation of resources under government schemes. The urban areas have pockets of urban poor*f* who have vastly unmet needs of healthcare.

Population Pyramid: Age Mix and the Demographic Dividend

The Indian population is poised for a demographic dividend. This is due to the proportion of working age people. As the number of people in the working age group is high, it is presumed that their productivity will contribute to the nation s GDP. This working age population is set to grow by 7% in the coming decade. Therefore, it is hypothesized that even though India is populous, it could also be prosperous. The Indian GDP growth rate is over 6%, which is in the top quartile in the world. However, this estimate will persist only if the overall population stabilizes and TFR slows further. If the overall population increases, the productivity of the working age group will not keep pace and the economy and infrastructure will suffer.

INDIA—PREVAILING CULTURAL AND SOCIAL ENVIRONMENT

Diversity and Multiculturalism

India can truly be defined as a multi-cultural nation. There is immense heterogeneity in the country and varied religions, cultures and traditional practices flourish here. The Indian constitution asserts that the Indian state is secular. This guarantees an equality of all religions and the freedom to practice the religion of one's choice. As in the rest of the world, the largest influence on culture comes from religion. About 80% of India are Hindus, 14% follow Islam and the remaining are Christians, Sikhs, Jains, Buddhists, Parsis, Jews and others.

Implications of Religion for Sexual and Reproductive Health

Almost the entire population follows some religion or another. Every religion imposes restrictions and boundaries on what women can and should be allowed to do. These vary by religion and community and therefore the range of problems to be addressed is large. The major implication of this for sexual and reproductive health is that the problems that women face are different. The common thread is that of restriction and suppression of women s rights (human, health, and reproductive) and opportunities (educational, financial and entrepreneurial).

The other implications for sexual and reproductive health apropos religion are the universality of marriage, taboos about menstruation, sexuality and contraception, and other religion-specific issues.

The only potential upside of religion is that if and when religious leaders are involved and can be convinced to work towards community improvement, mass involvement occurs and results can be seen rapidly.

Current Social Environment Apropos Women in India

There is gross inequality in the social structure amongst the genders. This begins before birth in the form of female feticide and prevails through the life cycle. The inequality is reflected in every parameter of health (infant mortality rate, under-5 mortality rate, immunization coverage, health spending), social development (literacy, education opportunities) and financial independence (wage gap).

Today, women in India have better opportunities than in any other time in recent history. Anecdotal stories and incidents such as India having a woman head of state, prime minister, armed forces heads, business chiefs and sporting stars abound. But it is the systematic promotion of women through gender equalizing measures that is bringing change at the ground level and closing the gap on the various parameters mentioned above.

As women are developing and fulfilling their fullest potentials, the cultural fabric of society is changing. These changes are more prevalent in urban areas and they mirror society in the West. Women are more open about sexuality, relationships are moving away from traditional marriages and health-seeking behavior is increasing. There is a rise in some risk factors for reproductive health (smoking, alcohol consumption, sexually transmitted infections, delayed child bearing leading to infertility).

The chapter will now further examine the most important issues related to sexual and reproductive health in the Indian context keeping the demographics and prevailing social cultural environment.

Violence against Women—Domestic

Violence in domestic settings is almost always directed towards the woman. There are various forms of such violence and definitions have evolved with time. The current definitions accepted in India by law are given by the Protection of Women from Domestic Violence Act 2005. The law now defines domestic violence against women to include sexual, physical, verbal, emotional and financial abuse. Even though reporting is low, the National Family and Health Survey in 2005 estimated that about a third of women experience domestic violence and of them, 8.5% have experienced sexual domestic violence. Other statistics prevail and anecdotal data based on rhetoric is often quoted in media. However, the reliability of such data is questionable.

Dowry

A common cultural practice in most communities in India is Dowry. This is the gift*f* given by the woman s family to the husband for accepting her as his bride. The burdensome arrangement and escalating expectations have lead to women/brides being subjected to violence in their newly wed homes and lives. This particular form of domestic violence is not unique to India. An extreme form of inflicting such violence involves setting the woman on fire under the guise of a kitchen accident. According to the National Crimes Records Bureau of the Ministry of Home Affairs of India, the last estimates of such deaths was published in 2012 and 8233 dowry deaths were reported. This translates to 1.4 deaths per year per 100 000 women in India. To put this into context, similar rates of homicides and violence against women prevail in the West. The worldwide rate of women s homicide is 3.6 per 100 000 women and in Northern Europe, it is 1.6 per 100 000 women per year.

The Dowry Prohibition Act was passed in 1961 and was made more stringent with the inclusion of Section 498A clause. This makes the law strongly in favour of women. Even with such laws, it is thought that the rates of reporting of dowry related violence is lower than the actual prevalence. The conviction rates are also proportionately lower. Families of women who are killed are intimidated, bullied and shamed into withdrawing complaints or they shy away from pursuing justice due to social pressures.

There has been substantial criticism of this clause by various groups, mostly comprising of men who have been subjected to false cases by women who have filed complaints with a malicious intent. However, these numbers are small.

Violence against Women—Workplace

In the workplace, women are subjected to violence in forms which are usually non-physical. Women face gender-based and systematic harassment at the workplace. This is prevalent in various workplace settings and across various strata of society. It is almost impossible to give an accurate rate of such occurrences. There are good grounds to believe that the prevalence is very high and some estimate it to be universal. Sexual harassment in the law is defined as per the Act passed in 2013 and is a broad umbrella that includes women in organized as well as unorganized sectors. Sexual harassment is a broad term which recognizes various gender-based discriminations, violations, and *quid pro quo* arrangements as being illegal.

Legal Status

The law mandates the setting up of Vishakha Committees in every workplace. This allows a channel for women to complain and be heard justly. The purpose is also to protect women from difficult legal procedures and ensure swift action. Complaints are to be addressed by the committee as per the Vishakha Guidelines and the process is time bound. The onus of constituting and conducting the proceeding lie on the employer. The committees have the powers of a civil court in terms of gathering evidence.

Social Media and #Me Too

In 2018, the issue of workplace based sexual harassment was in the spotlight. The origins of this are not clearly defined but are thought to be based on social media driven movements which operated under #Me Too and #Times Up. A number of famous personalities in entertainment, media and industry were named by various women in this regard. It is difficult to predict the long-term outcomes of such movements. There has been a raised awareness of the problem across strata and alertness on this issue in recent times. Women seem to be more vocal at expressing their angst and are speaking up more openly. Hopefully, this should translate into more gender sensitivity and lower prevalence of sexual harassment. There have been various criticisms of these media movements in terms of personal exposure, possibility of defamation and lack of penetration to the lower strata of society.

Rape

Indian law has recently broadened the definition of rape to include forms of sexual acts other than peno-vaginal intercourse. The current definition is more comprehensive and has also raised the age of valid consent for sexual intercourse to eighteen years from the earlier sixteen year limit. At present, marital rape is not recognized as a crime if a man and woman are married and are living together. It is a crime if they are married but live separately. Other forms of sexual violence such as voyeurism, stalking, and acid attacks have also been made punishable under the new amendments. The law for minors (male and female) is set by the Protection of Children from Sexual Offences Act (POCSO) of 2012. This was enacted to protect individuals below the age of eighteen years from sexual assault, sexual harassment, sexual violence and pornography.

Rape is a common occurrence in India. It is difficult to determine how common it is.

Western media has called India the rape capital of the world. On the other hand, official statistics show a very low incidence and India ranks amongst countries with the lowest incidence of sexual violence. The truth lies somewhere in between. There is under reporting of rape in India due to the difficult legal system, fear of further violation, shame brought to self and family and low conviction rates causing a sense of futility amongst survivors in going ahead with a complaint.

Nirbhaya Law and Fast-track Courts

There has been a concentrated effort in recent times since the country was shaken by a particularly violent, vicious and publicized sexual assault in 2013 which resulted in public outcry and protests. Legal systems for filing complaints with the police have been made easier. Police stations are now mandated to have women officers to receive sexual assault complaints. Gender sensitivity training has been widely disseminated amongst the police force and workers who come into contact with survivors of sexual assault. Standard procedures for consent and collection of evidence from survivors have been established and these have done away with antiquated tests such as the "two-finger test" which are demeaning and have no legal value. Conviction rates are still low, but it is hoped that with improved reporting and legal systems, these will change positively.

Genital Mutilation

Female Genital Mutilation hardly received any attention in India until this decade. There are practices in certain communities which could be construed as genital mutilation as per the international norms. However, these communities have taken a stand that there is no mutilation, but a physical religious ritual, akin to circumcision for men, which is widely prevalent and accepted.

Dawoodi Bohras practice removal of the clitoral hood (partial or complete) in a ceremony performed on preadolescent girls in non-standard health care settings. This is called *khafz* or *khatna*. The practice is thought to regulate sexuality and instill a moral temper in the girl as she grows up. A similar practice is also seen amongst some Muslim sects in Northern Kerala and is called *sunnathkalyanam*.

As per the definition given by the World Health Organization, these practices constitute Type 1 female genital mutilation. The practice exposes women to acute problems such as pain, bleeding, local infection and urinary tract infections. It may also have long-term implications in the form of chronic lower urinary tract symptoms, sexual dysfunction, abnormal vaginal discharge, dyspareunia and body dysmorphology. From the perspective of a professional gynecologist, it seems unlikely that removal of the clitoral hood alone without removing a part of the clitoris can be done by surgically untrained persons.

In India, a public interest litigation (PIL) has been filed in the Supreme Court contending that this practice is against the fundamental constitutional freedoms of right to life, right to equality and especially violates children s rights. The Dawoodi Bohra community has contested these claims. They have contested that restricting such practice is a restriction of the fundamental right to practice religion freely. The Government has taken a stand that there has been no official statistics on the prevalence of this practice. However, the Minister for Women and Child Development has expressed that such practice should be stopped voluntarily by the community or it would be banned by law.

SPECIAL SITUATIONS

SATI

This ancient custom has long stopped being practiced in India. The custom involved Hindu women sacrificing their lives by climbing the funeral pyre along with their deceased husbands. The practice was banned by the colonial government in 1829 in the Bengal province and it was further extended to the rest of the country in 1861. The Sati Prevention Act of 1988 criminalizes any type of aiding, abetting and glorification of this practice. The practice received some attention recently due to a Hindi film (Padmavat) depicting the event in a bygone era.

Child Marriage

The legal age for marriage in India is 18 years for girls and 21 years for boys. Due to a number of religious factors, traditions and cultural norms, it is common for girls, especially, to be married earlier. India has the largest number of girl brides globally. This has important implications for the girl in terms of exposing her to sexual intercourse and consequently infections and pregnancy at an early age. Pregnancy at an age younger than 15 years carries significant obstetric and medical risks. Child marriage and subsequently the burden of family responsibilities limits the opportunities that the girl has for education and financial independence. The cycle tends to repeat itself over generations.

The possible reasons behind such practices vary by religion and specific cultures. Child marriage is much more prevalent in rural areas, and amongst the socially and economically backward sections of society. The law is not implemented and there is protectionism by local leaders and tribal chiefs. The lack of action against such practices is largely a reflection of the lack of political will and fear of electoral backlash. The underlying thread in the prevalence of the practice on a national and possibly on a global level is the low social status that girls are accorded. They are usually looked upon as a burden to be passed on at the earliest to the husband s family in exchange for dowry. The other reasons for such a high prevalence is sham marriages used as a front for trafficking young girls.

Over the last decade, there has been a reduction in the proportion of women married by 18 years from 47% to 27%. This has largely been through the joint efforts of the central and various state governments, bodies such as UNICEF and UNFPA, and civil society. There has been a positive change coming from the community in response to the various initiatives launched by this joint effort. The thrust of the movement is towards empowerment. A positive legal and policy environment has been nurtured. Community leaders have been sensitized and through mass media, local and culturally appropriate programs, the message has percolated to the population. Girls are also being engaged into vocational courses to build skills that can make them financially self-sufficient such as training to work on computers, mechanics, nursing and self-defence. A key strategy has been to strengthen access to services through government programs such as the RKSK (Rashtriya Kishore Swasthya Karyakram National Adolescent Health Program). The institutionalization of such initiatives allows for a formalization and systematic change which is sustainable.

Honor Killings

Honor killing is the murder of a woman by her family members when she has chosen to marry or has married to a man outside of what is acceptable to the family.

This is usually accompanied by the murder of the man as well. The reason for this barbaric practice is the patriarchal mindset that the honor of a family is borne by the woman. She is looked upon as the guardian of the family s honor and if her choice does not match the expectations of the family (and broadly the community or tribe), she has committed adultery and therefore, should be punished and made a lesson for other women in the same situation. Approximately 100 of the global 5000 honor killings occur in India annually. An important reason for these is the caste system, the existence of very powerful and influential local bodies such as khap panchayats (which consider themselves to be above the laws of the land) and a lack of education in general.

There is no specific law which deals with honor killings in India. The Supreme Court, in 2018, has given guidelines for the state to implement specifically to prevent honor killings. This includes regulations on khap panchayats, protection of couples and measures for preventing their torture and abuse.

Trafficking

Human trafficking in India is a significant but understated problem. People are trafficked for different reasons. Most men and boys are trafficked for labour and crime related work. Girls and women are mostly trafficked for sex-related work. India, being a large and populous country, is a hub for human trafficking crimes in South Asia. A number of individuals may be willing entrants into the job market and may migrate, but are then misled and duped into exploitative work. Human trafficking of millions of individuals results in a huge financial gain for criminals and it is estimated that these gains could be as large as 7 billion USD. In India, the Government has introduced a bill which has been passed by the Lok Sabha (lower house of Parliament) to deal with Human Trafficking. The Trafficking of Persons (Prevention, Protection and Rehabilitation) Bill of 2018 sets out procedures and mechanisms for investigation, tracking and detection of human trafficking. It also looks at the penalties for the same, including aggravated trafficking. The stringent provisions (rigorous imprisonment of 10 years and/or fine of Rupees Fifty Thousand) are meant to be deterrents. It also provides for punishment of lessors and owners of premises where trafficking has been committed. There are some controversial features of the Bill. Some aspects are already covered under existing laws and there is a concern that there could be confusion on the correct criminal law that would apply. Also, there is a fear that there could be victimization of the trafficked individual.

Human trafficking, especially that of girls and women, is a complex problem. A number of measures have been taken over the years to combat it. Security forces have been sensitized on this problem, especially in border areas of India and Nepal. Help desks have been established at major railway stations. Security forces are also running awareness campaigns about the problem using mobile caravans going into villages and small towns. The Ministry for Home Affairs and the Ministry form Women and Children run an identification program called Track Child for missing children. There are various government lead initiatives such as Ujjwala and Swadhar Gruh which look after rehabilitation of trafficked women and providing shelter for women and children until they are independent. There have been increases in the allocation of funds towards these schemes. Besides law and government interventions, there is a need for social integration at the society and community level.

Refugees

Refugees have always been a source of political controversy. There is a fine line between an individual being an immigrant and a refugee in the international scenario. Within a given country, refugees are often referred to as internally displaced people. They face the common problems of a lack of livelihood, difficulty in accessing healthcare even in emergencies, poor social status and vulnerability to violence, hate crimes and exploitation. Each of these problems compounds the other and therefore, refugees (international and domestic) pose difficult problems to administrators, security forces and healthcare providers. Ever since India was partitioned in 1947, there have been refugees entering the country legally and illegally. The most recent influx has been the Rohingyas from Myanmar.

There are no specific laws on refugees in India. International refugees are dealt with on a case-by-case application basis by the Government on a bilateral basis. The United Nations Human Commission for Refugees (UNHCR) works with the Government on these issues. India has granted asylum to about 200000 refugees from across the world. The process of refugee status determination is followed. Refugees are then advised and integrated into local communities. The earlier practice of separate areas, known as camps, is now being given up except for the early internment.

Medical Issues in General

Women face gender inequality in seeking and provision of healthcare in India, just as in other walks of life and just as in other countries in the region. The proportion and extent is largely determined by the level of education, social background and financial independence. In India, about 80% of healthcare is through the private sector. The private sector is largely reimbursed on a pay-per-use model since insurance penetration in outside metro Therefore, the member of the India, especially cities is low, decision-making family for health matters is usually the one who controls the finances.

With improving healthcare facilities in the public sector, acceptability of going to public hospitals from a social standpoint and the recently launched Ayushman Bharat (Modicare) health insurance scheme of the Government of India, the healthcare scenario is set for a change. Women are important health beneficiaries under the scheme. Not only are they directly affected by access to quality maternity care, but they will also be able to influence child care substantially.

Health Rights

India is a signatory to various international treaties on human rights, such as the International Covenant on Economic, Social and Cultural Rights (ICESCR). These treaties have various clauses which make health a pre-requisite human right. The constitution of India does not make any special mention of individual health but does mention protection of public health. In modern times, courts have increasingly looked upon the right to health as a logical extension of the right to life. The National Health Policy, 2017, proposes an ambitious health agenda. The policy is directed towards moving the system towards a rights-based approach. However, it also acknowledges the lack of infrastructure and basic prerequisites (doctor–patient ratio, number of hospital beds, etc.) which stop the state from making this a legally enforceable issue. At present, every citizen is accorded equal access to public health facilities.

Consent

In terms of healthcare, consent should have three components—disclosure, capacity and voluntariness. According to the Indian Constitution, an individual has the right to self-determination and treatment should be administered only when consent (implied, verbal or written) has been given. The type of consent depends on the context in which it is being administered, the patient's condition and degree/extent of possible damage. The exception to seeking consent is, of course, emergency situations, with an immediate and imminent risk to life. Considering the ground realities of the level of education and health information available and the doctor–patient ratio, the courts in India accept the concept of "real" consent rather than "informed" consent.

As such, consent is valid only if it is given by the individual undergoing the treatment. The exception to this is in case of minors (age less than 18 years) and those of unsound mind.

Another area of exception is in reproductive healthcare. The Medical Council of India Code of Ethics and Regulation, 2002 states that for a married individual, if a surgery or procedure is likely to result in or intended to make the individual sterile, consent should be obtained from both partners. This is important from the point of view of surgical procedures of permanent sterilization. It is also important to note that from the legal point of view, consent for contraception (insertion of intrauterine device) and termination of pregnancy is to be obtained only from the woman undergoing the procedure.

Privacy

Privacy is a continuously evolving concept. There are cultural and ethical norms that apply to individual privacy and legal norms that apply to privacy of health data of individuals.

The extent to which individual privacy can be provided to an individual depends on the healthcare setting. The ideals of a private chamber for consultations, separate delivery rooms and isolated operation tables may not be feasible in public health settings. However, there is an increasing move towards respectful maternity care which is being carried over to other aspects of healthcare for women. In India, public maternity care facilities are being assessed and upgraded to meet the LaQSHYA standards. One of the key components of this is providing privacy to women during the intrapartum period by way of a separate labour room or at least in a curtained cubicle.

The law mandates that certain aspects of reproductive healthcare such as termination of pregnancy, prenatal ultrasound, HIV infection are strictly to be kept in confidence. However, there are concerns surrounding the increasing digitization of health systems and possibility of internet based unauthorized access (hacking) of such data on a large level. As more people are going to be covered by government insurance schemes which are largely digital record oriented, this concern is real. The Government has instituted steps in protecting digital data in healthcare under DISHA (Digital Information Security in Healthcare Act) 2018. The law is under formulation and implementation and robustness of the systems will be tested in real time as Ayushmaan Bharat will become more popular over the next few years.

STD and HIV

About 0.3% of India's population is infected with HIV. Even though it is a small percentage, due to the large population in general, this translates to 2.1 million people living with HIV (PLWHIV), which is the third largest epidemic in the world. Overall, the HIV epidemic is slowing down in India. In this decade, new HIV infections have reduced by a third and there has been a reduction of AIDS related deaths by more than half. Key population groups where there infection and deaths are concentrated are sex workers, men who have sex with men and intravenous drug users. Women sex workers have a reported incidence of HIV infection to the tune of 7% in some states of India. They face discrimination, stigma and hostility in reaching healthcare facilities.

HIV testing and counseling have been operationalized by NACO (National AIDS Control Organization). Due to the widespread messaging and access to antenatal care, women with HIV are more likely to be diagnosed (87% vs 68%) than men. The Indian government is committed to reducing HIV infections in children and has strengthened the PPTCT (Prevention of Parent to Child Transmission of HIV/AIDS) program since 2002. Based on the 2013 WHO guidelines, the program initiates antiretroviral therapy for all pregnant women and those who are breastfeeding diagnosed with HIV infection irrespective of clinical status and CD4 counts. This has led to more women starting and continuing on antiretroviral therapy than men.

Overall, about 56% of infected people are on antiretroviral therapy in India. This is nearly twice the proportion from about a decade ago. Antiretroviral therapy is free and available through the public health network at ART centers. However, there are issues with erratic supply, out of pocket expenses, stigmatization and lack of access by marginalized population which are barriers to treatment. The new challenges in the fight against HIV/AIDS are data collection, analysis of emerging resistance and countering the surge of co-infections with tuberculosis.

Contraception

India was the first country in the world to launch a national program for family planning in 1952. The commitment to contraception has been reiterated in various versions of health policy. The latest of these is the National Population Policy 2000. There has been decline in the total fertility rate from 3.2 to 2.3 over the last 20 years but we are still above replacement levels. The new efforts on contraceptive services are listed below.

Technological

- Introduction of injectable depot medroxy-progesterone acetate (DMPA) under the name Antara.
- Centchroman is being reintroduced under the name Chhaya
- IUCD placement in the postdelivery and postabortal period is being encouraged and health workers are being trained to do it safely and correctly
- More centers are being recognized as centers for excellence to train doctors to perform laparoscopic tubal ligations
- Shift from standard method to non-scalpel vasectomy
- Emergency contraception is available over-the-counter

Service Delivery

- Private providers are allowed to freely prescribe and dispense contraception.
- In public sector, every public health center is equipped to provide contraception services. There is an availability of fixed day static services at all centers. Laparoscopic tubal ligation is to be carried out only by qualified gynecologists in camp settings.
- Female health workers (ASHAs) are empowered to provide contraceptive services to the doorsteps of the couples to reduce the unmet need. They are incentivized to promote birth spacing.

Administrative

- Family Planning Logistics Information System (FP-LMIS) is a system to maintain the supply chain and ensure logistics in the contraceptive provision program.
- Clinical Outreach Team (COT) Scheme is for areas where personnel are not available and facilities are scant. These areas typically have the highest unmet need.
- Media campaign to emphasize the involvement of men, vasectomy acceptance. This is being done through various media platforms including television, films and social media.
- Quality assurance programs have been instituted to ensure high quality, assured availability, low failure and complication rates, which will eventually feedback into a favorable response to family planning services.
- Compensation and insurance schemes are available.

Abortion

India has some of the most permissive laws on abortion in the world. The MTP Act was perhaps, the most important women's health related legislation in independent India. This Act from 1972 is a protective umbrella for care providers. It allows pregnancy to be terminated for various indications including risk to maternal life (physical and mental), pregnancy resulting from rape, risk of physical or mental handicap in the child, socioeconomic conditions and failure of contraception in a married woman. A pregnancy can be terminated till 20 weeks of gestation. This limitation on time has been challenged on a number of occasions in courts and extensions have been granted. There are provisions for taking consent in prescribed formats. The woman's consent is mandatory. The exceptions are when the woman is less than 18 years old or those who are mentally ill. Only the woman's consent is needed. There is no requirement to take consent from the husband or partner. The Act describes the requirements of the place and practitioner in terms of infrastructure and training to legally provide pregnancy termination.

Comprehensive abortion care is now an integral part of the reproductive and child healthcare package. Guidelines and training programs are in place and all the major stakeholders are a part of the decision-making on this subject. A national media campaign has been undertaken to promote safe abortion. Recently, guidelines to separate the legal aspects of the MTP Act and the PCPNDT Act, which seeks prohibition of sex-selection and sex-selective termination, have been released.

A study published in 2015 has estimated that 15.6 million pregnancies are terminated annually in India. The major change over the last two decades has been the rise in numbers and the mode of pregnancy termination. The rise in numbers is probably an artifact. There are now more stringent requirements for reporting pregnancy termination and data is electronically available which reflects in the growing numbers. The mode of pregnancy termination is moving to an earlier gestation and about three quarters of pregnancies are terminated by medication, rather than a surgical procedure. Abortion related mortality has decreased faster and to a greater extent than the mortality related to other pregnancy related causes. Unsafe abortions have reduced significantly. In 2014, the government has proposed amendments to the MTP Act to further increase access to safe abortions in the country. The amendments seek to expand the provider base, increase the time limit for pregnancy termination, increasing access for unmarried women and clarifying technical and legal aspects.

CONCLUSIONS

The health scenario in India for women is improving. The sentinel parameter, maternal mortality has been decreasing significantly, but slower than envisioned in the millennium development goals. The National Health Mission has undertaken a number of measures encompassing the broad spectrum of reproductive, child and adolescent health care which bodes well for the times to come. It remains a work in progress as in other developing countries of the region.

BIBLIOGRAPHY

1. Abortion in India. 2017. Retrieved on 08-12-2018, from https://en.wikipedia.org/wiki/Abortion_in_India

2. Aggarwal KK. Real consent and not Informed Consent is Applicable in India. Ind J Clinical Practice 2014;25(4):392–3.

3. Anantnarayan, Lakshmi (31 January 2018). "The Clitoral Hood A Contested Site, Khafd or Female Genital Mutilation/Cutting (FGM/C) in India" (PDF). Retrieved 08-12-2018 from http://www.wespeakout.org/site/asset s/files/1439/fgmc_study_results_jan_2 018.pdf

4. Annual report of the National AIDS Control Organization, Government of India 2018. Retrieved on 08-12-2018, from https://mohfw.gov.in/sites/default/files/ 24Chapter.pdf

5. Antani M, Punnen D, Shukla A, Nishith Desai Associates. DISHA: The first step towards securing patient health data in India. Digital Health Legal, Cecile Park Media. 2018. Retrieved on 08-12-2018, from http://www.nishithdesai. com/fileadmin/user_upload/pdfs/NDA%20 In%20The %20Media/News%20Articles/180725_ A_DISHA-The-First-Step-towards-Securing-Patient-Health-Data-in-India.pdf

6. AVERT. HIV and AIDS in India. 2018. Retrieved on 08-12-2018, from https://www.avert.org/professionals/hi v-around-world/asia-pacific/india

7. Bhattacharya PC. (2013). Gender inequality and the sex ratio in three emerging economies. Progress in Development Studies, 13(2),117–33.

8. Constitution of India. Retrieved on 08-12-2018, from https://www.india.gov.in/sites/upload_files/npi/files/coi_part_full.pdf

9. e111-e120.

10. Economy of India (2018). Retrieved on 08-12-2018, from https://en.wikipedia.org/wiki/Economy_of_India

11. Female genital mutilation in India. 2018. Retrieved on 08-12-2018, from https://en.wikipedia.org/wiki/Female_genital_mutilation_in_India

12. Ganatra A, Joshi R, Tank PD. FOGSI Focus on Medicolegal Updates on Safe Abortion. FOGSI PSI Publication. Mumbai, 2015.

13. Gopakumar KM. 2017. National Health Policy 2017 and Right to Health: Negation of Reality. Retrieved on 08-12-2018, from https://www.livelaw.in/national-healthpolicy-2017-right-health-negation-reality/

14. Government of India, Rajya Sabha 2017. Retrieved on 08-12-2018, from http://164.100.24.219/Bills Texts/RSBil lTexts/AsIntroduced/MTP-4817-E.p

15. India Census 2011. Retreived on 08-12-2018, from http://censusindia.gov.in/2011Common/CensusData2011.html

16. India Population. (2018-09-18). Retrieved 08-12-2018, from http://worldpopulationreview.com/countries/india/

17. India Total Fertility Rate (2016). Retrieved on 08-12-2018, from https://niti.gov.in/content/total-fertility-rate-tfr-birth-woman

18. India, Parliament in the Fifty-sixth Year of the Republic of India, Protection of Women from Domestic Violence Act, 2005. Act. No. 43 of 2005. Retrieved on 08-12-2018, from http://chdslsa.gov.in/right_menu/act/p df/dom violence.pdf

19. International Institute for Population Sciences and Macro International, National Family Health Survey (NFHS-4), 2015-16: India Fact Sheet, IIPS, Mumbai, 2016. Retrieved on 08-12-2018, from

http://rchiips.org/NFHS/NFHS-4Reports/India.pdf

20. Ministry of Health and Family Welfare, Government of India 2014. Comprehensive Abortion Care - Provider's Manual. Retrieved on 08-12-2018, from http://nhm.gov.in/images/pdf/program mes/maternalhealth/guidelines/CAC_Providers_Manual.pdf

21. Ministry of Health and Family Welfare, Government of India 2017. Annual report on Family Planning component of National Health Mission. Retrieved on 08-12-2018, from http://nhm.gov.in/nhm_components/RMNCHA/family_planning/annual_report/Annual_report 2016_17.pdf

22. Ministry of Health and Family Welfare, Government of India, 2017. National Health Policy 2017. Retrieved on 08-12-2018, from http://cdsco.nic.in/writereaddata/National-Health-Policy.pdf

23. Ministry of Health and Family Welfare, Government of India, 2017. Digital Information Security in Healthcare Act, 2017 - Draft for public consultation. Retrieved on 08-12-2018, from https://mohfw.gov.in/newshighlights/comments-draft-digital-informationsecurity-health-care-actdisha

24. Ministry of Women and Child Development, India, 2018. The Trafficking of Persons (Prevention, Protection and Rehabilitation) Bill, 2018. Retrieved on 08-12-2018, from https://www. prsindia.org/sites/default/files/bill_files The % 20 Trafficking%20 of%20 Persons%20% 28 Prevention%2 C%20 Protection %20 and%20 Rehabilitation%29% 20Bill%2C% 202018.pdf

25. Naik AB. Impacts, Causes and Consequences of Human Trafficking in India from Human Rights Perspective. Social Sciences 2018;7(2):76–80.

26. Narayan D. India is the most dangerous country for women. Retrieved on 08-12-2018, from https://www.theguardian.com/comme ntisfree/2018/jul/02/india-mostdangerous-country-women-survey

27. National Crime Records Bureau, India. Crime in India 2012. Retrieved on 08-12-2018, from http://ncrb.nic.in/CDCII2012/Statistics2012.pdf

28. National Health Authority, Government of India, 2018. Pradhan Mantri Jan Arogya Yojana (PM-JAY) - Ayushman Bharat. Retrieved on 08-12-2018, from https://www.pmjay.gov.in/about-pmjay

29. National Health Mission, Ministry of Health and Family Welfare, Government of India. LaQSHYA Labour Room Quality Improvement Initiative 2017. Retrieved on 08-12-2018, from http://nhm.gov.in/New_Updates_2018/NHM_Components/RMNCH_MH_Guidelines/LaQshya-Guidelines.pdf

30. Shenoi KR, Pandiaraj S. Honor killing in India-a sociolegal study. International Journal of Pure and Applied Mathematics 2018; 120:4917-4929.

31. Singh S, Shekhar C, Acharya R, et al. The incidence of abortion and unintended pregnancy in India 2015. The Lancet Global Health 2017;6(1)

32. Sunita Kishor, Kamla Gupta. 2009. Gender Equality and Women's Empowerment in India. National Family Health Survey (NFHS-3), India, 2005-06. Mumbai: International Institute for Population Sciences; Calverton, Maryland, USA: ICF Macro. Retrieved on 08-12-2018, from https://dhsprogram.com/pubs/pdf/od57/od57.pdf

33. Supreme Court of India, 2018. Shakti Vahini v/s Union of India. Retrieved on 08-12-2018 from https://www.sci.gov.in/supremecourt/2 010/18233/18233_2010_Judgement_ 27-Mar-2018.pdf

34. The Criminal Law (Amendment) Act, 2013. Retrieved on 08-12-2018 from http://www.ycce.edu/admin/pdf/Anti-rape_bill_2013.pdf

35. The Nirbhaya Rape Case that rocked India. NDTV, 2014. Retrieved on 08-12-2018 from https://www.ndtv.com/india-news/the-nirbhaya-rape-case-that-rocked-india1880338

36. The Protection of Children from Sexual Offences Act (POCSO) of 2012. Retrieved on 08-12-2018, from https://web.archive.org/web/20150928 131849/http://wcd.nic.in/childact/child protection31072012.pdf

37. The Sexual Harassment of Women at Workplace (Prevention, Prohibition and Redressal) Act, 2013 Published in The Gazzette of India 2013. Retrieved on 08-12-2018, from https://www.prsindia.org/uploads/media/Sexual%20Harassment/Sexual %20harrassment%20bill%20As%20p assed% 20by%20Lok%20Sabha.pdf

38. The World Bank. World Development Indicators 2.12, 2017: India. Retrieved on 08-12-2018, from http://wdi.worldbank.org/table/2.12

39. Tumbe C. Migration persistence across twentieth century India. Migration and Development 2012; 1(1):87–112.

40. UNICEF, 2016. Ending Child Marriage in India. Retrieved on 08-12-2018, from https://www.unicef.org/protection/files/ Final_India_Unicef_Rosa_Online.pdf

41. United Nations High Commissioner for Refugees (UNHCR). What do we do in India? 2018. Retrieved on 0812-2018, from https://www.unhcr.org.in/index.php?o ption=com_content &view=article&id=8 &Itemid=130

42. United Nations Office on Drugs and Crime (2013). Global Study on Homicide. Retrieved on 08-12-2018, from http://www.unodc.org/gsh/en/data.htm l

43. US Department of State, 2018. Trafficking in persons 2018 report: Country Narratives-India. Retrieved on 08-12-2018, from https://www.state.gov/j/tip/rls/tiprpt/countries/2018/282672.htm

44. WHO. Female Genital Mutilation. 2018. Retrieved on 08-12-2018 from https://www.who.int/news-room/factsheets/detail/female-genital-mutilation

Situation Analysis of Nepal

Kusum Thapa, Sapana Amatya Vaidya, Saroja Pandey

BACKGROUND

Nepal is a South Asian country that lies between China and India. With an area of 147, 181 km², Nepal represents diverse topography ranging from the Himalayas in the North to the plains in the South. With the total population of 28,982,771, the country also represents diverse culture with over 125 ethnic groups and over 123 languages. The majority of the people follow Hindu religion (81.3%), followed by 9% Buddhists, 4.4% Muslim, 3% Kiranti, 1.4% Christian and 0.9% others.

Over the past two decades, Nepal has witnessed a lot of political instability and transitions, which has, directly and indirectly, affected the health system in Nepal. The country has transitioned from a unitary system of government under the monarchy to a federal republic state. The new constitution of the federal republic of Nepal was adopted in 2015 and the new federal structure was established recently following the provincial level elections in late 2017. At the central level, there are currently over 20 ministries. The development activities related to women's rights, health, and education are overseen by the Ministry of Women, Children and Senior Citizen, the Ministry of Health and Population, and the Ministry of Education respectively. According to the new federal structure, Nepal is comprised of 77 districts and 7 provinces. The current federal system in Nepal is a newly revised system that had replaced an older system where the country had 5 develop-mental regions, 14 zones and 75 districts. The country is ranked under the low-income countries as per the World Bank Classification. Majority of people continues to live in poverty and frequent natural disasters such as flood, landslide, fires, and avalanche affects thousands of lives every year. The country also ranks 11th for earthquake risks in the world. In April 2015, the country faced a devastating earthquake of 7.8 magnitude followed by numerous aftershocks. The earthquake killed over 8,000 people and over 6,000 were severely injured. Over 400,000 homes and 16,000 schools were damaged across the country. The earthquake had damaged a total of 83.5% public health facilities in 14 severely hit districts in Nepal. Moreover, the 2015 earthquake in Nepal affected 2 million women of reproductive age and 126,000 pregnant women.

Despite the challenges faced by the country, the living standards of the people, their access to education and health care and their health indicators have improved over the years. The life expectancy in Nepal has been on increasing trend. The aging index has increased from 7.78 in 1971 to 15.50 in 2011, which indicates the number of old people has been consistently increasing compared to children.

DEMOGRAPHIC INDICATORS IN NEPAL

The population census of Nepal 2011 suggests that the population in the country is in declining trend. The population growth rate has decreased from 2.25% to 1.35% between 2001 and 1.35% in 2011. The population decline in the country has been attributed to the reduction in fertility rate and migration of the youth to foreign lands. The mortality rate of the country is also in declining order with 7.3 per thousand crude death rates in 2011 as compared to 10.3 in 2001. The life expectancy at birth has increased to around 70 years as compared to around 50 years in 1981. The life expectancy among females has increased to 67.9 years in 2011 from 48.1 in the past 3 decades.

The literacy status has improved remarkably over the past decade. However, the gender disparity persists with the literacy rate of 57.45 among females as compared to 75.1% in males. Nevertheless, the Nepal Demographic Health Survey 2016 indicated an increase in the median number of years of schooling from 3.5 to 5.0 between 2011 and 2016.

The main occupation in Nepal continues to be agriculture with the higher proportion of female working in this sector (70%) as compared to males (33%). The employment status in other sectors remains lower in females (57%) as compared to males (78%). Moreover, a majority of the youth has opted for foreign employment in the past decade with the increase in external migration over the years with the male population exceeding female population. According to NDHS, 32% of the women had responded that their husbands were working in foreign lands leading to temporary spousal separation. It has been suggested that migration has also attributed to the decline in overall birth rate and the fertility rate of the country.

MARRIAGE AND SEXUALITY

NDHS indicated the median age of marriage to be 17.9 among the women of age group 20 to 29. Similarly, the median age for sexual initiation was also found to be 17.9 which is 3 years earlier as compared to men.

FERTILITY AND CONTRACEPTION

The overall fertility rate has declined in the country remarkably from 4.6 in 1996 to 2.3 in 2011. The largest declined was observed from 2001 of 4.1 to 2006 of 3.1. However, adolescent childbearing has remained consistent for the past 5 years at 17%, after declining between 2001 (21%) and 2011 (17%). This highlights the need to address adolescent pregnancy more carefully.

The contraceptive prevalence rate has remained stagnant for the past decade in Nepal. Various factors were considered for the stagnation such as separation of spouses as a result of migration, increase in the use of traditional methods, and abortion services. According to NDHS, more than 50% of married couples use family methods of which modern contraceptive methods are used by 43%. Among the married couples, a total of 15% married women are estimated to have opted for female sterilization which remains the most used option. The injectable is estimated to have been used by 9% married women, 6% married men estimated to have opted for male sterilization and the 5% married women to have used oral contraceptive pills. Around 3% of married women are estimated to use implants and IUD by just 1% of the married women.

MATERNAL HEALTH

The overall coverage of antenatal care (ANC) services from skilled health providers have improved remarkably from just 28% in 2001 to 84% in 2016. Women having a minimum of 4 ANC visit has also improved from 14% to 69% between 2001 and 2016. The proportion of women having institutional delivery has also increased over the past two decades from just 9% in 2001 to 57% in 2016. These improvements could be attributed to the government's program on safe motherhood called *Aama program,* which promoted free of cost services for ANC and childbirth across the nation in government facilities and a few academic and not-for-profit institutions. According to NDHS estimates, the maternal mortality ratio (MMR) has also reduced significantly over the past decades from 415 in 2001 to 239 in 2016. The remarkable decline over the past two decades could be attributed to the improved MNH health service coverage.

Abortion

The legalization of abortion was introduced in 2002 in Nepal. The government has introduced the comprehensive abortion care since 2004. Based on the abortion law in Nepal, women are allowed to have a safe abortion in an authorized health center by a trained and licensed health provider within 12 weeks of gestation according to her own decision. Whereas, in case of rape and incest, the pregnancy can be terminated until 18 weeks of pregnancy by an authorized health provider. The authorized health provider can terminate the pregnancy of the mother at any time of the gestation, if her life is at risk, if her physical and mental health is impaired, and if the abnormality in the fetus such as deformity is identified. However, it is illegal to perform abortion without the consent of the women and abortion based on sex selection of the fetus. It is also illegal for unauthorized person and institution to perform an abortion.

According to NDHS, 41% of women of reproductive age groups have knowledge about abortion being legal in Nepal and 48% know a place where safe abortion service is provided. NDHS 2016 indicated that 72% of the women who had abortion opted for medical abortion, 17% opted for manual vacuum aspiration, and 7% dilation and evacuation or dilation and curettage. Majority of them in the survey responded to have obtained the abortion service from the doctor for their most recent abortion.

HIV/AIDS

The key population of people living with HIV (PLHIV) in Nepal includes injecting drug users, sex workers and their clients, male labor migrants and their wives, men who have sex with men, and prison inmate. The major source of transmission is heterosexual and the prevalence is below 1% in the country. As of 2017, it was estimated that 1,200 women had HIV. The annual new infection in male to female ratio is 2:1. Women of reproductive age groups accounts for 31% of all PLHIV and an estimated number of 304 pregnant women are infected every year. There are 175 service sites providing HIV testing and counseling, including 136 government sites as of July 2018. The comprehensive PMTCT service started in Nepal since 2005 and the community-based PMCT program has been expanded to all 77 districts. The coverage of PMTCT has improved from just 6% in 2006 to 63% in 2017.

VIOLENCE AGAINST WOMEN

According to NDHS, 22% of reproductive-aged women have started suffering from physical violence from a young age of just 15 years. Moreover, 7% of women have ever experienced sexual violence. Furthermore, 6% women of have experienced violence during their pregnancy. The most common form of reported violence among married women includes physical violence reported by 23% of women. This is followed by emotional violence in 12% and sexual violence in 7% of the women suffered from violence.

The government of Nepal considers violence against women a criminal act and the helplines are established through the National Women Commission in Nepal through a 24-hour toll-free line to provide survivors of violence. The survivors or anyone who have witnessed the violence can call the number to receive psychosocial support, shelter, child support and legal aid. There are also many women activists and human rights organization as well as health-related non-profit organizations working actively in the field of gender-based violence. Despite these efforts, 66% of the women who have suffered violence from the NDHS did not seek any help to protect themselves against violence.

WOMEN EMPOWERMENT AND GENDER EQUALITY

Nepal continues to be a highly patriarchal society where women empowerment and gender equality remains a challenge. Female literacy, employment, the age of marriage, ownership of property are lower among women than in men.

However, there has been an improvement on women paid in cash from 14% in 2006 to 24% in 2016. The women who have the authority to decide independently on spending the cash too has remained constant at 53% since 2011 but had increased from 31% in 2006.

Over 50% of women had mentioned of their participation in decision making of the household and in their own health care. The women who participate more in making decisions were also more likely to use contraceptives and have better MNH health-seeking behaviors such as ANC visits, institutional delivery, and postnatal care. Moreover, the women's choice of contraceptive use was determined by the women's perception of her sense of empowerment and ability to control sexual behaviors and fertility.

SUSTAINABLE DEVELOPMENT GOALS

As suggested by the health indicators, Nepal has been making significant progress in uplifting the health status of the people. To sustain the progress and continue to uplift the people, Nepal too has set its specific goals. SDG 3 and SDG 4 specially focused on the health and women's position in the society.

For SDG 3, Nepal aims to promote well-being and safeguard healthy lives for all. The SDG goal outlines reducing the MMR to 70 per 100,000 live birth by 2030. The decline in MMR has been encouraging so far but additional effort is necessary to achieve the projected target for MMR. By 2030, Nepal also aims to eradicate the epidemic of AIDS, TB, malaria and other neglected diseases. The HIV prevalence currently is 0.2% and further efforts such as prevention of mother to child transmission could help halt the transmission to great extent in the newer generations. Nepal is also committed to integrate sexual and reproductive health (SRH) issues into the national programs in order to accomplish the universal access to SRH throughout the country.

The proposed targets for SDG 5 focuses on eliminating gender disparities at all levels including education disparity, wage disparities, violence of all forms including physical, and sexual, and harmful practices such as forced and child marriage. The targets also aim to improve representation of women in parliament. The indicators from NDHS suggest the progress in achieving these targets remains slow and a collective effort is needed to address the issues of gender inequality and women empowerment.

In conclusion, the overall demographic and health indicators of women in Nepal have improved remarkably. However, increase in rise of adolescent pregnancy, stagnation of contraceptive prevalence rates, violence against women and slow decline in gender gap still remains huge challenges for the country. To achieve the targets of health and women related SDG, health sector including the specialized fields such as obstetrics and gynecology could play a crucial role in not just improving the women's health but also in uplifting their social status.

BIBLIOGRAPHY

1. Central Bureau of Statistics, Government of Nepal. National Population and Housing Census 2011. Kathmandu, Nepal: Central Bureau of Statistics, Government of Nepal; 2012.

2. Central Bureau of Statistics, Government of Nepal. Nepal in Figures 2016 Kathmandu, Nepal: Government of Nepal; 2016 [Available from: http://cbs.gov.np/image/data/2017/Nepal in Figures 2016.pdf.]

3. Central Bureau of Statistics, Government of Nepal. Population Monograph of Nepal (Social Demography). Kathmandu, Nepal: Central Bureau of Statistics, Government of Nepal; 2014.

4. Gaire S, Castro Delgado R, Arcos González P. Disaster risk profile and existing legal framework of Nepal: floods and landslides. Risk Manag Health Policy. 2015;8:139-49.

5. Government of Nepal. Nepal earthquake 2015 Postdisaster needs assessment. National Planning Commission, Government of Nepal; 2015.

6. Government of Nepal. The Official Portal of Government of Nepal Kathmandu, Nepal: Government of Nepal; 2018 [Available from: https://http://www.nepal.gov.np/National Portal/home.]

7. Ministry of Health Nepal NE, ORC Macro. Nepal Demographic Health Survey 2001. Kathmandu, Nepal: Ministry of Health Nepal, New Era, ORC Macro; 2002.

8. Ministry of Health Nepal, New Era, Macro International Inc. Nepal Demographic Health Survey 2011. Kathmandu, Nepal: Ministry of Health Nepal, New Era, Macro International Inc.; 2011.

9. Ministry of Health, New Era, ICF. Nepal Demographic Health Survey 2016. Kathmandu, Nepal; 2017.

10. National Center for AIDS and STD Control, Government of Nepal. 2018 World AIDS Day Fact Sheets Kathmandu, Nepal: National Center for AIDS and STD Control, Government of Nepal; 2018.

11. National Planning Commission, Government of Nepal. Sustainable Development Goals, 2016-2030, National Preliminary Report. Government of Nepal, National Planning Commission; 2015.

12. National Women's Commission, Government of Nepal. Helpline Kathmandu, Nepal: National Women Commission; 2017 [Available from: new.gov.np/en/helpline.

13. UNFPA. Nepal earthquake:women and girls in need Kathmandu, Nepal: UNFPA; 2015 [Available from: https://http://www.unfpa. org/resources/nepal-earthquake-women-and girls-need.]

14. Upreti SR, Lamichhane P, Khanal MN, et al. Rapid Assessment of the Demand Side Financing Schemes: Aama program and 4 ANC. 2012.

15. World Bank. World Bank Country and Lending Groups country classification [cited 2018 February 1]. Available from: https://datahelpdesk. world bank.org/knowledgebase/articles/906519-world-bank-country-and-lendinggroups.

6

Situation Analysis of Maldives

Madeeha Rashid, Noreen Rasul, Aqeela Abbas

The Maldives is a land for sunshine, warm seas with clear blue waters, coral oceans, scuba diving, surfacing and sailing. Anyone can come here to escape from worldly problems. Annually 600,000 tourist visit Maldives. By the end of this century, it is likely that due to climate change Maldives will be submerged underwater. Consequently, the southern tip of Maldives, Villngili, is only 240 cm above the sea being the world's lowest high point. In ancient times, Maldives was known as Mahiladiva meaning Land of women.

HISTORY

Maldives is the smallest Asian country, both by land area and population. It is an isolated and peaceful nation. Buddhist sailors and seamen from India and Sri Lanka in 5th century BC settled Maldives islands. In 1153, people accepted Islam. Initially, the islands were under the suzerainty of Ceylon (now Sri Lanka). They came under British protection in 1887. An independence agreement with Britain was signed on July 26, 1965.

POPULATION AND POPULATION DENSITY

It consists of 1,190 coral islands grouped into 26 Atolls in the Indian Ocean on south—southwest of India. In 2019, Maldives has an estimated population of 451,738, which ranks 175th in the world. The Maldives Islands has a high population density of 1,102 people per square kilometer, making it the 11th most densely populated country on earth. The youth cohort (15–29 years) comprise 31.5% of the population. While Male', the capital island, has a population of roughly 38 percent of the total population, about 62 percent live in the islands of the Atolls.

COMPONENTS OF POPULATION CHANGE

1. One birth every 72 minutes
2. One death every 360 minutes
3. One net migrant every 288 minutes
4. Net gain of one person every 69 minutes

DEVELOPMENTAL SUCCESS STORY OF MALDIVES

The Maldives was one of the world's 20 poorest countries in eighties, with a population of 156,000. In 2018, with a population of more than 448,966 it is a middle-income country with a per capita income of over $9,100. The country has impressive improvements in health and education with a life expectancy of 74.8 and a literacy rate 98.4%. However, still the country faces challenges in environmental sustainability, policy uncertainty and service delivery. Maldives ranks at 105 out of the 188 countries in the UNDP Human Development Index.

MALDIVES DEMOGRAPHIC PROFILE

Indicators	Demographic profile
Population	449,113
Population growth rate	–0.06%
Birth rate	16.1 births/1,000 population
Death rate	16.1 births/1,000 population
Urbanization	Urban population: 47.5% of total population Rate of urbanization: 3.52% annual rate of change
Children under the age of 5 years underweight	17.8%
Mother's mean age at first birth	23.9 years
Contraceptive prevalence rate	
Total fertility rate	1.73 children born/woman
Life expectancy at birth	**Total population:** 75.8 years **Male:** 73.5 years **Female:** 78.3 years
Infant mortality rate	**Total:** 22 deaths/1,000 live births **Male:** 24.4 deaths/1,000 live births **Female:** 19.6 deaths/1,000 live births

Source: https://www.cia.gov/library/publications/the-world

LEGAL SYSTEM OF MALDIVES

Maldives judicial system consist of Islamic and English common Law. Mostly Islamic Sharia is incorporated in Maldivian legislation.

GENDER FRAMEWORK

Maldives is among one of the first South Asian countries to finish gender disparity and discrimination in their society as shown by high literacy rates for women, then for men and equal opportunities of employments for females.

The Maldivian Government signed at the Convention on the Elimination of All Forms of Discrimination (CEDAW) in 1993 and the CEDAW Optional Protocol in 2006. Reservations include Article 7 (a) and Article 16.

Article 7 (a) "States Parties shall take all appropriate measures to eliminate discrimination against women in the political and public life of the country and, in particular, shall ensure to women, on equal terms with men, the right: (a) To vote in all elections and public referenda and to be eligible for election to all publicly elected bodies."

Article 16: "The Government of the Republic of Maldives reserves its right to apply Article 16 of the Convention concerning the equality of men and women in all matters relating to marriage and family relations without prejudice to the provisions of the Islamic Sharia, which govern all marital and family relations of the 100 percent Muslim population of the Maldives."

There are four guiding principles and four policy goals that underlie the vision:
1. Equality of women
2. Recognition that traditional, customary and cultural practices that negatively affect women and girls are a violation of human rights
3. Recognition that public and private are not separable spheres of life
4. Women's entitlement to the right of integrity and security of person

STATUS OF WOMEN IN THE MALDIVES GENDER ROLE

Maldives cultural framework is influenced by South Asian traditions and Islamic morals. These values help Maldives, developed diverse lifestyle and culture in which men considered to be head of family. This culture of gender inequalities effects social behavior of boys and girls at early age. In old areas of Maldives still girl child is trained to be submissive and family oriented while boys are strengthen to be sociable, progressive and self-confident to future head of the family. The environment of safety and tenderness towards female gender is in their valves.

MARRIAGE AND FAMILY STRUCTURE

The minimum age of marriage for women and men is 18 years. Females are responsible for domestic chores and functioning while male members take over public, social and political domains. Domestic liabilities on rural women are high due to large extended families, as by culture decision making is carried out by male family members.

Divorce

In Maldivian society nuclear family is of vital importance even then divorce rate is highest among world but there is no stigma associated with divorce in the society. Half of households in the Maldives are headed by women (42% of households), including 40% in Male' and 44% in the Atolls.

Education

Maldives ranked at 30 numbers in countries with high literacy rate. Maldives has adult literacy rate of 98.61% by UNESCO. In Maldives female literacy rate is more than males. Girls primary and secondary school enrolment (Primary school: 97% female, 96% male, Secondary school: 71% female, 67% male) is better than boys. From 1995 to 2000 a total of 876 students were awarded government scholarships to study abroad, 42% of which went to girls. From 2001 to 2005, 39% of undergraduate scholarships went to girls, 38% of postgraduate scholarships and 22% of doctorate scholarships.

Women's Political Participation

The Maldives Gender Empowerment Measure (GEM) is 76. The share of ladies seats in national parliament and other decision-making bodies is considerably little. Only 15 percent females are working as legislators, senior officials and managers. Only 6.5% and 14% of women are parliamentarians and ministers respectively. First female judge was appointed in 2007 and only one female magistrates till now. In civil services commission they have now female representative and two out of three members of national human right commission are females.

Poverty

There is no official or Asian Development Bank poverty data in Maldives. In Maldives, a "low" poverty line of Rf10 ($0.78) per person per day, and a high poverty line of Rf15 ($1.17) per person per day are in use.

As in most of countries here also poor families have larger household with lower education and bad health. Women ownership in property is low, only 31.3% of females are property holder as compared to 65.5% of male counterpart.

Women in the Economy

Percentage of female employs in government setup is rising. It is an encouraging change and way towards gender equality. But mostly women are employed in supporting roles and have little influence in decision-making. Departments like finance, tourism, and economic development are still dominated by males.

Towards north islands level, women are involved in hatch weaving while in south mostly they are employed as sales worker, cleaning (resort work) and have their own business like cake selling. In Male, mostly females are employed in white collar jobs including government administration.

Attitudes

Society shows varied attitudes towards working women. Most generations are in view that it is preferable for woman to sit in home to upbring children and do household chores rather than joining workforce.

Violence against Women

Lifetime physical/sexual intimate partner violence is 20% in Maldives. In last 12 months physical or sexual intimate partner violence is 6% while non-partner violence is 6% despite a lot of government measures, violence against women is prevalent in society.

Ministry of gender and family in 2007 conducted a survey and found that 1 in every 3 women aged between 15 and 49 years had underwent physical or sexual abuse or both at some part of life. Every 1 in 5 females of same age group had suffered from physical or sexual abuse by an intimate partner.

Every 1 in 8 females were sexually abuse before the age of 15.

The Maldivian Police Services statistics indicate that domestic violence is increasing at alarming rate. Number of cases has been increased from 187 in 2014 to 341 in 2015 and in 2016 it was 300 victims. According to police department the exact number of cases is underreported.

CHALLENGING SOCIAL NORMS OF HIDING VIOLENCE

Maldivian society has culture of hiding violence as they believe that it is family matter and will effect reputation of community. The general idea of society is that women should stay at home and male is head of family and bread earner, gives less importance to female counterpart. In Male where high and expensive living standards females have to work with their male counterpart. Women are given less important jobs while administrative and managerial post are given to males. Government is working to finish this gender disparity and inequality. Over the decade female education is markedly improved and girls are enrolling for tertiary levels of studies. Women situation in the Maldives is much improved now as compared to past. Empowerment of female gender is possible in Maldives if females are allowed to contribute at parliamentarian and cabinet level.

STAND AGAINST VIOLENCE BY ENFORCING LAW

Current government is determined to finish this gender discrepancy and will have zero tolerance against sexual and physical violence. They will finish the root cause of violence by promoting equality and equal employment.

Government will reinforce and support Sexual Abuse and Harassment Prevention Act, the Sexual Offences Act and the Domestic Violence Prevention Act

In Domestic Violence Act, Act Number 3/2012, the prohibition and prevention of domestic violence, including measures to be taken against those committing acts of domestic violence; protecting and supporting victims of domestic violence. The law also covers children as potential victims, creating a legal framework for protecting children who face incidences of domestic violence.

ROLE OF SOCIETY IN PREVENTING VIOLENCE

1. It is imperative to understand that to finish violence, it is vital to say no to violence. The women need to understand that it is not the right of the husband to be violent with the wife.
2. Every individual of society should be responsible enough and report any case of violence.
3. Rather than tolerating, victim should step forward and take help of law enforcing departments.
4. NGOs and human right activities should identify the victims and work in their betterment in order to avoid tragic losses.

Dowry

According to family law in Maldives the woman contracting a marriage shall in accordance with the principles of Sharia be entitled to dowry upon solemnization of the marriage. It shall be obligatory for the man contracting the marriage to give the dowry in accordance with the principles of Sharia. (27th December 2004 5b). It shall be the right of the woman contracting a marriage to receive the dowry, and to determine its nature and amount. No other person shall have any right in deciding any of the foregoing.

Rape

The 2013 world crime data shows rape rate of Maldives was lowest with 1.4 cases per 100,000 population. Now the government official sites are not providing basic statistics on rape and sexual assault. However, 355 cases of sexual violence were reported in police in 2017.

Female Genital Mutilation

Non-governmental organizations in the Maldives have confirmed that FGM/C has been a societal tradition for generations. There is no official data on the frequency of FGM/C, but religious leaders asked general public to revive this practice. In 2011, Dr Iyaz Abdul Latheef, the Vice-President of the Fiqh Academy, the primary religious academy in the Maldives, spoke on a live MNBC (the nation's public broadcast television channel) Radio program, encouraging more FGM/C be done on girls. Many Maldivian citizens, women included, believe and abide by the opinions and directions given by these leaders and scholars.

The lack of statistics on the number of FGM/C procedures performed each year is a major hurdle to bringing the prevalence of FGM/C to light in the Maldives.

SPECIAL SITUATIONS

Child Marriage

Child marriage rate is lowest in Maldives in South Asia, according to UNICEF. Only 4% girls are married before 18 years of age.

Human Trafficking

Human trafficking is common in Maldives and according to United Nations lots of females, males and minors are subjected to trafficking every year. These people become victim of slave trade and illegal sex exploitation. Approximately one hundred thousand documented and sixty thousand undocumented foreign workers mostly Bangladeshi and Indians are subjected to involuntary prostitution, domestic salve trade and debt bondage. Maldives government is doing substantial efforts in eliminating trafficking but still does not meet minimum standards. The Government has launched more effective management system and anti-trafficking units with greater funding and resources.

MEDICAL ISSUES IN GENERAL

Universal Health Coverage Asandha

Maldives health system has made tremendous improvement and admirable achievements in health indicators over 2–3 decades. Universal health coverage insurance scheme Asandha is a great relief for Maldivians who have been facing difficulties due to increasing health care cost.

Maldives and SDGs

Maldives is the only South Asian nation to achieve five out of eight MDGs before 2015. No doubt, Maldives has been facing number of economic, social and environmental challenges but still made noteworthy advancement in areas of eliminating grave poverty, universal education, health care, maternal health, and protecting terrestrial and marine biodiversity. Few areas need special attention like women empowerment, minimizing economic disparity and strengthening mechanism of governance. Maldives was successful in achieving most of MDGs and now implementation of sustainable development goals (SDGs)in Maldives will be built upon the successes of the Millennium Development Goals (MDGs) in the country.

Health Rights

To ensure good standard of health care for population government has implemented.

The Public Health Act (2012), the Health Services Act (2015) and the Health Professionals Act (2015) in society. These laws ensured protection from hazardous agents for health by prevention, and by providing appropriate care of a reasonable quality. The Gender Equality Act (2016) mandates government to provide SRH information and services to all.

Government specifies in Health master plan 2016–2025 promotion of safe sexual and reproductive health behaviors and practices for adolescents and young adults. In the National Reproductive Health Strategy 2014–2018, the government recognizes that reproductive health is a crucial component of the general health.

Health Situation

Maldives has shown conspicuous improvement in dipping maternal mortality rates, infant mortality rate and increased life expectancy. Most of the communicable diseases have been eradicated or controlled. World Health Organization has certified Maldives as Malaria free country in 2015. Polio, diphtheria, whooping cough and neonatal tetanus are non-existent in country. Tuberculosis and HIV prevalence have been maintained at very low level. Primary health care approach is based on good quality health care with dire importance to protective and promotional health. The good educational status and economic development in country help achieved government these parameters.

With regard to health issues, the United States Central Intelligence Agency (CIA) reports 1.6 physicians per 1000 people (2007), 4.3 hospital beds per 1000 people (2009), and that the state spent 11.5% of its GDP on health expenditures.

Maternal Mortality Rate

Over the last 25 years, there is magnificent decrease of 90 percent in maternal death rate and this is the largest drop in the world over this time period. In 1990 maternal mortality rate was 677/100,000 live births which dropped to 68/100,000 live birth. It shows 9.2% decline in maternal mortality ratio every year in last 25 years, while during same time period globally, it was only 2.3% annual decline.

Nutritional Status

The Maldives has made significant improvement in maternal and child health over the last decade. Rate of underweight children in under five has been decline from 43% in 1990 to 17% in 2009, stunting from 30% to 18% and wasting from 17% to 10.6 % (MDHS, 2009).

Breastfeeding

Exclusive breastfeeding is essential for child's health, growth and immune system. In Maldives 64% of newborn are breastfed within first hour of life and 92% of newborns within the first day. But this decreased to 48% infants at 6 month of age. Government is promoting absolute breastfeeding by constructing baby-friendly hospital initiative. Many awareness campaigns have been started. Stronger incentives and increased flexibility for working mother will bring change.

NUTRITIONAL STATUS OF WOMEN

46% of women in Maldives are obese while underweight females are only 8%.

Thalassemia

The Republic of the Maldives has one of the highest carrier rates of the beta thalassemia in the world:

   i. Beta thalassemia carriers 16–18%
   ii. Alpha thalassemia carriers 2.1%
   iii. HbE carriers 0.9%
   iv. HbS carriers 0.13%
   v. HbD carriers 0.43%

A national register of thalassemia patients has been kept over many years, which includes 563 currently living—this is roughly 1.6/1000 of the total population. 288 are living in the capital Male while roughly the other half live in Atolls.

Antenatal Care

Antenatal visit in 1st trimester of pregnancy is 90%
85% of women had 4 or more ANC visits, as recommended.
No ANC visits is less than 1%
More than 99% of women received antenatal care from a skilled provider (gynaecologist, doctor, nurse, midwife, or community/family health worker) at least once
Components of Antenatal Care
i. 87% took iron tablets or syrup during last pregnancy ii. 52% were informed of signs of pregnancy complications iii. More than 99% had blood pressure measured iv. More than 99% were weighed v. 98% had blood samples taken vi. 97% had urine samples taken

Source: MDHS 2009

Delivery and Postnatal care

95% of women in the Maldives deliver in a health facility.
95% of births were delivered by a skilled provider (skilled provider includes gynaecologist, doctor, nurse, midwife or community/family health worker)
46% of mothers had a postnatal check-up within 4 hours after delivery.
21% of mothers had a postnatal check-up within 2 days after delivery.
6% of mothers had no postnatal check-up within 41 days of delivery.

Source: MDHS 2009

STD and HIV

Maldives government take HIV/AIDS as serious public health problem and is making every effort in reducing high risk behaviors and is all out to spread prevention of HIV throughout country. Government has devised national strategic plan for HIV/AIDS control. Prevalence of HIV and AIDS in Maldives is very low. In 2009 UNAIDS found less than 100 people were infected with virus. Everyone in the Maldives has free to the service of testing,

counseling and ARV treatment once diagnosed with HIV/AIDS including expatriate migrant workers with a valid work permit. The country has high rates of hepatitis B and C, while STI rates are average for the region.

Contraception

In 1986, the Republic of Maldives adopted a policy to promote and implement family planning programs in the country. By 1990, all the islands were covered under the programs.

Family planning services are provided for free in all government hospitals and health centers. It is also covered in universal health coverage Aasandha. All family planning methods and counsellors are available in the islands except long-term method, implants and intrauterine devices can only be provided in atoll hospital where specialists are employed.

Abortion

Abortion is considered illegal in Maldives as it follows Islamic laws. Abortion is permissible in following five conditions only:

1. Abortion is permissible if a woman is pregnant as a result of rape, either by persons who the woman is prohibited to, or lawful to marry. In both cases, the council ruled that the fetus must be aborted within 120 days of conception.

2. Pregnancy of a minor through rape, whose body is too weak or not developed enough to sustain the fetus.

3. If the fetus is determined to have a major disease that would result in a medical deformity. In this case, the parents must be legally bound by marriage.

4. "If a woman comes to conceive through legal wedlock and if a doctor can confirm for a certainty that the fetus is a thalassemia major, or a sickle cell major, or if the fetus carries a disease that might result in a major permanent deformity to its body or its brain, and if the disease cannot be cured through medical treatment or medication, it is

permissible for her to abort the fetus within 120 days of conception.

5. If the fetus threatens the life of the mother.

It is challenging to understand the degree of problem as not much data is available on abortion, also no significant research has been carried out in this respect. Despite being illegal, Sex outside of marriage mainly among young adolescents is common occurring. Also it is not uncommon for married men to have affairs with unmarried girls. These people then go for illegal abortions. Now health ministry is devising strategies to create awareness and educate the public about the health risks involved. Government is also developing mass media campaigns.

EXISTING DEVELOPMENTAL CHALLENGES

Maldives existing development challenges ranges from climate variations, disaster management and environmental sustainability with rising levels of solid waste. About two-thirds of country infrastructure is located 100 meters above sea level and are at threat from rising sea levels. Country's topography leads to a scattered population across many small islands, which makes service delivery difficult and can limit opportunities for job creation and economic diversification. Higher rates of youth unemployment 25.3% and limited job opportunities for females will lead to negative effect on society like drug abuse and rising theft rate.

However, new political government of Ibrahim Mohamed Solih after coming to rule are determined to overcome these challenges by beginning Greater Male developmental strategy, bringing economic reforms by investing in larger islands. This will improve basic service delivery, job creation and protection from climate changes. Government will promote tourism more as it is a major contributor to economic development.

New elect government is determined to reinstate democratic organizations and the freedom of the press, re-establish the justice system, and protect fundamental human rights.

CONCLUSION

Maldivian Gender Development Index (GDI) is 0.767 and Gender Empowerment Measure (GEM) is 0.430 which is highest in all south Asian countries showing they have done considerable work in improving women life indicators of country. Currently women and men have equal access to education and health services. Government is introducing policy reforms for making women empowered and start their own small setups to overcome economic constrains. Still there are difficulties due to in skill shortage and human resource development. More vocational and technical institutes are needed for better training of youth which will improve their employment opportunities. It is necessary to change customary and old-fashioned thinking of society on female gender. A robust law-making is required to protect the rights of women.

BIBLIOGRAPHY

1. Abortion permissible in five circumstances, rules Fiqh Academy https://english.sun.mv/18588
2. ADB, September 2007, Maldives: Gender and Development Assessment, Manila, Philippines
3. Central intelligence agency US https://www.cia.gov/library/publications/the-world-factbook/geos/mv.html
4. Central Intelligence Agency, The World Factbook, https://www.cia.gov/library/publications/resources/the-worldfactbook/geos/mv.html
5. Challenges faced by Maldives goverment https://thediplomat.com/2018/10/the-maldives-new-government-mission-impossible/
6. Family Law Act 2000; Maldives law, http://suoodanwar.blogspot.com/ HYPERLINK "http://suoodanwar.blogspot.com/2015/03/family-law-act-2000.html"2015/03/family-law-act-2000.html
7. Gender Advocacy Working Group, Press Release: Statement on International Day against Female

Genital Mutilation, 06.02.2014 http://hopefor women.org.mv/wp

8. Gender based violence in the Maldives: What We Know So Far A report on the findings of qualitative research on GBV carried out by the Ministry of Gender, Family Development and Social Security in 2004.

9. Global Database on Violence against Women-http://evaw-globaldatabase.unwomen.org/en/countries /asia/Maldives

10. Government of Maldives, 2010, Common Core Document Forming Part of the Reports of States Parties, 16 February 2010.

11. Government of the Maldives, 2010, Common Core Document Forming Part of the Report of State Parties, Republic of the Maldives, 16 February 2010.

12. Health Information Research Section Planning and International Health www.health.gov.mv ppd@health.gov.mv

13. http://worldpopulationreview.com/countries/maldives-population/

14. http://www.worldbank.org/en/results/2013/04/10/maldives-development-success-story

15. https://borgenproject.org/top-10facts-about-poverty-in-maldives/

16. https://sustainabledevelopment.un.org/memberstates/maldives

17. https://trvl.com/maldives/maldives

18. https://www.infoplease.com/world/co untries/maldivesinundation. Marine Geodesy 25:133–43.

19. Human Development Indices and Indicators: 2018 Statistical Update Briefing note for countries on the 2018 Statistical Update Maldives UNDP.

20. Ibid.

21. June 1999 23 UN CEDAW, Reservations, http://www.un.org/womenwatch/daw/ cedaw/reservations country.htm#N35, accessed 9 Sept 2010. 23 June 1999

22. Maldives and family planning overview https://www.scribd.com/document/59355780/Family-Planning-Fact-Sheets-Maldives

23. Maldives overcoming the challenges of a small island state, country diagnostic study. Asian Development Bank 2015

24. Maldives, Rape rate, https://knoema.com/atlas/Maldives/Rape-rate

25. Maldives,https://www.unicef.org/maldives/hiv_aids.html

26. Maldives: Gender and developmental assessment Strategy and program assessment, Sept. 2007.

27. Maternal mortality in 1990–2015 WHO, UNICEF, UNFPA, World Bank Group, and United Nations Population Division Maternal Mortality Estimation Inter-Agency Group Maldives

28. Ministry of Health, The Maldives Health Statistics 2012.

29. Ministry of Planning and National Development, March 2007, National Population and Housing Census, Maldives, 2006.

30. National Strategic Plan for the Prevention and Control of HIV/AIDS Republic of Maldives 2014-2018 Ministry of Health Republic of Maldives 2013.

31. Office to monitor and combat trafficking in persons; Maldives, 2018 Trafficking in Persons Report https://www.state.gov/j/tip/rls/tiprpt/countries/2018/282702.htm

32. SAIEVAC, South Asia Initiative to End Violence Against Children, [website], 2018, http://www.saievac.org/ (accessed February 2018)

33. Sexual and Reproductive Health and Rights in Maldives: Policy Brief Report from United Nations Population Fund Published on 13 Mar 2018. https://reliefweb.int/report/maldives/sexual-and-reproductive-health and-rights-maldives-policy-brief

34. TMA, DA Quadir. 2002. Relative sea level changes in Maldives and vulnerability of land.

35. Thalassemia International Federation Maldives World Mission Report 2014 http://www. searo.who.int/maldives/mediacentre/thalassaemia-report-august-2014.pdf

36. The GEM-gender empowerment measure-is a composite indicator that captures gender inequality in three key areas: Political participation and decision-making, as measured by women's and men's percentage shares of parliamentary seats; Economic participation and decision-making power, as measured by two indicators-women's and men's percentage shares of positions as legislators, senior officials and managers and women's and men's percentage shares of professional and technical positions; Power over economic resources, as measured by women's and men's estimated earned income (PPP US$).

37. To the extent that the provision contained in the said paragraph conflicts with the provision of Article 34 of the (previous) Constitution of the Republic of Maldives. UN CEDAW, Reservations, http://www.un.org/womenwatch/daw/cedaw/reservationscountry.htm#N35, accessed 9 September 2010

38. UN, 2000, Gender and Development in the Maldives, A review of Twenty Years, 1979–1999, by Husna Razee.

39. UNDP Maldives—Women in Public Life—Situational Analysis/Baseline Assessment—August 2010.

40. Universal Health Coverage and Quality of Care in the Maldives, Issue 23 https://adkteamtalk. wordpress.com/2012/02/01/universal-health-coverage-and-quality-of-care-in-the-maldives/

41. World Economic Forum. 2008. The Global Gender Gap 2008 Report: Country Profiles. http:// www.weforum.org/pdf/genderg ap/ggg08_ maldives.pdf,

42. World Economic Forum. 2009. The Global Gender Gap 2009 Report: Country Profiles. http:// www.weforum.org/pdf/gendergap/ggg09_ maldives. pdfhttps://countryeconomy.com/ demography/literacyrate/maldivas

43. Zaheena Rasheed, Figh Academy VP endorses female genital mutilation, Minivan News: Independent News for the Maldives, February 6, 2014 http://minivannews.com/politics/figha cademy-vp-endorses-female-genitalmutilation 77037#sthash.Uo0ksLmI.dpbs

44. Zubair S, D Bowen, and J Elwin. 2011. Not quite paradise: Inadequacies of environmental impact assessment in the Maldives. Tourism Management 32:225–34.

7

Situation Analysis of Pakistan

Sadia Ahsan Pal, Rubina Sohail, Asifa Naureen

COUNTRY INTRODUCTION AND DEMOGRAPHICS

Violence against women is not a new phenomenon but prevalent in the sub-continental culture through centuries. Approximately 60 to 90 percent women in Pakistan have suffered from different forms of abuse such as rape, marital rape, domestic violence, psychological abuse, emotional abuse, honour killings, dowry violence, acid throwing, forced marriages, mob violence, stalking, sexual harassment and human trafficking. An estimated figure shows that more than 5000 women are killed and buried every year, suffering from domestic violence, while others are left mutilated. Even more alarming is that instead of a decline, there is a 20-25 percent increase in cases of violence against women reported every year.

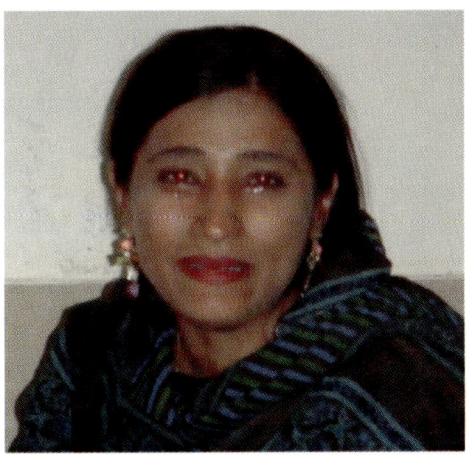

During 2015, International NGOs recorded that 6 women were kidnapped, 4 raped, 3 committed suicide and 6 murdered every day in Pakistan.

Problems

There are numerous issues relating to gender-based violence (GBV) against women in Pakistan. It occurs at the workplace, domestic and all walks of life, both in the form of physical and verbal/psychological abuse. Rape, child abuse, "honour" killing in the form of "Karokari", "satti", "wattasatta", "swara" are prevalent in all four provinces.

EARLY AGE MARRIAGE

Old tribal customs are still prevalent especially in rural areas. The legal age for marriage is 18 years, but still not implemented as conflicting federal and provincial laws make child marriage socially and legally permissible with customs like "paitlikhi", "vani", swara", etc. Factors which contribute to it are poverty, socio-religious teachings, protecting girls and their honour, gender discrimination, lack of importance given to female education and limited legal protection against child marriage. The result is early childbearing, restricted mobility, high infant and maternal mortality, limited access to family planning, poor reproductive health and vulnerability to sexual and physical abuse. This in turn causes emotional distress, inability to make decisions, economic dependency, psychological and verbal abuse. There exists a Child Marriage Restraint Act, but there is a need for advocacy, awareness and stronger implementation of the law using the CNIC and birth registration.

TEENAGE PREGNANCY AND MOTHERHOOD

The issue of adolescent fertility is important for both health and social reasons. Children born to very young mothers are at increased risk of sickness and death. Teenage mothers are more likely to experience adverse pregnancy outcomes and to be constrained in their ability to pursue educational opportunities than young women who delay childbearing.

According to the latest Pakistan demographic health survey (PDHS) 2018, the median age of first birth for women age 25–49 is 22.8 years, an increase of 0.6 years in the past 5 years since the 2012-13 PDHS, which was 22.2 years. Overall, 8% of women age 15–19 had begun childbearing. The proportion of teenagers who had begun childbearing rises rapidly with age, from 1% at age 15 to 19% at age 19. Rural teenagers tend to start childbearing earlier than urban teenagers. Teenagers with more than a secondary education and those in the highest wealth quintile tend to start childbearing later than those with no education or with lower levels of education.

Fifteen percent of teenagers in Khyber Pakhtunkhwa had begun childbearing as compared with only 6% in Punjab (PDHS 2017–18)

Female genital mutilation (FGM) is not common in Pakistan, limited to the Bohri community, a few clusters from Baluchistan and a few with African connections. It is said to be on the decline through generations. It is kept very private and not talked about even within the community, and not seen by gynaecologists.

Natural Disasters

Crisis situations have occurred during massive floods, earthquake (2005) and internal displacement of people (IDP) due to terrorist activities and government operations (Migrants and IDPs) where women and children are at risk.

MEDICAL ISSUES

Unsafe Abortion accounts for 5.6% of maternal deaths (PDHS 2007) while 2.2 million abortions occur every year (Population Council Study 2014). The number of abortions have more than doubled in 10 years, as it was 896,000 per year in the 2004 Population council study.

Women are mostly unable to make decisions about their own health issues like contraception, tubal ligation, abortion without husband's/family's consent. Even in the wake of dire emergency like postpartum hemorrhage, repeated cesarean sections, consent is denied by the husband or family. The woman is reluctant herself because of fear that her husband will take another wife if she is unable to bear children. Polygamy is legal and four wives are permissible at a time, with 4% of couples in polygamous relationships (PDHS 2007).

Women in Pakistan have a high level of unmet need for contraception—estimated at 17% in 2017 (PDHS 2017–18)). This results in high rates of unintended pregnancy, unplanned births and induced abortions. Out of a total of approximately 9 million pregnancies in Pakistan in 2012, 4.2 million (46 percent) are unintended. Of these, 4.2 million unintended pregnancies, 54 percent end in induced abortions. These abortions carry huge costs, as safe abortion services are severely restricted in Pakistan.

The abortion law in Pakistan provides exceptions in the criminal code for abortion in cases of threat to health and in early pregnancy for "necessary treatment." It does not explicitly allow abortion on grounds of rape, nor in cases of fetal impairment but some providers do allow under necessary treatment. However, the phrase "necessary treatment" is not clearly defined or widely understood. Most clinicians are unaware of the law as it is not taught in medical schools and hence do not offer services, as a result, safe and legal abortion care is not widely accessible. Women are also unaware of the law. Under the law, both women and providers, as well as anyone assisting the woman can be punished for a term of 3 years imprisonment.

The narrow legal grounds for abortion, lack of knowledge of the law, religion and the lack of understanding in interpreting and implementing the law by both women and healthcare providers means that women often resort to clandestine and unsafe abortion procedures that result in death or adverse health consequences. Despite some positive steps, the state has taken to address unsafe abortion, it still accounts for at least 6% of maternal mortality in Pakistan, this might be an underestimate given the sub regional average of 13% and the high number of unreported abortions.

In addition to the restrictive law, underlying economic, social and cultural factors, including stigma, also play a role in the high maternal mortality rate as well as concerns over receiving post-abortion care. Abortion like other public health concerns that are related to sex, gender and sexuality, has engendered stigma and discrimination against both those seeking and those providing services. As a result, women are not only obstructed from obtaining legal abortion in its limited circumstances, but also push women away from seeking even post-abortion care service.

It is in this context, one study found that in 2012 there were a reported 2.2 million abortions, performed in Pakistan, of which more than 85% of women accessed untrained service providers or quacks and resorted to life-threatening complications (*almost 700,000 each year*) due to use of outdated and unsafe approaches and methods (Population Council 2014). Many factors become a barrier when a woman with post-abortion complications needs treatment at a health facility. These barriers include fear of criminal law, stigma, costs, availability, distance and level of family support. Usually women seek care only when complications have become more serious.

SOCIAL ISSUES

The Nikahnama, marriage is a social union, a legal contract, a journey towards mutual happiness with equal rights, obligations and expectations.

Why a girl MUST get married, the issue of dowry; need for compatibility assessment of the man and the woman; choice of partner—who has the right to choose? Inequality in social and financial status, education, nature of employment, earning capacity; previous marriage; joint family system—interference from mother-in-law, other family members, decision-making for household expenditure, housework.

Anti-woman practices like Watta Satta, Vanni, Swara, Chatti and the prevention of anti-women practices.

Marriage and domestic violence: PPC does not discriminate between marital and out of marriage rape (leverage point: Broadly framed laws). Figures are meaningless because rape is taboo, under-reported and internalized (Fig. 7.1).

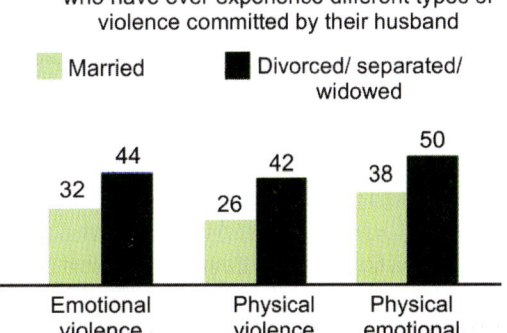

Percent of ever-married women age 15–49 who have ever experience different types of violence committed by their husband

Fig. 7.1: Spousal violence by marital status
Source: PDHS 2014

There were total 289 cases of domestic violence reported in last six months of 2012 (Aurat Foundation) and domestic violence increased by 25.51 percent.

The Nikahnama (marriage certificate) is a Prenuptial contract. Conditions can be outlined for dowry, polygamy, delegation of right of divorce, maintenance, etc. It is the duty of the Nikahkhwan (Registrar) to ascertain the age of the bride, obtain explicit consent, explain the clauses and provisions clearly, i.e. nature of the nikahnama, delegate the right of divorce, dower (timely delivery of prompt dower amount); fair evaluation of deferred dower, Nikah registration; to ascertain whether it is the first marriage; if married before, to obtain written consent of the wife/wives and concerned Union council of the wife (compliance with MFLO). However, informed consent is rarely taken in these matters and often the right to divorce (khula) is crossed off in the Nikahnama form, without knowledge of the bride.

STD

According to an estimate by UNAIDS, Pakistan contains approximately 130 000 people living with HIV. Several factors, including low literacy, high poverty, and unsafe blood transfusions have made Pakistan more vulnerable to HIV spread than other countries.

Lapses in basic health facilities have worsened the situation. In March, 2018, another HIV outbreak was reported in a village near to Kot Momin, Sargodha, situated in central Punjab 175 km from Lahore. Initially, the unusual disease was mistakenly diagnosed either as hepatitis B or C or tuberculosis at basic health units in the area.

Pakistan is registering approximately 20,000 new HIV infections annually, the highest rate of increase among all countries in the region, warns the World Health Organization (WHO). Mortality among Pakistanis living with the virus, which causes the deadly AIDS disease, is also rising, in spite of the availability of life-saving antiretroviral therapy.

The latest government figures show that only 16 percent of the estimated 150,000 people living with HIV had been tested and only nine percent have access to life-saving treatment.

"The remaining 135,000 people are walking around in the communities as carriers of (HIV) infection who are ready to transmit infections to those who are not infected, even to their unborn babies," the HIV epidemic in Pakistan remains largely concentrated among the key populations, including people who inject drugs, the transgender community, sex workers and their clients and men who have sex with men.

Other STDs are also on the rise but it is difficult to get reliable figures/studies.

Contraception access is not universal, especially in the rural areas resulting in a high incidence of abortions.

PREVAILING CULTURAL AND SOCIAL ENVIRONMENT

Earlier in 2018 according to the Thompson Reuters Foundation survey, Pakistan ranked as the sixth most unsafe country for women. Sexual violence, non-sexual violence, human trafficking and discrimination remained some top of the list sources of violence inflicted upon women. In January 2018, a day after eight-year-old Zainab's murder, a 16-year-old was raped and murdered in Punjab. The victim's body was recovered from an agricultural field in Sargodha district. A report by the Human Rights Watch, revealed that about 1,000 honour killings happen in Pakistan every year. According to Aurat Foundation, in 138 cases of this year, 51 women and 25 men were killed. Thirty women and 19 men were killed in the name of 'honour'. Fourteen women committed suicide over domestic dispute while 21 women and eight men had been tortured to death in Balochsitan.

By February 2018, data collected by a local NGO revealed that at least 18 major incidents of violence against women had been reported across Khyber-Pakhtunkhwa (K-P). While there were more than 54 cases of violence against women perpetrated in the province, only some of whom drew attention of the Supreme Court of Pakistan. In July, a woman was beaten by her father and relatives in court over a domestic spate. Another alarming instance was reported about a woman being allegedly blackmailed and raped in Islamabad by Capital Development Authority (CDA) officials inside a public park for accompanying a boy. In September 2018, a woman was allegedly thrashed for shoplifting in Lahore.

30 Women Killed in the Name of Honour in 2018: Report

Zia Ahmed Awan, founder of Madadgaar National Helpline 1098 and national commissioner for children, during a news conference in 2017 maintained that 70% women and girls in the country experience physical or sexual violence by their intimate partners and 93% women experience some form of sexual violence in public places in their lifetime.

In May 2018, the National Assembly passed 'The Acid and Burn Crime Bill 2017'. It promises free medical treatment and re-habilitation for acid attack victims and also expedites conducting trials of accused.

While women constantly undergo violence in the society, the K-P cabinet in November passed a domestic violence bill which shall be tabled before the provincial assembly. The bill criminalises offences against women and promotes creating district protection committees to safeguard women.

In November, National Commission on the Status of Women (NCSW) Chairperson Khawar Mumtaz underlined the need to implement the Violence Against Women (VAW) law in the federal capital, following its implementation in all other provinces.

She mentioned earlier that this law was implemented in Punjab, Sindh and Balochistan while it was recently approved in K-P. "Now, it is time to implement the bill at capital level so that women's protection in the country can be ensured." Strict implementation of such laws is required for empowering these segments of the society out of school in rural Sindh.

MAJOR NEW LAWS PASSED IN PAKISTAN SINCE 2004

Criminal Law Amendment Act 2004

Made killing on the pretext of honor equivalent to homicide or pre-meditated murder (Men could no longer use "sudden and grave provocation" as a mitigating circumstance or as a plea for reduced sentence). It increased punishment to life imprisonment, and removed discretion of the court to decide where, according to the injunctions of Islam, the punishment of qisas was not applicable. It also removed the possibility of the murderer being the wali (guardian), and allowed the State to take the responsibility of wali, if necessary. Only higher rank police officers can investigate matters of honor-killing and adultery.

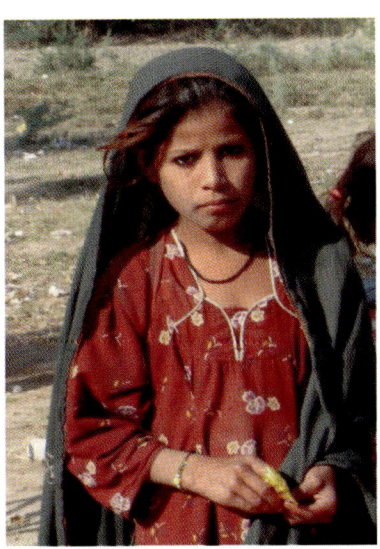

Protection of Women, Criminal Law Amendment Act 2006

Introduction of the principle of statutory rape. Amendment was made to evidence requirement, for 4 male, Muslim eye-witnesses to provide testimony. Zina became a bailable offence. Rape became a non-compoundable offence (litigants could not settle amongst themselves). Space was created for bringing charges of marital rape (no marital exception for rape). Case of rape could not be converted into zina for want of evidence.

Criminal Law Amendment Act 2010

Criminalized sexual harassment at the workplace and public spaces and defined various means (written, verbal, stalling of promotion, deprivation from increments, interference of sexual harassment (SH). Called for immediate setting up of inquiry committees in public and private institutions to look into complaints of SH. Created the role for provincial ombudsman to look into cases of SH above inquiry committees and to ensure compliance.

The Acid Control and Acid Crime Prevention Act

PPC Section 332: Inclusion of words "disable" and "disfigures, defaces". New insertion, PPC Section 336-A. Hurt caused by corrosive substance "Whoever with the intention or knowingly causes or attempts to cause hurt by means of a corrosive substance or any substance which is deleterious to human body when it is swallowed, inhaled, comes into contact or received into human body or otherwise shall be said to cause hurt by corrosive substance." PPC Section 336-B: Punishment for hurt by corrosive substance "Whoever causes hurt by corrosive substance shall be punished with imprisonment for life of imprisonment of either description which shall not be less than fourteen years and a minimum fine of one million rupees." Explanation: Disfigure means disfigurement

of face or disfigurement of any organ or any part of the organ of the human body which impairs or injures or corrodes or deforms the symmetry or appearance of a person.

Prevention of Anti-Women Practices (Criminal Law Amendment) Act 2011

Criminalized forced marriages and inheritance deprivation of women in the name of customary practices such as watta-satta, wanni, swara, and Quran marriage. It allowed women the right to inherit moveable and immovable property and prescribe major punishments for such offences. Forced marriage, inheritance deprivation are, however, non-cognizable offence (police cannot take action with a Magistrates order or a warrant).

The Women in Distress and Detention Fund 2011

Calls for the establishment of a fund to help women inmates in jail financially and legally funds to be held by the Human Rights Ministry.

Sindh Child Marriage Authority Act 2011

Persons under age of 18 to be considered minors and under the protection of this law. Protects children at risk of violence, abuse, exploitation, labor, begging, trafficking substance abuse, armed conflict, and children without family or alternative care, and those affected by HIV. It mandates setting up a Child Protection Authority [CPA] at provincial level and Child Protection Units [CPUs] at district level—12 units established across Sindh so far. The state assumes responsible for providing or referring children at risk to appropriate services, whether existing or newly set-up, to tackle the issues holistically.

Sindh Human Rights Commission Act 2011

Inquire, *suo moto* or on a petition presented to it by a victim or any person on his behalf, into complaint of violation of human rights or abetment thereof and negligence in the prevention of such violation, by a public servant. It is recommend to Government the remedial measures including action to be taken against the persons involved in violation of human rights, formulate, implement and regularly update policies with a view to protect human rights, visit under intimation to Government, any jail or institution under the control of Government where persons are kept or detained or admitted for purpose of treatment, reformation or protection. To see the living conditions of the inmates and make recommendations thereon, review the safeguards provided by or under the Constitution or any law for the time being in force for protection of human rights and recommend measures for their effective implementation. Study treaties and other international instruments on human rights and make recommendations for their effective implementation. Undertake and promote research in the field of human rights. Spread human rights literacy among various sections of society and promote awareness of the safeguards available for protection of human rights through print and electronic media, seminars and other available means. Encourage the efforts of non-governmental organizations and institutions working in the field of human rights.

Sindh Prevention and Protection from Domestic Violence 2013

Provides women, children (biological, adopted, foster children, etc.), elderly, tenants and other vulnerable persons (such as mentally or physically disabled persons) with protection against domestic abuse. It is not necessary that concerned people may be living together at the time of violence, and may have lived together at some point in time. It criminalizes physical, mental, sexual, emotional and economic abuse/ violence, and provides protection against stalking and trespassing. Anyone can report on behalf of the affected, including any "informer" or any person authorized by the affected person. Protection Orders can be acquired by affected persons. Resident Orders can be acquired [court can order an alternate accommodation to be arranged/supported by the accused]. Temporary custody in cases involving children's abuse . Protection Committees to be made across the province. Provincial Officers to be appointed across the country. Service Providers may be approached for assistance [whether they be public or private entities. Court summons date must be set within 7 days of complaint. Case to be disposed within 90 days. Calls for awareness raising campaigns and trainings for law enforcement officers.

Sindh Child Marriage Restraint Act 2014

The age of marriage for both boys and girls has been identified as 18. Previously, the age of marriage for girls was 16 under Federal Laws (Child Marriage Restraint Act, 1929). The identified perpetrators remain the same, i.e. adult male marrying a female child; parents, guardians or any person having lawful or unlawful charge of the child; the person who solemnizes the marriage. Punishment: Three years but not less than two years and a fine (undefined). No time limitation has been placed on the reporting of the offence of child marriage. Courts (Judicial Magistrate of the First Class) may issue a ruling prohibiting a child marriage on the basis of an application laid before it. While there is a requirement for a notice to be given to any person against whom a ruling is to be issued, the Court is allowed to dispense with this, if necessary. Punishment for any person who disobeys a ruling shall be punished with imprisonment for a maximum of one year, a fine or both. Offence is cognizable (police can make an arrest without a warrant), non-bailable and non-compoundable (cannot compromise with the injured party). The case must be concluded within 90 days.

KP Child Protection and Welfare Act, 2010

Elimination of Custom of Ghag, Act, 2013. Where ghag has been described as :"A custom, usage, tradition or practice whereby a person forcibly demands or claims the hand of a woman, without her own or her parents' or wali's will and free consent, by making an open declaration either by words spoken or written or by visible representation or by an imputation, innuendo, or insinuation, directly or indirectly, in a locality or before public in general that the woman shall stand engaged to him or any other particular man and that no other man shall make a marriage proposal to her or marry her, threatening her parents and other relatives to refrain from giving her hand in marriage to any other person, and shall also include obstructing the marriage of such woman in any other manner pursuant to such declaration" [Italics by author]. Ghag is a criminal offence punishable with up to seven years imprisonment or Rs 500,000 fine or both.

Balochistan Domestic Violence (Prevention and Protection) Act, 2014

The Punjab Fair Representation of Women Act, 2014

North-West Frontier Province Establishment of a Commission on the Status of Women Act, 2009

Punjab Commission on the Status of Women Act 2014.[4]

Year 2015

The Anti-Honour Killings Laws (Criminal Laws Amendment) Act, 2014 (passed by the Senate only—Editor)

The Anti-Rape Laws (Criminal Laws Amendment) Act, 2013 (passed by the Senate only—Editor)

The Torture, Custodial Death and Custodial Rape (Punishment) Act, 2014 (passed by the Senate only—Editor)

Year 2016

The Criminal Law (Amendment) Act, 2016 (Act No.VI of 2016)

The Minimum Wages for Unskilled Workers (Amendment) Act, 2016 (Act No.VII of 2016)

The Civil Servants (Amendment) Act, 2016 (Act No. IX of 2016)

The Criminal Law (Second Amendment) Act, 2016 (Act No. X of 2016)

The Pakistan Health Research Council Act, 2016 (Act No. XII of 2016)

The Civil Servants (Amendment) Act, 2016 (Act No. XVII))

The Delimitation of Constituencies (Amendment) Act, 2016 (Act No.XXVI of 2016)

The Prevention of Electronic Crimes Act, 2016 (Act No.XL of 2016)

The Criminal Law (Amendment) (Offences Relating to Rape) Act, 2016 (Act No. XLIV of 2016)

The Criminal Law (Amendment) (Offences in the Name or on pretext of Honour) (Act No. XLIII of 2016)

Year 2017

The Elections Act, 2017 (Act No. XXXIII of 2017)

The Criminal Laws (Amendment) Act, 2017 (Act No. IV of 2017)

The Hindu Marriage Act, 2017 (Act No.VII of 2017)

The Representation of the People (Amendment) Act, 2017 (Act No.XXIV of 2017)

The Senate Secretariat Services Act, 2017 (Act No. XXII of 2017)

The Witness Protection, Security and Benefit Act, 2017 (Act No. XXI of 2017)

The National Counter Terrorism Authority (Amendment) Act, 2017 (Act No. XXVI of 2017)

The Elections Act, 2017 (Act No. XXXIII of 2017)

The Right of Access to Information Act, 2017 (Act No. XXXIV of 2017)

The Elections (Amendment) Act, 2017 (Act No. XXXV of 2017)

The Elections (Second Amendment) Act, 2017 (Act No. XXXVII of 2017)

Year 2018

The National Commission on the Status of Women (Amendment) Act No.II 2018

The Transgender Persons (Protection and Rights) Act, 2018 (Act No. XIII of 2018)

The Juvenile Justice System Act, 2018 (Act No. XXII of 2018)

The Prevention of Smuggling of Migrants Act, 2018 (Act No.XXVIII of 2018)

The Islamabad Capital Territory Child Protection Act, 2018 (Act No. XXI of 2018)

The Criminal Laws (Amenment) Act, 2018 (Act No.XXVII of 2018)

The Women in Distress and Detention Fund (Amendment) Act, 2018 (Act No.XIX of 2018)

Life Skills Based Education (LSBE) has become mandatory in schools in Sindh and Baluchistan (2018)

Suggested National Policy on Ending Violence Against Women and Children

These suggestions provide:

a. Guiding principles to provide minimum requirements, and support for provincial and local governments to develop plans, strategies or laws to deal with present cases and raise greater awareness to prevent future acts of violence.

b. Policy directions in order to guide policy and law makers in areas of common concerns at national, provincial and local levels. The Objectives are:

It should survive political change: Ensure that the policy's overarching framework draws the consensus of all major political parties and other stakeholders and survive with changes of government or political direction.

Budget allocation: A dedicated and conti-nuous budget allocation should be ensured for violence against women and children awareness, with rapid relief to the victim/survivor

GBV seamless service model: Women and Girls Centres which deal with violence victims should be introduced in all districts of each province. Facilities should be promptly provided to the victim/ survivors including first aid, police reporting, FIR lodging, medical examination, collection and analysis of forensic and other evidence, psychologist evaluation and post-trauma rehabilitation.

Address sex discrimination: The gender gap between men and women, which inevitably leads to sex discrimination, should be narrowed/closed. This is one of the most effective ways of addressing violence against women and girls.

Strengthen structures and institutions: Enhance support mechanisms and response. These would include National Commission on the Status of Women, Ministry of Human Rights and Ministry of Law and Justice.

Future plans: Any action plan or legislation must ensure that it is ethical, culturally and gender sensitive, accountable, comprehensive and sustainable.

Future amendments to existing legislation: Future legislation or review and eventual amendment of existing legislation must adhere to the basic principles of this policy. This includes addressing issues of language or content that are directly or indirectly gender discriminatory.

Standardized, accredited and comprehensive training: It is essential that all relevant professionals across sectors and jurisdictions, such as health sector workers, teachers education institutions, police and judiciary and all those that respond to violence against women and girls receive standardized, accredited and comprehensive pre-service and in-service training on the issues surrounding violence against women, its causes and consequences. It should be ensured that training is not an isolated event but an ongoing process, which is part of the requirement of the job.

Public–private partnerships: Establish public private partnerships forums to promote coordination and establish legitimacy of collective efforts of government and non-governmental bodies.

Guiding principles: The policy will guide the State and various stakeholders to achieve the purpose and objectives of the policy on the basis of the following principles:

- *Zero tolerance* towards any form of violence against women and girls. The state does not accept any caveat that allows for and covers up violence against women and girls. This shall be incorporated through coordinated, sustained and meaningful action, which challenges and deconstructs the prevalent deep rooted and entrenched social attitudes. Ensure good practices and inter-agency coordination across all relevant sectors, structures and institutions, formal and informal, be gender equitable and provide shift response and justice to the victim/survivor, throughout the process.
- *Justice and equality*: The policy will guide the State and its various organs in accordance with the fundamental rights as enshrined in the Constitution of Pakistan, in particular, the principles of justice and equality. Every person, regardless of sex or other difference, is equal before the law and shall be entitled to their basic human rights and facilities, including protection and recourse to free and fair legal protection.
- *Human Rights Framework*: Viewing violence against women and girls within a human rights framework shifts responsibility for prevention from the private to the public sphere and focuses on public bodies' responsibility for the rehabilitation of the abused and punishment of the abuser. No person in authority should use his/her discretion subjectively from punishing a

person accused of a gender based crime. The human rights framework broadens the realm of various state and private institutions and the inter-link between violence and public health, education and gender equality. This policy establishes its directions within the overall human rights framework, which entails a strategic guide to the national and provincial governments.

- *Political will and leadership*: The policy aims to build on a wide consensus between all relevant stakeholders, public and private, in order that it embeds itself in political will and survives party politics.

Political will is imperative for societal change towards violence. Swift, just and confidential response to the victim. Successive governments have accepted nationally and internationally, that violence against women and girls can have long-term economic and public health costs to society. Additionally, the victim experiences long-term negative health consequences (medical and psychological), loss of security, quality of life and loss of agency in her own life. It is also widely accepted that there are wide-reaching potential damaging implications for children, families and communities and burdens the health care system further.

All national, provincial and local bodies must ensure that gender sensitive, accountable and transparent structures and institutions exist to provide immediate relief and response to the victim/survivor, including police, health care providers and the judicial system.

Provincial responsibility: The 18th amendment has devolved powers to the provinces where policymakers and legislators have greater autonomy. Provinces should note that more allocation to areas for the emancipation of women and girls would result in greater progress as a whole. In particular it would in terms of women's and girl's development and education. This in turn will ensure less discrimination, better understanding of women and girls to access facilities and institutions, such as police and the judiciary and eventual equality and safety of women and girls.

Education: Education is the backbone of a successful country and the strongest primary violence prevention mechanism. The Government of Pakistan, under its constitutional obligations under Article 25A, is fully committed to education for girls, recognizing that education is the only long- term solution to help bridge the discriminatory gap and for the future success of this policy. It is the responsibility of all provincial and local governments to further consolidate efforts and enhance mechanism to ensure that all school-age going girls are enrolled and stay in school. The state through its various organs should guide all levels of government to revise curriculum and teacher training to incorporate gender sensitive curriculum for both boys and girls. This should be made compulsory across all disciplines from primary to college level. Gender sensitive concepts and underlying reasons should be incorporated. Education including community education and legal literacy should be invested in and disseminated from all relevant government platforms.

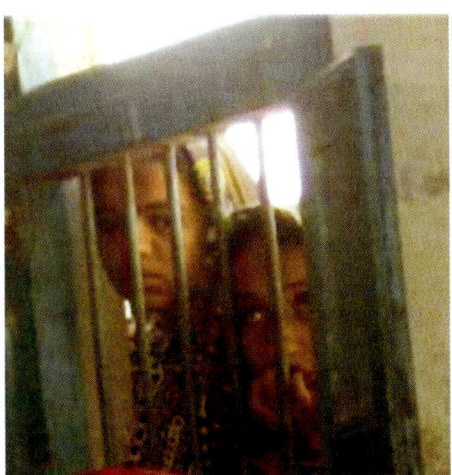

Sindhi village women

Ethical, cultural and gender sensitive plans: Any future strategy, action plan or legislation resulting from this policy should be ethical, culture and gender sensitive, accountable, comprehensive and sustainable.

Future legislation or review, and eventual amendment of existing legislation, must adhere to the basic principles of these suggestions.

ROLE OF THE MEDICAL PROFESSION

Doctors and nurses lack training and are guilty of maintaining silence on the issue of sexual violence and child abuse that they deal with, or refuse to deal with. The solution lies in Life skills and sex education in schools and educational institutions of Pakistan, as well as education of Parents. Structured training on management of sexual violence should be part of the curriculum. This should be taught and implemented during undergraduate education of doctors and nurses, as well as in Postgraduate training.

Improved access to quality contraceptive services should be a priority, especially in rural areas. Contraceptive counseling should be a routine part of post-abortion care. This will reduce the trauma of unsafe abortions.

The restrictive abortion law should be brought in compliance with international human rights standards, and ensure clarification regarding 'necessary treatment', address the stigma around abortion and post abortion care and the barriers women face in accessing such services.

Gynecologists have a special highly respected position in Society, and are capable of bringing about a change in the mindset of people about the importance of addressing these very important issues. They should take part/arrange advocacy programs, and counsel their clients and families; form linkages with other professional bodies/societies to disseminate information.

BIBLIOGRAPHY

1. http://hrcpmonitor.org/ (accessed 11.2.19)
2. https://nation.com.pk/03-Dec-2018/hiv-epidemic-spreads-at-alarming-rate-in-pakistan-who (accessed 15.2.19)
3. https://tribune.com.pk/story/10134 68/lets-talk-about-stds/ (accessed 15.2.19)
4. Kaukab Tahir Shairani, https://tribune.com.pk/story/1867614/1-2018-witnesses-no-respite-violence-women/(accessed 11.2.19)
5. Legislation at Federal level since 2002. Aurat Foundation. https://www.af.org.pk/legislation_Federal.php
6. Mohammad aid, Mohammad Sohail Afzal; HIV Outbreak in Pakistan,The Lancet Infectious diseases Vol 18 Issue 6, pg 601, June 1 2018 https://www. thelancet.com/journals/laninf/article/PIIS147 33099(18)30281-0/fulltext (accessed 15.2.19)
7. Muhammad Bakhtiar, https://nation.com.pk/02-Oct-2018/violence-against-women (accessed 11.2.19)
8. National Institute of Population Studies (NIPS) [Pakistan] and ICF International. 2013. Pakistan Demographic and Health Survey 2012-13. Islamabad, Pakistan, and Calverton, Maryland, USA: NIPS and ICF International.
9. PAPAC Oral Statement to the Human Rights Committee 120th Session July 2017
10. PDHS 2017-18. Key Indicators https://dhsprogram.com/pubs/pdf/PR109/PR109.pdf (accessed 13.2.19)
11. Sadiah Ahsan Pal, Premarital Health and social Issues JPMA Vol. 67, No. 7, July 2017 pg 973974
12. Sarah Zaman 09 March 2015 (WAF IWD Program-SZABIST)

Situation Analysis of Sri Lanka

Udagamage Don Puspananda Ratnasiri, Athula Kaluarachchi

SRI LANKA—DEMOGRAPHICS

Sri Lanka, officially known as the Democratic Socialist Republic of Sri Lanka, is an island situated off southern coast of India in the northern Indian Ocean of South Asia, separated from the Indian sub-continent by a narrow strip of shallow water, known as Palk Strait. Sri Lanka lies between northern latitudes 50 55′ and 90 50′ and eastern longitudes 790 42′ and 810 52′. It has total area of 65,610 square kilometers including 2,905 square kilometers of inland water. The island has a central mountainous region, 'Hill country' with peak as high as 2,524 meters above the sea level and is surrounded by a plain known as 'Low country' which is narrow in East, West and South, broadens in the North. A number of rivers spring up from the mountain peaks and flow towards the sea through low lying plains following a radial pattern.

For the purpose of administration, Sri Lanka is divided into 9 provinces, 25 districts and 331 divisional secretary areas. The provincial administration is vested in the Provincial Councils. Local government which is the lowest level of government in Sri Lanka is responsible for providing supportive services for the public.

Sri Lanka has a population of 20.3 million (2011) of whom the majority are Sinhalese (74%). Other ethnic groups are made up of Sri Lankan Tamils (12.6%), Indian Tamils (5.5%), Moors, Malays, Burghers (of Portuguese & Dutch descent) and others (7.9%). Although Sri Lanka is a multi-religious country, Buddhists constitute the majority with 69.3%. Other religious groups are Hindus 15.5%, Muslims 7.6% and Christians 7.5%. Sri Lanka's literacy rate of 92.7% (2003 estimated) is one of the highest in Asia.

Life expectancy at birth is 76.4 females, 71.7 males (2001 est), urban population (%) 2012, 18.2, census of population and housing, 2012. Sex ratio (no. of males per 100 females) 2012, 93.8. Child population (under 5 years) % 2012, 8.6. Women in the reproductive age group (15–49 years) % 2012, 51.0. Average household size (number of persons per family) is two (Fig. 8.1).

Nearly 50% of the total government hospital deaths in Sri Lanka in 2016 were due to major non-communicable diseases.

- Over 50% of total deaths in Sri Lanka, reported through vital registration, were due to major chronic non-communicable disease.
- Ischemic heart disease has been the number one leading cause of hospital deaths for more than a decade.

Singulate mean age at marriage (years) Female is 23.4 in 2012, census of population and housing, 2012.

It is noticeable that dependency ratio, which is an approximation of the average number of dependents that each person of working age must support, has decreased from 71.8 in 1981 to 60.2 in 2016, due to relative decline in the

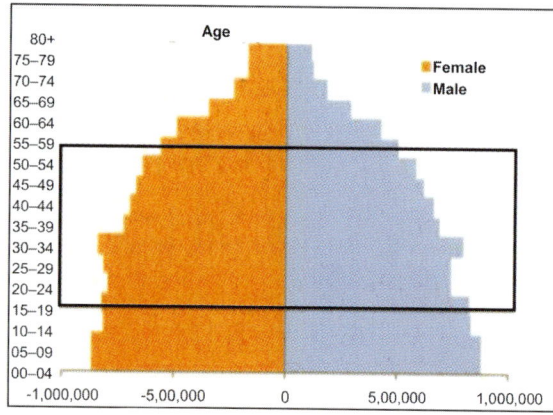

Fig. 8.1: Age–sex pyramid: Sri Lanka 2012

proportion of children. It is important to note that working age population was 62.4 percent in 2012 and shows an increase from 58.2 in 1981, i.e. the working age population was significantly larger than the dependent population.

Population Density

Population density for the year 2016 was 338 persons per square kilometre which shows an increase of 47 percent from 230 persons per square kilometre since 1981. Population densities among districts show marked regional variations. Colombo district shows the highest density of 3,543 persons per square kilometre in 2016. The next highest density of 1,769 was recorded from the adjoining district Gampaha.

Sex ratio was 93.8 in Sri Lanka for the year 2016, i.e. an excess of females over males. Up to age 14, sex ratio was over 100, and afterwards all age groups have a female-biased population. In other words, younger age groups and older age groups have more females.

The public health sector is organized as two parallel streams: Community health services focusing mainly on promotive and preventive health—curative care services ranging from non-specialized primary care to specialized care delivered through a variety of hospitals.

Maternity Services

The registration of pregnant mothers has been more than 90% over the years and in 2016 it was 99.1%. Out of them, over 78.5% registered for care before 8 weeks of amenorrhea and this number has been rising over the last few years from 72% to 78%. Protection for rubella with immunization before pregnancy, protection for tetanus, antenatal screening for syphilis and testing for blood group at the time of delivery has achieved almost universal coverage of 99.1%.

Pregnancy outcome was reported for 94.5% of pregnancies registered with the PHM. Almost all reported deliveries in 2016 had taken place in institutions and the percentage of home deliveries has decreased to a very minimum level (0.1%) over the years. The cesarean section rate has gradually increased to 36.3% in 2016. In-depth analysis is needed in the future. Due to obstetric transition, indirect maternal mortality causes and over-medicalisation have been recognized as emerging issues in maternal care. Out of total deliveries in government hospitals 65% occurred in teaching, provincial general hospitals and district general hospitals. Cesarean rate is 37.3% out of total deliveries occurred in government hospitals in 2017. A number of cases of placental adhesive disorders are seen due to this increasing cesarean rates.

Respectful maternity care to all pregnant mothers were introduced in 2016 by a ministry circular and it is being practiced in most of the maternity units of the country at the moment. A female labour companion is allowed to stay with the mother in labour in the labour room. Early breastfeeding is promoted and Sri Lanka achieved the first in the world regarding this achievement in 2018.

During the important postpartum period, approximately 85% of mothers were visited at home by PHMs at least once during the first 10 days, and 66% during the first five postpartum days. On average, most mothers received two postpartum home visits.

Government has launched an emergency pre-hospital medical care ambulance service (emergency telephone number 1919) in partnership with the Government of India in all the districts in the country in 2018.

Maternal Mortality

"Sri Lanka carries best health indices in the south Asian region." Maternal mortality rate 37.2 per 100000 live births in 2017 (Fig. 8.2). Though it has shown a decline for last 10 years, the rate remains at a static level and measures need to be taken to reduce further. Sri Lanka College of Obstetricians and Gynaecologist with the help of Family Health Bureau taking further steps to develop highly specialised centres of excellence in health regions to deal with major causalities of maternal deaths, e.g. heart disease, respiratory disease and hemorrhagic deaths due to placental adhesive disorders. Infectious diseases like dengue and influenza also contributes to maternal deaths as a major contributor in the last few years.

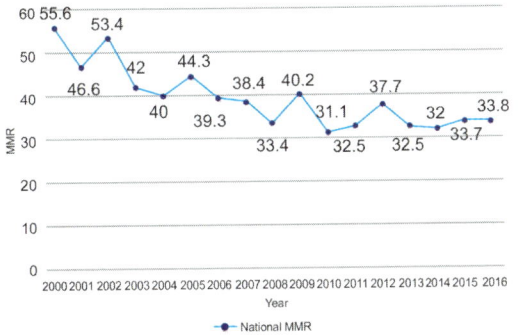

Stillbirth Rate

During 2016, a total of 303,593 live births and 1,823 stillbirths took place in government hospitals (Table 8.1). This was a decrease of 4.7% in stillbirths when compared with 2015. According to the Medical Statistics Unit, stillbirth rate in the state sector hospitals of Sri Lanka was reported to be 6.0 per 1000 (total births occurred in government hospitals) in 2016. The highest stillbirth rate was reported

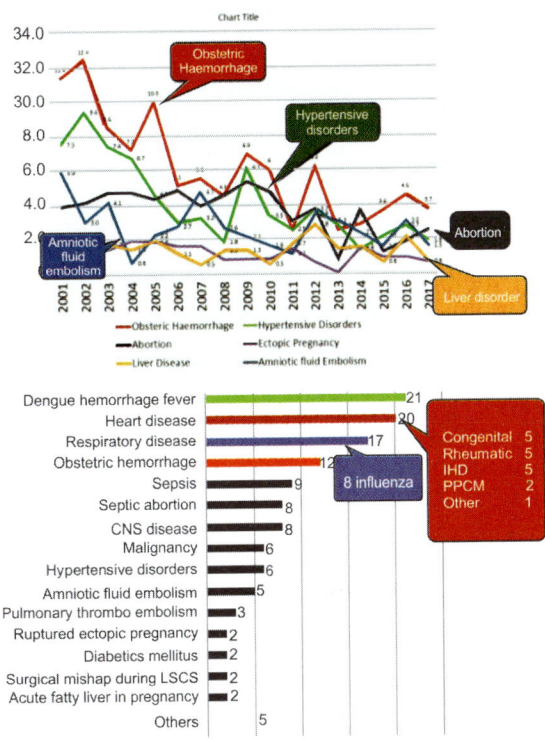

Fig. 8.2: Cause specific MMRs (2001–2017) direct causes (*Source:* Details obtained with the permission of Family Health Bureau).

from hospitals in Nuwara Eliya district, and it was 11.5, which is close to twice the national figure. This may be due to the fact that, Nuwara Eliya district is different from other districts in climate, sector distribution and many other demographic and socio-economic factors. The lowest stillbirth rate was from Trincomalee which was 2.8. According to RHMIS, stillbirth rates have been falling over the years. In order to reduce the stillbirth rate from 6.4/1000 (births reported from RHMIS system) in 2013 to 3.5/1000 total births by the end of 2025, as given in Every Newborn Action Plan (WHO 2014), a stillbirth rate of 4.5/1000 total births by 2020 must be achieved. Given that the stillbirth rate showed an annual decline of 4.6% for the period of 2007–2013 (SLENAP, 2017), it appears that the country was on course to achieve the goals for stillbirths.

Table 8.1: Live births, maternal deaths, stillbirths and low birth weight babies in government hospitals by districts 2016

District	Live births	Maternal deaths		Stillbirths		Low births[4]	
		No.	Rate[1]	No.	Rate[2]	No.	Rate[3]
Colombo	36,285	12	33.1	263	7.2	5,371	14.8
Gampaha	20,606	8	38.8	139	6.7	3,104	15.1
Kalutara	14,270	1	7.0	79	5.5	1,935	13.6
Kandy	24,826	12	48.3	168	6.7	4,207	16.9
Matale	9,013	-	-	62	6.8	1,489	16.5
Nuwara Eliya	9,234	3	32.5	106	11.3	2,250	24.4
Galle	17,446	1	5.7	108	6.2	2,334	13.4
Matara	10,428	-	-	72	6.9	1,500	14.4
Hambantota	10,453	-	-	41	3.9	1,157	11.1
Jaffna	7,209	-	-	767	9.2	904	12.5
Killinochchi	2,178	1	45.9	12	5.5	233	10.7
Mullaitivu	841	-	-	3	3.6	102	12.1
Vavuniya	3,404	-	-	14	4.1	458	13.5
Mannar	1,687	-	-	8	4.7	170	10.1
Batticoloa	7,984	-	-	49	6.1	1,222	15.3
Ampara[5]	13,217	1	7.6	46	3.5	1,919	14.5
Trincomalee	7,844	-	-	22	2.8	1,100	14.0
Kurunegala	22,119	10	45.2	67	3.0	3,356	15.2
Puttalam	13,100	-	-	74	5.6	2,047	15.6
Anuradhapura	15,121	1	6.6	106	7.0	2,256	14.9
Polonnaruwa	7,015	2	28.5	31	4.4	1,179	16.8
Badulla	15,885	8	50.4	109	6.8	3,125	19.7
Monaragala	6,659	-	-	29	4.3	1,111	16.7
Ratnapura	17,731	1	5.6	101	5.7	2,958	16.7
Kegalle	9,038	-	-	47	5.2	1,431	15.8
Sri Lanka	**303,593**	**61**	**20.1**	**1,823**	**6.0**	**46,918**	**15.5**

[1]Per 100,000 live births; [2]Per 1,000 total births; [3]Per 100 live births; [4]Birth weight less than 2500 grams; [5]Includes Kalmunai RDHS division 2 per 1000 total births. *Source:* Medical Statistics Unit

Primary Health Care Coverage Indicators: Percentage of pregnant women attended by skilled personnel 2016 is 99.5 (Demographic and Health Survey, 2016).

Percentage of live births occurred in government hospitals is 91.7 in 2016, Medical Statistics Unit.

Current contraceptive usage of currently married women age 15-49 years (%): Modern method 2016, 53.6 (Demographic and Health Survey, 2016). Traditional method, 11.0.

Population with access to safe water is 81.1% in 2012 (Census Population and Housing, 2012).

Total Fertility Ratio

TFR declined steadily from 2.8 in the year 1987 to 1.9 in the year 2000, which was below the replacement level of fertility. (Replacement level of fertility is defined as an average of 2.1 children per woman.) Afterwards it increased to above the replacement level of fertility during the period 2003 to 2012. Currently TFR is 2.2 children per woman according to the Demographic and Health Survey (DHS) 2016.

STI and HIV Status

Situation of HIV epidemic in Sri Lanka during 2016, a total of 249 HIV cases were newly reported in Sri Lanka (Fig. 8.3). This was the highest number reported in a year since the identification of the first HIV infected

Sri Lankan in 1987. However, the reported numbers do not represent all HIV infected people in the country as many infected persons may perhaps not be aware of their HIV status. In addition, stigma and discrimination towards HIV hinders seeking HIV testing services. Since 2011, the proportion of males with HIV has been gradually increasing (Fig. 8.4). The male to female ratio of cumulative reported cases up to end of 2016 was

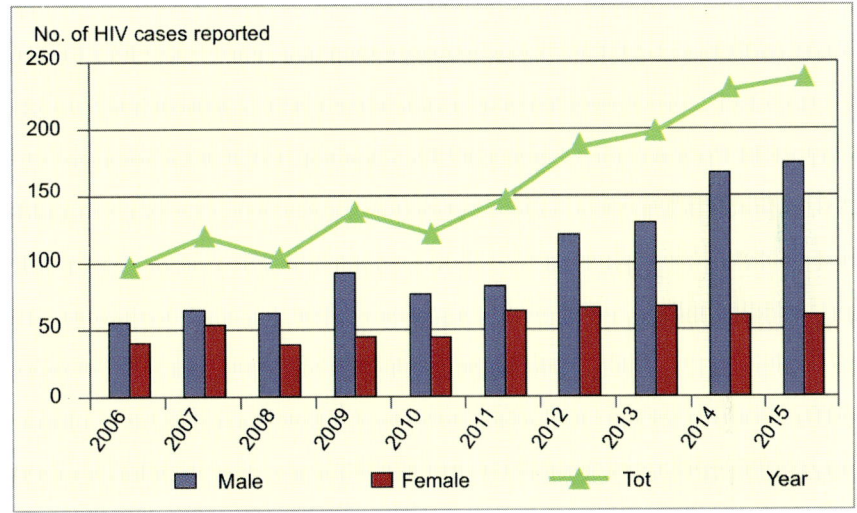

Fig. 8.3: Number of HIV cases reported

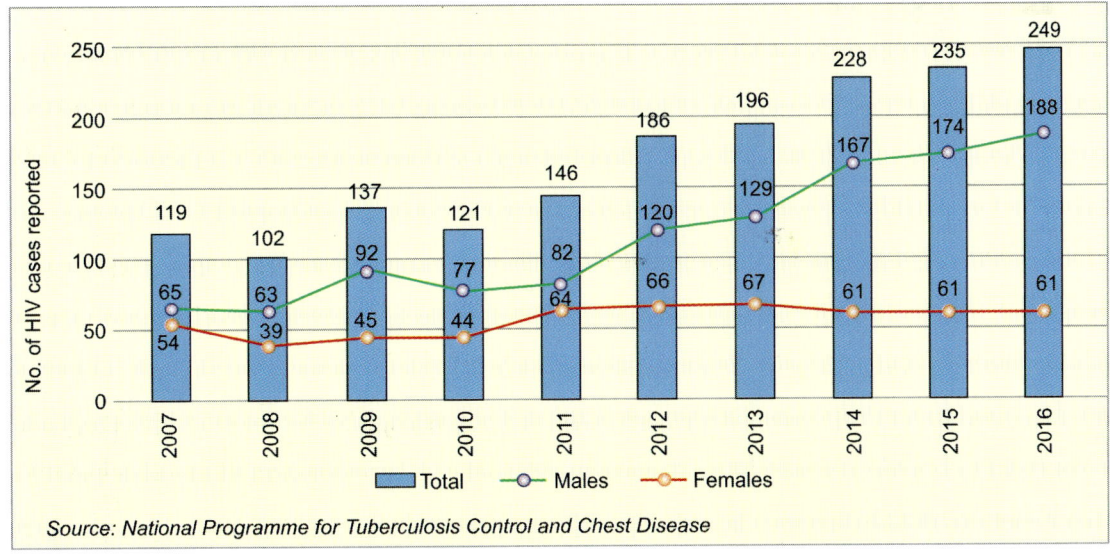

Source: National Programme for Tuberculosis Control and Chest Disease

Fig. 8.4: Trends of reported HIV cases by sex 2007–2016

1.8:1. However, among newly reported HIV cases during 2016, the male to female ratio increased to 3.1:1. HIV testing services in 2016: HIV testing services are critical in national response to HIV epidemic in the country. Over the years the number of HIV tests carried out in the country has been increased. However, total number of HIV tests done may be under-reported in the private sector as there is no formal mechanism established to report all the HIV tests. However, all confirmed positive HIV results are reported to NSACP as confirmatory test (Western Blot) is available only at the national reference laboratory of NSACP. Diversification of testing and service delivery methods were attempted during 2016 (Table 8.2). HIV treatment and care services: Globally there is consensus that activities for HIV prevention and care services need to be accelerated to reach the targets of ending AIDS by 2030. Early enrollment in ART services contributes significantly to reducing HIV transmission while minimizing morbidities and mortality related to HIV/AIDS. A total of 21,973 new patients had received services from the National STD/AIDS Control Program during 2016, while a total of 65,820

clinic visits were made by all STD attendees. Among them 9,129 STI diagnoses were made as summarized in Table 8.2. Genital herpes has been reported as the commonest STI presentation.

Elimination of mother to child transmission (EMTCT) of syphilis and HIV: The elimination of mother to child transmission (EMTCT) of syphilis and HIV program was scaled-up to cover the whole country in 2016. During 2016 the EMTCT program was carried out mainly with government funds while UNICEF assisted in printing IEC (Information Education and Communication) material, conducting review meetings and purchasing safe delivery kits. Sri Lanka has achieved the required status in relation to indicators for validation of EMTCT of syphilis by the end of 2016 and is likely to satisfy indicators for EMTCT of HIV by the end of 2017.

VIOLENCE AGAINST WOMEN: DOMESTIC

Prevalence

Domestic violence is an identified problem in Sri Lanka. Violation against women is direct in various forms including sexual, physical,

Table 8.2: Relative productivity of HIV testing methods and testing details in 2016

Type of blood samples screened for HIV	Number tested	Percentage of samples	Number positive	Percentage of positives	Positivity rate (%)
Blood donor screening (NBTS and private blood banks)	417,428	37	23	9	0.01
Antenatal mothers	323,518	29	11	4	0.003
Private hospitals, laboratories and Sri Jayewardenepura GH	225,047	20	40	16	0.02
STD clinic samples	90,271	8	160	64	0.18
Tri-forces	29,236	3	4	2	0.01
Survey sample	23,615	2	1	0	0.004
Prison HIV testing programme	12,776	1	6	2	0.05
TB screening	7,896	1	4	2	0.05
Total	**1,129,787**	**100%**	**249**	**100**	**0.02**

spiritual, mental, symbolical, verbal, emotional and financial threat against women. Nowadays reporting of these cases are not lower than past decades.

In Sri Lanka, 17 percent of ever-married women age 15–49 have suffered from domestic violence from their intimate partner. Two percent of ever-married women who suffered from domestic violence, experiences in any form of domestic violence daily. Prevalence of domestic violence by an intimate partner increases with the age of the women. Urban residents also reported the highest percentage of domestic violence (20 percent). Kilinochchi and Batticaloa districts have the highest level of domestic violence (50 percent). Ever-married women who belong to the lowest wealth quintile and those with primary education reported the highest percentages in domestic violence (28 and 30 percent respectively). Among women who suffered from domestic violence, only just over one-fourth of women (28 percent) have sought help, with three-fourth of them (75 percent) seeking help from their family members, 27 percent from friends or neighbours and only 18 percent seeking help from the police. Half of the ever-married women age 15–49 (50 percent) indicated to know about the Sri Lanka Women Bureau to combat violence, while 26 percent mentioned the midwife

and Women Help Line. For the purpose of counseling and supporting of victims of GBV, 60 Mithuru Piyasa centers have been established in the country. The numbers of attendance to these centers have shown a dramatic increase over the years.

VIOLENCE AGAINST WOMEN: WORKPLACE

Prevalence

There is no reliable data regarding this issue. Gender-based violence and harassment at the working places is another identified problem. This problem is reported from various workplace settings and across various levels of society.

Legal Status

The Prevention of Domestic Violence Act addresses domestic violence and provides with civil remedies.

The Act itself provides the person who is affected by domestic violence (aggrieved person) with protection by means of Interim Protection Order or a Protection Order. The person who is affected by domestic violence is introduced as an "aggrieved person" in order to avoid treating them same as other victims.

Certain ways of domestic violence can also be a part of general criminal offences under the

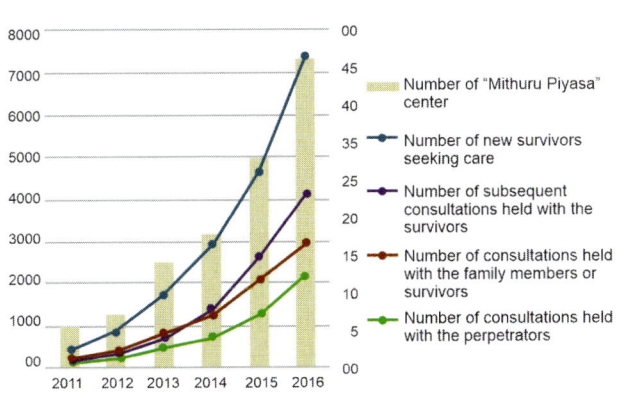

Source: Women's Health Unit, Family Health Bureau

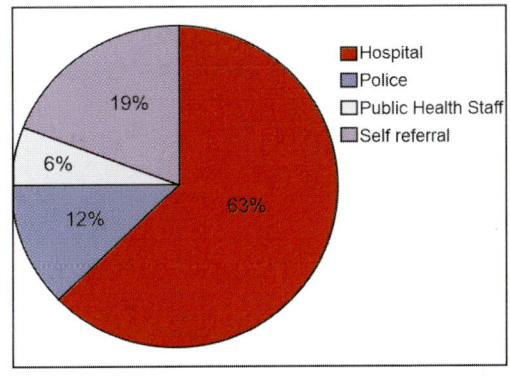

Source: Referral to Mithuru Piyasa (FHB)

Performance statistics of Mithuru Piyasa 2011–2016

penal code such as hurt, offences against human body and grievous sexual abuse.

Magistrate court carries the jurisdiction of hearing cases under the Domestic Violence Act.

In circumstances where either party is not satisfied with the decision, an appeal can be made to the High Court.

Rape

In terms of Section 363(e) of the penal code, sexual intercourse with a woman under 16 years of age is rape whether committed with or without the consent of the woman. The provision is based on the legal principle that a girl below 16 years has no legal capacity to grant consent to sexual intercourse. Section 364 (e) provides for the imposition of a minimum sentence of 10 years imprisonment for those convicted of rape where the woman is under 18 years of age.

Prevalence

In 2013, rape rate for Sri Lanka was 10.6 cases per 100,000 population. Rape rate of Sri Lanka increased from 7.4 cases per 100,000 population in 2004 to 10.6 cases per 100,000 population in 2013 growing at an average annual rate of 6.57 %.

Genital Mutilation

The government has issued a circular banning Female Genital Mutilation by medical practitioners and it is illegal in Sri Lanka.

A number of Sri Lankan Muslim groups have called on the government to medicalise female circumcision.

In representations made to the Parliamentary Committee on Women and Gender, members of the All Ceylon Jamiyathul Ulama, All Ceylon YMMA Conference, Centre for Islamic Studies and United Religions Initiative urged the Health Ministry to withdraw a recent circular prohibiting medical professionals from carrying out female circumcision.

In their submission, the joint Muslim groups stated that the Muslim community is very concerned about moves to ban this obligatory Islamic duty on the grounds that it is Female Genital Mutilation (FGM).

Child Marriage

In Sri Lanka the legal marriage age is 18. Sri Lanka plans to reform its constitution and so activists believe now is the moment to act.

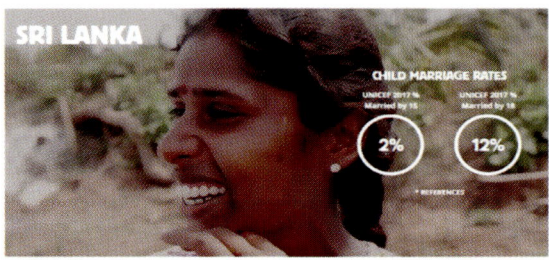

Honor killing is the murder of a woman by her family members when she has chosen to marry or has married to a man outside of what is acceptable to the family. This is not practiced in Sri Lanka.

Human Trafficking

Human trafficking is not a significant problem in Sri Lanka. It is hardly heard girls and women are mostly trafficked for sex-related work.

Refugees

Due to 30 years internal war number of internal refugees had increased till 2009 in Sri Lanka. Most of these displaced refugees were resettled in the recent years.

Refugees have always been a source of political controversy. There is a fine line between an individual being an immigrant and a refugee in the international scenario. Within a given country, refugees are often referred to as internally displaced people. They face the common problems of a lack of livelihood, difficulty in accessing healthcare even in emergencies, poor social status and vulnerability to violence, hate crimes and exploitation. Each of these problems compounds the other and therefore, refugees (international and domestic) pose difficult problems to administrators, security forces and healthcare providers. There were few Rohingyas refugees came to Sri Lanka from Myanmar.

Medical Issues in General

There is no gender inequality in seeking and provision of health care in Sri Lanka, in comparison with other countries in the region. This is because the proportion and extent of level of education is high in Sri Lanka in comparison with other countries of south Asia. In urban areas social background and financial independence is higher than rural areas in Sri Lanka. Health care is free to all citizens in Sri Lanka.

With improving health care facilities in the public sector, acceptability of going to public hospitals from GP set up has been increased. Women are important health beneficiaries under the scheme. Not only are they directly affected by access to quality maternity care, but they will also be able to influence child care substantially.

Elderly population is increasing in the country. Non-communicable diseases (NCD) are more prevalent among elders. Promotion of active healthy ageing concept focusing more towards control of modifiable risk factors to prevent NCDs is implemented through life course approach.

- Active healthy elders are an asset to the society and they are a resource group to the youth.
- Promotion of accessibility facilities and promotion of availability, affordability and correct usage of recommended assistive devices enhances productivity of persons
- With disabilities. Disability rehabilitation is complex. Therefore multi-disciplinary team care and right-based holistic approaches are to be considered for disability rehabilitation.

Health Rights

Sri Lanka is a signatory to various international treaties on human rights in UNHRC (United Nations Human Rights Commission). These treaties have various clauses which make health a prerequisite human right. The constitution of Sri Lanka mention protection of public health. Nowadays, courts have increasingly looked upon the right to health as a logical extension of the right to life. The law is directed towards moving the system towards a rights-based approach. However, it also acknowledges the lack of infrastructure and basic prerequisites (doctor–patient ratio, number of nurses, number of hospital beds, number of government medical schools, etc.) which stop the state from making this a legally enforceable issue. At present, every citizen is granted an equal access to public health facilities.

Consent

In terms of healthcare, consent should have three components—disclosure, capacity and voluntariness. According to the Sri Lankan law an individual has the right to self-determination and treatment should be administered only when consent (implied, verbal or written) has been given. The type of consent depends on the context in which it is being administered, the patient's condition and degree/extent of possible damage. The exception to seeking consent is, of course, emergency situations, with an immediate and imminent risk to life. Considering the ground realities of the level of education and health information available and the doctor–patient ratio, the Sri Lankan law accept the concept of "real" consent rather than "informed" consent.

As such, consent is valid only if it is given by the individual undergoing the treatment. The exception to this is in case of minors (age less than 18 years) and those of unsound mind. Another area of exception is in reproductive healthcare. The SLMC (Sri Lanka Medical Council) states that for a married individual, if a surgery or procedure is likely to result in or intended to make the individual sterile, consent should be obtained from both partners. This is important from the point of view of surgical procedures of permanent sterilization. It is also important to note that from the legal point of view, consent for contraception. (insertion of intrauterine device), termination of pregnancy is illegal in Sri Lanka.

Privacy

Privacy is a continuously evolving concept. There are cultural and ethical norms that apply to individual privacy and legal norms that apply to privacy of health data of individuals.

The extent to which individual privacy can be provided to an individual depends on the healthcare setting. The ideals of a private chamber for consultations, separate delivery rooms and isolated operation tables may not be feasible in public health settings. However, there is an increasing move towards respectful maternity care which is being carried over to other aspects of healthcare for women. In India, public maternity care facilities are being assessed and upgraded to meet the international standards.

One of the key components of this is providing privacy to women during the intrapartum period by way of a separate labour room or at least in a curtained cubicle.

The law mandates that certain aspects of reproductive healthcare such as termination of pregnancy, prenatal ultrasound, HIV infection are strictly to be kept in confidence. However, there are concerns surrounding the increasing digitization of health systems and possibility of internet-based unauthorized access (hacking) of such data on a large level.

Contraception

Sri Lanka is a south Asian country that has made heavy investments in the public health system. The results of this are seen in the form of a steep reduction in mortality rates, specially maternal and infant mortality. About 25% of

Sri Lanka's population are below the age of 15 years, and therefore have yet to enter the reproductive lifespan (Population Reference Bureau, 2012). Sri Lankan government began its programmatic initiative into the family planning arena in 1965, when family planning was integrated with the national maternal and child health programme. The national population policy was formulated in 1977 and focused on population reduction as a means to sustainable development. The very first Sri Lanka DHS was carried out in 1987, followed by two more in 1993 and 2000. The latest DHS was conducted in 2006–2007, in which the respondents were ever-married women 15–49 years of age and children under the age of 5 years.

Data Contraceptive Prevalence Rate (CPR)

National level CPR is 65 percent. In the district of Mannar have the lowest at only 18 percent.

Modern contraceptive use: Female sterilization is the most commonly used contraceptive method, used by 14 percent of currently married women. IUD is the most popular non-permanent contraceptive method, which is used by 11 percent of currently married women.

Source of contraception: More than 90 percent of current users of female sterilization, IUD, and implants obtain their services from government sector institutions.

Informed choice: Only 53 percent of ever-married women currently using modern contraceptive methods were informed about the potential side effects or other problems associated with the method prior to use and just over half (51 percent) were informed about what to do if they experienced such side effects. Merely 42 percent of them were informed on the available other methods that can be used.

Contraceptive discontinuation: At the time of the 2016 SLDHS, 35 percent of currently married women indicated no use of contraceptive methods in the 5 years before the survey and another 29 percent of those women who began using a contraceptive method, discontinued the method in less than 12 months. The leading reasons for discontinuation is reported as their "desire to become pregnant" (42 percent).

Percentage of demand and unmet need for family planning: Total demand for family planning is 72 percent. Ninety percent of demand is satisfied, (74 percent by modern methods.) Unmet need is reported as 7.5 percent.

Abortion

Abortion is generally illegal in Sri Lanka under the Penal Code of 1883 and provides that anyone voluntarily causing a woman with child to miscarry is subject to up to three years imprisonment and/or payment of a fine, unless the miscarriage was caused in good faith in order to save the life of the mother. A woman who induces her own miscarriage is subject to the same penalties. The penal code contains no procedural requirements for the legal termination of pregnancy, except that the pregnant woman's consent is necessary. There are no provisions specifying the qualifications of those authorized to perform abortions nor the type of facilities in which the procedures are to be performed. A rural survey suggests that 54 abortions per 1,000 population are performed each year.

In Sri Lanka Misoprostol is available in government hospitals for the use of post-partum hemorrhage and for termination of missed miscarriages. But this drug is brought to the country illegally and used for the termination of pregnancies. With the availability of this as a smuggled drug from India in baggage brought by people, the number of septic abortions have come down. In the year 2017 there were 7 maternal deaths due to septic abortions out of 127 maternal deaths according to statistics from Family Health Bureau.

SRI LANKA—PENAL CODE

303. Whoever voluntarily causes a woman with child to miscarry shall, if such miscarriage not be caused in good faith for the purpose of saving the life of the woman, be punished with imprisonment of either description for a term which may extend to three years, or with fine, or with both; and if the woman be quick with child, shall be punished with imprisonment of either description for a term which may extend to seven years, and shall also be liable to fine.

CONCLUSIONS

The health sector of Sri Lanka for women is dramatically improving.

The most important parameter, "maternal mortality" has been decreasing significantly. Sri Lankan Health Mission has undertaken a number of measures including the broad spectrum of reproductive, child and maternal health care. It remains a work in progress as in other developing countries of the region.

BIBLIOGRAPHY

1. Annual health Bulletin 2016 Ministry of Health, Nutrition and Indigenous medicine, Sri Lanka.
2. Country profile of Gender Based Violence in Sri Lanka. WHO.
3. Demographic and health survey 2016, Sri Lanka.
4. Global abortion policies data base.
5. Ministry of child development and women's affairs. Sri Lanka law directory on protection of women and girl children 2012. Colombo; Ministry of Child Development and Women Affairs;2012
6. The Lancet Volume 391, Issue 10126, P1121, March 24, 2018.
7. women waves.org/en/page/4894/abortion law in Sri Lanka

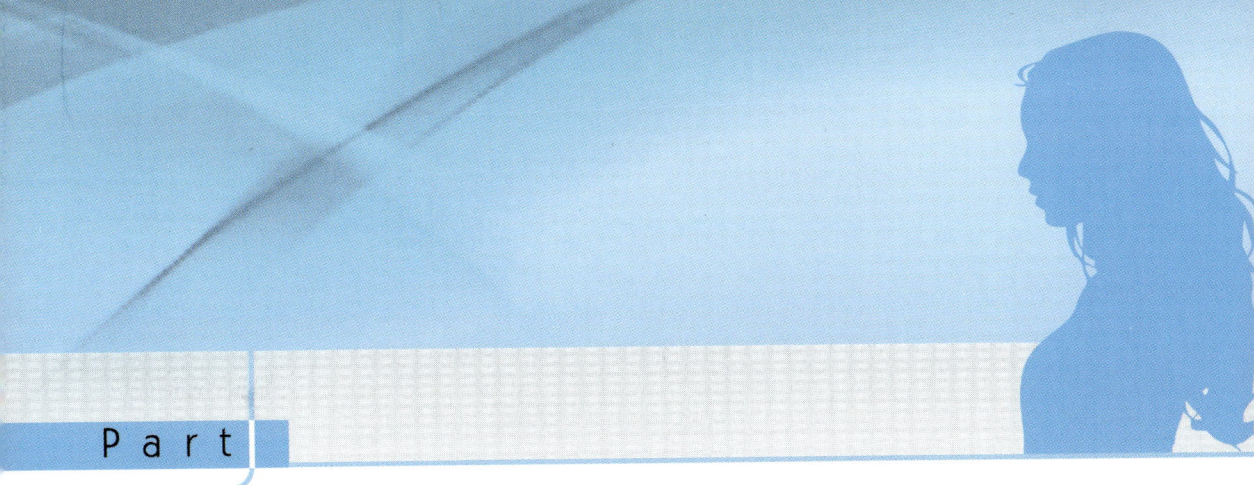

Part

2

Issues and Solutions

9

Lack of Women Empowerment

Kusum Thapa, Saroja Pandey, Sapna Vaidya

BACKGROUND

United Nations Summit in 2015 adopted the "Agenda 2030 for Sustainable Development Goals (SDG)" which comprised of 17 goals and 169 targets. Among the 17 goals, Goal 5 addresses women empowerment. The SDG 5 targets to "end all forms of discrimination, eliminate all forms of violence against all women and girls, eliminate all harmful practices, such as early child and forced marriage, female genital mutilation, recognizing and valuing unpaid care and domestic work through the provision of public services, infrastructure and social protection policies, ensuring women's participation at all areas and levels of decision making, and universal access to sexual and reproductive health (SRH) rights". It also includes "enhancing the use of enabling technology for information and communications and strengthening policies to promote gender equality at all levels in the societies". Kofi Annan, the 7th UN Secretary General, had rightly quoted, "There is no tool for development more effective than the empowerment of women. Hence, empowering of the women and children should be the first and foremost priority for human rights, social justice, poverty alleviation, economic growth, peace, security and for overall development.

The United Nations Guidelines on the empowerment of women consist of five components comprising of self-worth of women; their right to have choices; to have access to resources and opportunities; to be able to control their own lives in their own home and beyond; and their ability to influence the social change for uplifting the economic and social environment.

Hence, the empowerment of women facilitates women to overcome the barriers of their gender roles and allow them to have equal access to the opportunities in the personal and professional worlds as the men. It also allows women to have a louder voice and an undeniable presence in the societies that were ruled by men for ages.

In general, women empowerment can be broadly divided into economic empowerment and political empowerment. Economic empowerment enables women to step outside the barriers of their own homes, allows them the financial freedom and enhances their purchasing decision. Formal education for women is a stepping stone to prepare women for economic empowerment as it develops their capacity for better employment opportunities in the job market. It also strengthens their ability to make the decisions that would benefit their financial capacity. Micro finance is an example of economic empowerment for women across all education and socio-economic statuses.

Political empowerment, on the other hand, refers to the process of policy reforms that allow women's prominent representation in the decision-making position such as in politics. Policies that define women's presence in parliament, allocated women's quota in professional spheres and women's welfare and property rights are all examples of political empowerment.

The health sector is often the first interaction for most women to share their problems. Women tend to discuss the issues such as violence and the barriers they face indirectly to the health providers. Thus, the health providers such as the obstetricians and gynecologists who directly deal with women's health issues every day could have a crucial role to help empower women. They also have a crucial role in achieving some of the SDG targets such as addressing violence and harmful practices against women and enabling them to have universal access to SRH rights.

Problem

Despite the global recognition of the importance of women empowerment, women across the world continue to face barriers with their fundamental rights being violated every day. Globally, 1 in every 5 women and girls has experienced violence (physical and/or sexual) from their own intimate partner. Globally, 700 million women still alive were married under 18 years of age and 50% of all the child brides globally are from South Asia. Women are often discriminated by the laws of their own country and 49 countries do not have laws that protect women from domestic violence, while 39 countries are still lack the laws for the equal inheritance rights for daughters and sons. Women are almost three times more likely to have domestic work than men which is often unpaid.

In South Asia patriarchal society at large, women face far more challenges. The measures of gender equality such as the global gender gap and gender development index show a high level of gender inequality in South Asia. While Sri Lanka and the Maldives have performed better in terms of these indicators, Pakistan and Afghanistan had poorer rankings in gender equality. In 2015, the political representation of women in South Asian countries was at 18% which was below the global average of 22%. The paid employment of the women outside the agricultural sector was 21% which was also below the global average of 41%.

Most of the South Asian countries have a female literacy rate of less than 50% which is much lower than their male counterparts. The only exception to this disparity is in Sri Lanka and Maldives. In the Maldives, the female literacy rate is at 92.9% and male literacy rate at 93.1%. Similarly, in Sri Lanka, the literacy rates for female and males are 89.1% and 92.7% respectively. Whereas for Bangladesh, literacy rate for female is at 48% and for male are 58.7%. In Nepal, the female literacy for a female is just 43.6% and for a male is 70.1%. Pakistan has female literacy rate as low as 39% while Bhutan had the lowest female literacy rate at 38.7%.

In terms of political empowerment through the representation of women in the parliament, Nepal has the highest proportion of women in the parliament with 33%. In Bhutan and Pakistan, women represent 14% of the parliament, in the Maldives women occupy 12% seats and in India 9%. The least representation is in Bangladesh and Sri Lanka where women held only 6% of the parliament.

The representation of women in the professional and technical sphere is the highest for the Maldives at 49% followed by Sri Lanka at 46%. The women representation for Bangladesh and Nepal were 22% and 20% respectively. For Pakistan, the representation is estimated to be as low as 3%.

All these indicators on gender equality and empowerment highlight the seriousness of the situation in South Asia and the urgency to address to women empowerment in the region.

Relation of Lack of Women Empowerment to Poor Health Indicators

Lack of women empowerment in South Asia is also reflected by the poor health indicators in the region. South Asia accounts for the highest level of female child mortality rate in the world and the violence against women and girls remain prevalent across the countries. The probability of survival in the first five years of life for girls in most South Asian countries is less than that for boys.

This gender inequality is largely reflected by the unbalanced sex ratio. In some parts of South Asia, the sex ratio has reduced to 770 women per 1000 men. It has been surmised that an estimated 60–100 million girls are missing globally.

The maternal health indicators in South Asia also remain to be one of the poorest in the world. South Asia along with Sub-Saharan Africa attribute to 85% maternal deaths in the world.

Moreover, the socioeconomic disparity is very high in South Asian countries such that the poorer women are less likely to give birth with a skilled birth attendant as compared to their richer counterparts. Moreover, violence against women and girls remains very prevalent in the region. In South Asia, one in every five women in general and one in every two married women are affected by the violence from their own intimate partner. The violence starts early at home and it has detrimental and long-lasting effects on the health of these survivors, whilst very few of them have access to health care.

It has also been estimated that women from South Asia are more likely to have worse health as they age and suffer loss of daily activities. The fact that they are more likely to be illiterate, less or less educated, unemployed and dependent on others makes them even more vulnerable to poorer health outcomes.

What are the Issues?

The underlying gender discrimination at each stage of the girl's and women's life cycle has contributed to the huge gender inequality. The major underlying issues of gender inequality begin from the day she conceives which puts her at risk of sex-selective abortions. The ones who survive continue to face neglect of being a girl child, denial of equal rights to education and other opportunities as she grows followed by early marriage, violence by intimate partners and complications with pregnancy and childbirth.

The deep-rooted prejudice against the girl child and the preference for a son, which is worsened by the widely practiced dowry system in South Asia, has been contributing to this cycle of gender inequality for generations.

The lack of freedom over sexual reproductive health rights is also an important underlying factor which could be addressed by improving the knowledge of women and men on sexual reproductive health rights and improving access to contraceptives. Having control over fertility has been proven to be an important empowering factor for women. It allows the women time and space to focus on her own personal growth which eventually would prove beneficial on empowering her.

Moreover, the lack of autonomy in health-seeking behaviors during pregnancy and childbirth has also contributed to reproductive health and maternal health morbidities. Delay in seeking health care services has attributed to the high maternal mortality ratio over the region. Moreover, the ones who survive the obstetric complications often have to spend the rest of their lives with life-long debilitating conditions such as pelvic organ prolapse and obstetric fistula. Such morbidities further aggravate the cycle of discrimination by isolating these women.

Though the progress over the years in educating and empowering girls and women has been promising in South Asian countries, the issue cannot be solved entirely until the changes take place within the societies creating a cultural shift and changing of the attitude towards women.

How do they Present?

Health service providers have an important role in addressing women's health by improving their SRH rights and improving their overall health condition. Majority of the women lack access to health care services entirely. However, those who have access may come to the health service providers with a wide range of symptoms implying their daily struggle as a result of gender disparity. Studies from South Asian countries such as India has indicated that many women from low income household often present vague symptoms of the stress due to poverty, excessive household chores, poor education, lack of empowerment, violence of different forms and problems in marriage.

Many women often complain of a wide range of generalizing body aches and weaknesses, dizziness, and chronic fatigue. Many women often present to the obstetrics and gynecology outpatient clinics with the complaints of white vaginal discharge and lower abdominal pain. Besides, the underlying patho-physiology of a physical cause, these symptoms have been linked to psychosocial factors such as gender disparities, gender-based violence, pressures due to social and cultural norms, and low level of empowerment leading poor self-esteem.

While many symptoms reflect the underlying problems, the women are facing in their daily lives, many times, women present with complications as an obvious result of low empowerment. The majority of the obvious SRH problems and maternal morbidities are a direct result of the low women empowerment.

HANDLING THE SITUATION

There are several paths to improve women empowerment by improving their health and quality of life and vice versa. Empowered women are more likely to have better control over their fertility and have more access to health care services. Thus, policy reforms in educating women, introducing SRH to school curriculum early and timely, and initiating

discussions in the communities can enable women to be better informed and prepared to make decisions about these issues later in life. Improved health status of these women eventually would again help empower them further. Healthier women are also more likely to be able to attend the schools and work in the professional and other sphere. Therefore, the inter-sectoral and collaborative approach involving the health sector, education sector, and others can help make the most of the impact of gender policies on health and vice versa.

The best example the South Asian countries have about women empowerment and better health indicators is through the success story of Sri Lanka. Sri Lanka has the lowest gender inequality in terms of education and work-force, and it also has the best health indicators for health in South Asia including women's health. Sri Lanka has demonstrated leadership in reducing the maternal mortality which reflects the positive changes in the country and society at large. The country provides an excellent example of inter-sectoral collaboration.

As health service providers, it is also imperative not just to judge the symptoms based on its physical nature but also to make an effort to understand the layered complexities of the psychosocial status of the women presenting to the health facilities. It is essential for every health service providers to listen carefully and observe closely to the underlying factors, unspoken words and the hidden symptoms of the women presenting to the health facilities since they are often going through the issues of low empowerment, violence, neglect, and many others.

Health training programs that build the capacity of the health service providers in South Asia must also focus on women empowerment in their objectives.

Women empowerment should be a tool to fight for SRH right for which the health service providers need to be informed so as to train themselves. Women empowerment needs to be a part of the curriculum of different training modalities such as on reproductive morbidities, adolescent health, family planning, health response to gender-based violence and many others.

Further, the medical education curriculum for the clinicians must also incorporate the social aspects of health. It is even more important for the clinicians who are directly dealing with the women's health such as obstetricians and gynecologists to have a sound understanding and widening of their horizon on the underlying social implications of their specialty.

Community engagement and mobilization by empowering the front line female community health workers would also be crucial to reach out to the inaccessible, in the deepest corners of the communities. Economic and social empowerment of these female representatives in the communities would be a stepping stone of empowering the women in the entire community as a whole.

The Pakistan Lady Health Workers (PLHW) program in Pakistan, the female community health volunteers (FCHV) program in Nepal, the accredited social health activists (ASHA) program in India are some of the major health initiatives that built the capacity of hundreds of thousands of women in the communities. These programs succeeded in addressing the health needs of women by providing them information, basic services and access to further care. These programs also had a significant positive impact on improving family planning coverage, immunization coverage, and the uptake of health care services for pregnancy and childbirth. The initiatives in these countries have earned them respect allowing them in turn to empower many others in the communities. The success of these initiatives was possible only due to the commitments from the government and for the recognition of their work. Thus, governments of South Asian countries must address the empowerment by first empowering the front line workers in the communities.

ASSOCIATIONS WORKING IN SOUTH ASIA

The South Asian Federation of Obstetrics and Gynecology has been the pioneer and key player of bridging the gap between the core clinical world of obstetrics and gynecology and human rights issues such as women empowerment. Some of the core objectives of the federation is focused on social aspects of health and women empowerment by bringing the obstetricians and gynecologists of the same region together for better cooperation and understanding, this is through using and developing the reproductive health as instruments towards social and health development, by endeavoring to provide SRH care across the region, by improving the access to safe motherhood, and by enhancing the process of decision making of obstetricians and gynecologists in the health policies of the region.

The National Health Professional Societies though started initially as professional bodies for enhancing the professional development, over the years have evolved in taking up more social responsibilities demonstrated by the wide range of health programs they have initiated in the region. The health professional societies of the obstetricians and gynecologists of each country in SAARC region has made invaluable contributions and continue to work tirelessly in uplifting the health status of their country and ultimately facilitating in the women empowerment. The Federation of Obstetrics and Gynecological Societies of India (FOGSI) aims at promoting the betterment of the women's and children's health, the community health and advocating SRH rights of the women in India while collaborating with the government for policy reforms. Similarly, the Society of Obstetricians and Gynecologists Pakistan has prioritized improving of health and rights of women, and enabling access and adequate care for every woman to the reproductive and maternal-newborn health care services in Pakistan. Nepal Society of Obstetricians and Gynecologists is widely known as a key advocate of SRH rights of women in the country over the years. Likewise, Obstetrical and Gynecological Society Bangladesh in Bangladesh, Afghan Society of Obstetrician and Gynecologists in Afghanistan, Bhutan Society of Obstetrics and Gynecologists in Bhutan have also been consistently working in elevating the health status of women in their countries.

The United Nations agencies have also been working on improving the health rights and empowering the women in the region through its regional and country offices. In particular, UN agencies such as UN Women, UNFPA and UNICEF have prioritized the SDG 5 in improving the women empowerment, encouraging universal access to SRH rights and uplifting the maternal and child health in the region.

There are thousands of local organizations working in each country to address the issues of women's health and gender inequity at national levels as well as community levels. Each of these associations has played a crucial role. However, mentioning each and every association working in this sector from all the South Asian countries is beyond the scope of this chapter and their specific roles will be explained under specific topics in other chapters.

Examples of Women Empowerment

Addressing the empowerment of women as part of health care practices is essential but complex at the same time. Any health care setting should provide the enabling environment to women's autonomy and a decision over their own health which is a core aspect of empowering women.

Scenario 1

An example of the health initiative leading to the empowerment of women could be from Nepal. The NESOG is implementing a postpartum family planning (PPFP) initiative with the support from the Federation of International Gynecologists and Obstetricians (FIGO). Though it is a clinical health professional society, over the years, it has embraced a holistic approach to approach the social aspects of health. The PPFP initiative is one such example, where the society has incorporated various activities such as careful counseling of women during antenatal care about postpartum family planning options, proper training of health service providers including the obstetricians and gynecologists and nurses, mobilization of the communities through FCHVs to enhance the knowledge of the people in the communities, and enabling women to make informed decision to choose the contraceptives of their choice after the childbirth. This initiative has improved the uptake of postpartum intrauterine device in the selected project sites over the years exceeding the national average. To achieve and sustain the progress, the initiative has constantly focused on understanding the barriers women face in the communities at a deeper level.

In a qualitative research conducted by the initiative in Nepal, an eighteen-year-old mother said, "I got married soon and also gave birth soon. But now I want to plan my life and complete my education. Understanding the contraceptive options after childbirth has now made me take the right decision and take control of my life. I want to become a teacher or a nurse someday."

Another 20 years old mother said, "understanding the family planning options after childbirth and using one has helped me focus on my personal growth as well as to raise my child the best I can."

These responses from the women are a true reflection of how the health provider's role in educating them about family planning has eventually helped in empowering them.

Scenario 2

Another example includes capacity building of health service providers which helped women suffering from sexual violence in Nepal. JHPIEGO in Nepal and UNFPA had provided technical support for the initiative on health response to gender-based violence. The initiative aimed the sensitizing the health providers on gender-based violence, and enable them to timely recognize, treat, and refer to other sectors for holistic care. After the training, a doctor from a peripheral facility indicated that the training helped him to look minutely to the presenting symptoms of the women coming to his clinic.

He shared an experience with a female patient, "I recall a female patient who came to our outpatient clinic every three months with the same symptoms of lower abdominal pain. Before the training, I treated her physical symptoms only. But after the training, I realized that there was more to her than just the obvious physical symptoms. She was actually seeking help from me all this time indirectly. I came to know that he was in fact sexually abused by her husband every three months, who lives abroad and comes home every three months. I then addressed her problem by informing her of the legal support she can seek, about the help lines. I even invited her husband and counseled him. I tried my best to treat her holistically. As a result, the woman was better informed of her choices and made aware of the steps she needs to take protect herself in the future." This is an example of how building the capacity of health service providers enable them to empower women and how this empowerment can be integrated into the daily practice of OBGYN.

CONCLUSION

Empowering women in South Asia can help to reduce gender bias and improve the financial status of women and family, for this a strong political will is required, supported by legislated and out lock discrimination against women both in social and economical sector. Providing equal opportunity for girls to get educated, in this context civil society and media can play a significant role.

Empowerment of women begins at home with parents providing equal opportunities to girls and boys in terms of education, respect, inheritance and job opportunities.

The health service providers have a crucial role in improving the SRH rights and address empowerment of women. Thus, health training programs that build the capacity of the health service providers in South Asia must also sensitize them about their role in empowerment of women.

Moreover, policy reforms in South Asian countries must continue to prioritize educating women, introducing SRH to school curriculum, and identifying solutions in the communities to empower women and girls.

It is imperative to strengthen the inter-sectoral and collaborative approach involving the health sector, education sector, and other sectors to address the gender inequality and empowerment of women.

Further, the medical education curriculum for the clinicians must also elaborate on their social responsibility, social determinants of health, and their role in empowering women and society at large.

The health policies of each South Asian countries must also continue and strengthen community engagement by building the capacity of the front line female community health workers, who then have the capacity to become role models of women empowerment in their own communities.

Lastly, all South Asian countries must learn about the best practices on empowerment of women from each other and from global evidence, and implement them in their own countries after customizing it to their local needs.

BIBLIOGRAPHY

1. Akseer N, Kamali M, Arifeen SE, Malik A, Bhatti Z, Thacker N, et al. Progress in maternal and child health: how has South Asia fared? BMJ. 2017;357: j1608.

2. Anwar I, Nababan HY, Mostari S, Rahman A, Khan JA. Trends and inequities in use of maternal health care services in Bangladesh, 1991–2011. PLoS One. 2015;10(3):e0120309.

3. Bank W. South Asia's Quest for Reduced Maternal Mortality: What the Data Show [Available from: http://blogs.worldbank.org/health/south-asia-s-quest-reduced-maternal-mortality-what-data-show.

4. Bhuiyan AB, Goodall D. The role of the South Asia Federation of Obstetrics and Gynaecology (SAFOG) in South Asia. BJOG. 2011;118 Suppl 2:22–5.

5. Bhutta ZA, Gupta I, de'Silva H, Manandhar D, Awasthi S, Hossain SM, et al. Maternal and child health: is South Asia ready for change? BMJ. 2004;328(7443):816–9.

6. Bonomi AE, Anderson ML, Rivara FP, Thompson RS. Health care utilization and costs associated with physical and nonphysical-only intimate partner violence. Health Serv Res. 2009;44(3): 1052–67.

7. Chaban S, et al. Regional Organizations, Gender Equality and the Political Empowerment of Women. International Institute for Democracy and Electoral Assistance, Permanent Secretariat of the Community of Democracies, United Nations Development Programme 2017.

8. Davis J, Vyankandondera J, Luchters S, Simon D, Holmes W. Male involvement in reproductive, maternal and child health: a qualitative study of policymaker and practitioner perspectives in the Pacific. Reprod Health. 2016;13(1):81.

9. Fikree FF, Pasha O. Role of gender in health disparity: the South Asian context. BMJ. 2004; 328(7443):823–6.

10. Fulu E, Miedema S. Violence Against Women: Globalizing the Integrated Ecological Model. Violence Against Women. 2015;21(12):1431–55.

11. Holland J. Empowerment in Practice: From Analysis to Implementation. Washington DC: The World Bank; 2006.

12. International Labour Organization. Small change, Big changes:Women and Microfinance. Geneva: International Labour Organization; 2007.

13. Jejeebhoy SJ, Santhya KG, Acharya R. Violence against women in South Asia: the need for the active engagement of the health sector. Glob Public Health. 2014;9(6):678–90.

14. Khatri RB, Karkee R. Social determinants of health affecting utilisation of routine maternity services in Nepal: a narrative review of the evidence. Reprod Health Matters. 2018:1–15.

15. Khatri RB, Mishra SR, Khanal V. Female Community Health Volunteers in Community-Based Health Programs of Nepal: Future Perspective. Front Public Health. 2017;5:181.

16. Kostick KM, Schensul SL, Jadhav K, Singh R, Bavadekar A, Saggurti N. Treatment seeking, vaginal discharge and psychosocial distress among women in urban Mumbai. Cult Med Psychiatry. 2010;34(3):529–47.

17. Mehata S, Paudel YR, Dariang M, Aryal KK, Lal BK, Khanal MN, et al. Trends and Inequalities in Use of Maternal Health Care Services in Nepal: Strategy in the Search for Improvements. Biomed Res Int. 2017;2017:5079234.

18. Moonzwe Davis L, Schensul SL, Schensul JJ, Verma RK, Nastasi BK, Singh R. Women's empowerment and its differential impact on health in low-income communities in Mumbai, India. Glob Public Health. 2014;9(5):481–94.

19. Nepal Society of Obstetricians and Gynaeco-logists. Mission Vision And Goal [Available from: http://www.nesog.org.np/mission-vision-and-goal.html.

20. Obstetrical and Gynecological Society of Bangladesh. Obstetrical and Gynecological Society Bangladesh in Bangladesh [Available from: http://www.ogsb.org/].

21. Oxfam International. OXFAM Women's Economic Empowerment Conceptual Framework. Oxford, UK: Oxfam International; 2017.

22. Partnership for Maternal NaCH. Promoting women empowerment for better health outcomes for women and children. Geneva: Partnership for Maternal, Newborn and Child Health; 2013.

23. Saprii L, Richards E, Kokho P, Theobald S. Community health workers in rural India: analysing the opportunities and challenges Accredited Social Health Activists (ASHAs) face in realising their multiple roles. Hum Resour Health. 2015;13:95.

24. Shobhana N. A Study on Women Empowerment in South-Asian Countries: A Contemporary Analysis. Mediterranean Journal of Social Sciences. 2012;3(16):37–45.

25. Society of Obstetricians and Gynaecologists of Pakistan. Vision of SOGP [Available from: http://sogp.org/].

26. The Federation of Obstetric and Gynaecological Societies of India. Mission & Vision [cited 2018 24 December]. Available from: https://http://www.fogsi.org/fogsimission-vision/.

27. Tripathi V, Elneil S, Romanzi L. Demand and capacity to integrate pelvic organ prolapse and genital fistula services in low-resource settings. Int Urogynecol J. 2018;29(10):1509–15.

28. UN Women. SDG 5: Achieve gender equality and empower all women and girls [Available from: http://www.unwomen.org/en/news/in-focus/women-and-the-sdgs/sdg-5gender-equality.

29. UNESCAP. Achieving the Sustainable Development Goals in South Asia: Key Policy Priorities and Implementation Challenges. 2016.

30. UNICEF. Ending child marriage progress and prospects. New York: UNICEF; 2013.

31. United Nations Sustainable Development Goals [Available from: https://http://www.un.org/sustainabledevelopment/gender-equality/

32. United Nations.Guidelines On Women's Empowerment. [Available from http://www.un.org/popin/unfpa/taskforce/guide/iatfwemp.gdl.html

33. WHO, Global Health Workforce Alliance. Country Case Study: Pakistan's lady health worker program. Global Health Workforce Alliance, World Health Organization.

34. WHO. Global and regional estimates of violence against women: prevalence and health effects of intimate partner violence and non-partner sexual violence. Geneva: WHO; 2013; 129.

10

Women in Crisis Situations

Madeeha Rashid, Asifa Naureen, Rubina Sohail

BACKGROUND

South Asia is world's most populous and ethnically, culturally and linguistically diverse area. It is one of the most conflict prone regions in the world and after Iraq it is the second most violent place on earth.

The political, social and financial growth of South Asia has been utterly slowed down by external, internal conflicts and internal displacements. These conflicts, civil unrest and insurgencies keep South Asia as one of the poorest and underdeveloped region of world. Since ages it had hosted deep-seated ethnic aggression, political violence and many wars. Many of these conflicts, like those in Kashmir, Afghanistan and Sri Lanka have involved global attention while parts of India, Nepal, and Bangladesh have experienced long-running conflicts. The result is human misery, destruction of infrastructure and social cohesion, and death. The knock-on effects are huge.

Who are Refugees and IDPs?

A refugee is someone who is forced to leave his country in order to avoid ill-treatment, violation of the fundamental, social and cultural rights and consequences of war. Conventions relating to status of refugees, such as the 1951 Refugee Convention and 1967 Protocol, protect the rights of a refugee at the international level. In these conventions, a refugee has been defined as a person who has fled his country of origin due to fear of being persecuted and is not being protected by any other State. Fear of persecution could be due to religion, race, and nationality and for being a member of a particular group or for having a political opinion.

On the other hand, a person who is forced to flee his home but remains within the borders of his country, is an internally displaced person. An internally displaced person is forced to flee his places of habitual residence due to a number of reasons including 'refugee-type' reasons or 'man-made' events. These include war, conflicts, earthquake, famine, political strife, drought, climate change or some development projects, e.g. building of a dam.

Contributing Factors

The political, social and financial growth of South Asia has been utterly slowed down by external, internal conflicts and internal displacements. These conflicts, civil unrest and insurgencies have contributed in keeping it as one of the poorest and underdeveloped regions of world. Since ages, it has been host to deep seated ethnic aggression, political violence and many wars. Many of these conflicts, like those in Afghanistan, Kashmir and Sri Lanka have involved global attention. They have all resulted in human misery, destruction of infrastructure and social cohesion and death. The knock-on effects are huge.

Refugees and internally displaced persons are increasing due to discrimination against minorities, violence, war, ethnic hatred, state repression, demands for self-determination, natural and man-made disasters such as famines and floods, ill-judged development projects such as highways and dams—all have contributed massively to internal displacement. More than five million refugees and IDPs reside in India, Pakistan and Nepal put together with two millions of these being innate to the area.

Effects of Refugees and IDPs

Since World War II, the earth has face 160 wars and armed conflicts leading to 30 million deaths and 90 million injuries. Wars and terrorism in South Asia has resulted in poor economic growth, human wretchedness, ruining of infrastructure and countless deaths. South Asia consists of countries who already have limited resources and financial constraints. Over and above the huge economic impact there are law and order issues, administrative issues, and difficulty in provision of services. One of the challenges is to provide the basic amenities, provision of reproductive health care services, protection of vulnerable groups, providing education and to protect the infringement of rights specially of vulnerable population.

Refugees and Internally Displaced Persons (IDPs) in South Asia: How Big is the Problem?

Currently, there are around 65.5 million displaced persons in the world, including asylum seekers, irregular migrants, returnees and internally displaced persons. Almost 50% of these are women. More than five millions refugees and IDPs reside in India, Pakistan and Nepal. Around two millions of these are innate to this area.

India

According to UNHCR more than two hundred thousand refugees are in India. They have come from Afghanistan, Bangladesh, Myanmar, Iran and Iraq. India has accommodated refugees from Tibet since 1959, refugees from Bangladesh since 1971, Chakmas, a Buddhist ethnic minority from the former East Pakistan, since 1963, and refugees from Sri Lanka since 1983, 1989 and 1995 due to the civil war. Conflict in Afghanistan since the 1980s and Myanmar's instability of the 1990s prompted further waves of migration.

Pakistan

Pakistan is a country which has been affected by a number of natural hazards such as earthquakes, floods, cold waves, droughts, heat waves and avalanches in addition to the huge problem of terrorism. Comprehensive military and civilian operations were launched in 2005 in Federally Administered Trial Areas (FATA) and in 2009 in Swat. As a result of these counter insurgency operations, huge population of internally displaced people (IDPs) were produced. The largest population of refugees in the world has been hosted by Pakistan. Out of this large refugee population, Pakistan hosted 1.45 million refugees from Afghanistan. In 2005 earthquake, there was a death toll of 100,000 people, 138,000 were seriously injured, whereas 3.5 million were rendered homeless due to the destruction of buildings. Operation Black Thunderstorm was a military operation against the talibans which resulted in the 2009 refugee crisis in Pakistan. Under this operation, over 1.2 million civilians were rendered homeless and were further joined by 555,000 displaced people. Floods in 2010 affected 20 million people and the death toll reached to almost 2000 people. Infrastructure was also largely damaged and the livelihood of the people was also affected. Overall impact on the economy was estimated to be $43 billion. In 2012 floods, over 465,000 houses were destructed, 14,720 villages and 1.1 million acres of crops suffered heavy losses due to floods. Relief camps were set up and approximately 270,000 people were moved to

478 such camps. In 2013 Balochistan earthquake over 300,000 people were affected, communication system came to a halt. Again, the humanitarian partners responded and supported the government in providing relief to the victims. In 2014 Zarb-e-Azab was started by the Pakistani army, due to which a lot of people were internally displaced. Approximately 787,888 IDPs were officially registered. Additionally, the total number of families that were reported to be displaced were almost 62,493. Data released by United Nations Office for Coordination of Humanitarian Affairs (OCHA) revealed that till 5th September 2014, almost 961,000 people were displaced from North Waziristan.

Afghanistan Pakistan Refugee Crisis

The Afghan immigrants in Pakistan are primarily the refugees who have left their country due to wars in Afghanistan. However, there are small number of Afghanis who have migrated to Pakistan for work, asylum, trade, business or as exchange students. Majority of them are considered citizens of Afghanistan, although they were born and raised in Pakistan and are under 30 years of age. They are protected by the United Nations High Commissioner for Refugees (UNHCR) and Pakistan provided them a legal status till the end of 2017.

It was during the Soviet-Afghan War in the late 1970s when the Afghan refugees migrated to Pakistan for the very first time. There were over 4 million afghan refugees in Pakistan by the end of 2001. Although majority of them returned back to their country in 2002, but as per UNHCR, it was reported in February 2017 that almost 1.3 million Afghan citizens were still residing in Pakistan; Khyber Pakhtunkhwa accounted the largest share of 81%, followed by Punjab, i.e. 10%, Baluchistan, i.e. 7% and Sindh with the smallest share of 1%. In September 2018, it was announced by lmran Khan, Prime Minister of Pakistan, to provide citizenship to 1.5 million Afghan refugees residing in Pakistan.

Bangladesh–Rohingya Refugees

There has been extensive damage and suffering due to outbreak of violence in the Myanmar's Rakhine State. The further escalation of violence resulted in the refugee crisis. As result of these violent attacks and discrimination, over 727,000 Rohingya refugees were forced to move to Cox's Bazar, Bangladesh. The migration of Rohingya refugees became the fastest growing refugee crisis in the world because of two reasons. Firstly, Rohingya refugees moved to Cox's Bazar very rapidly and secondly such large concentration of refugees made Cox's Bazar as one of the densest regions in the world. Most of the refugees, especially women and children, migrating to Bangladesh were not only traumatized but they were also suffering from injuries due to gunshots, shrapnel, fire and landmines. In 73rd United Nations General Assembly Summit, Bangladeshi prime minister Sheik Hasina, informed that 1.1 million Rohingya refugees were residing in Bangladesh.

PROBLEMS FACED BY REFUGEES AND IDPs

War and Conflicts Effects on Human Life

Wars are humiliating for welfare of human beings. Wars lead to devastating effects in form of land destruction, displacement of people, shattered economies and long-term destruction of families. History shows that wars and conflicts influenced women, girls and children more than men. Not only they are killed, injured, tortured and sexually abuse, they also bear the psychological trauma of losing loved ones.

Impact of Warfare and Conflicts on Women Life

Women's sexual and reproductive health is related to multiple human rights, including the right to life, the right to be free from torture, the right to health, the right to privacy, the right to education, and the prohibition of discrimination. In conflicts and displacements, all these rights are infringed upon.

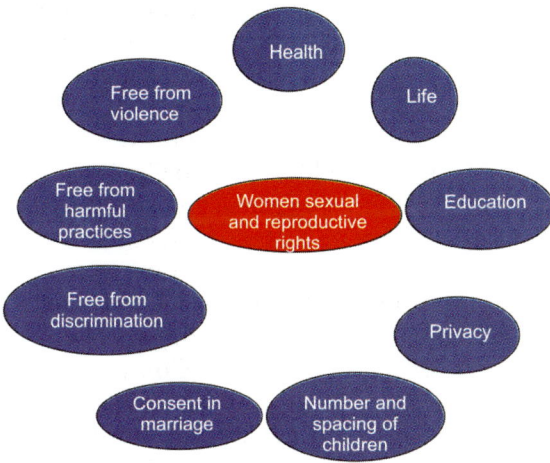

Distressing effects of forced migration and war:
1. Forced to participate in acts of violence and armed conflicts
2. Exposure to killing, disability and prison
3. Poverty
4. Malnutrition
5. Worsening health situation
6. Displacement of women during war
7. Separation from the rest of the family and homelessness
8. Trafficking of women
9. Sexual exploitation and rape

Women's Position in Armed Conflict Situation

It has been divided in three phases:
1. **Pre-conflict phase:** In this phase nonexistence of law and order, corruption, power abuse, economic crisis make their life miserable further promoting to gender inequality and disparity.
2. **During conflict phase:** During armed conflicts the danger of violence, abuse, panic and anxiety, the annihilation of incomes and death of near ones are among their sufferings.

3. **Post-conflict phase:** Despite all sufferings female gender is very strong and committed, after war they not only promote peace but also take part in the rehabilitation and reintegration developments.

Barrier and challenges women and girls face in refugee/IDP camps

IDPs and refugees face many impediments upon entering to their camps. They are subjected to insecurity, loss of livelihoods, lack of shelter and financial hardships.

Economic Hardship

IDPs and refugees have a lot of fiscal limitations. They are enforced to concentrate on day-to-day living. Financial hardships and economic burden forced their children and women's to work as laborers.

Sexual Violence/Rape

Refugees and internally displaced persons are highly vulnerable to sexual violence during conflict and subsequent displacement. In camps men, women, boys and girls all sleep together, without any privacy. Bathing shelters are common for men and women, latrines cannot be locked or lit. Also the camp borders are not guarded. These conditions are conducive to harassment, abuse and killings. Sick women and girls often remain inside the camp unattended while other go out to earn for their family in the daytime. Most rape cases are never investigated. In many cases the culprits may be soldiers and police officers.

Early and Child Marriages

In order to overcome economic constraints and avoid sexual abuse girls are subjected to early marriages.

Lack of Employment

IDPs and refugees have difficulty in getting employments due to language barriers and social inequalities. They do not have sufficient support to look after children and older peoples. In jobs also they suffer from unfair wages and unsafe environments. They lack in networking and interpersonal relations which hinder their progress.

Discrimination

Being outsiders they face high level of discrimination, despite good qualifications, they are facing considerable barriers in getting respectable jobs.

Lack of Education

Giving education to girl child is not a priority, meanwhile children have no access to host school systems. Parents cannot bear the cost and mostly they forced their children to work to earn livelihood.

Cultural Constraints

In a new country the society norms may be different and the refugees have to face lots of cultural barriers.

Camp Constraint

Refugees in camps cannot work legally outside the camp.

Reproductive Health Care

Reproductive health care has been an abandoned component in rehabilitating refugees and IDPs.

Access to Family Planning Services

Many refugees and IDPs face unwanted unplanned pregnancies due to poor access to family planning services. Proper demand–supply chain is not maintained, no education and counseling is provided to them due to overburdened staff. Sexual exploitation and rape exposes the women and adolescent girls to the risk of becoming pregnant.

Antenatal Care

Many refugee women and their newborns face health problems related to pregnancy and delivery, including pregnancy complications and miscarriages. During flight and early settlement, women may be forced to give birth in temporary shelters or odd places, with conditions hazardous both to them and their newborns.

Complications of pregnancy and childbirth, such as severe bleeding, obstructed labor, and unsafe abortion, may be more serious for displaced women, and may lead to serious morbidity and death. A refugee woman who wants to end her pregnancy and has no access to safe abortion services may seek an unsafe abortion and end up requiring emergency care and counseling. According to the United Nations Population Fund (UNFPA), post-abortion complications alone account for up to 50 percent of maternal deaths in refugee situations.

Sexually Transmitted Diseases

STIs, including HIV/AIDS, can spread quickly in refugee settings, because of limited contraceptive supplies, such as condoms. They have greater vulnerability to sexual and gender violence and sex work, greater exposure to inadequately screened blood transfusions and the presence of populations with HIV.

Menstrual Hygiene Challenges

A common and significant challenge that the currently displaced girls and women face is the inability to manage their menstruation safely, comfortably and with dignity. In many emergency contexts, women and girls lack access to basic materials, such as sanitary pads, clothes and underwear that are needed to manage monthly blood flow. Privacy is often non-existent while in transit, or in camps or informal settlements, and they often lack easy access to toilets, which even if available, may lack doors, locks and lighting and are inadequate to manage menses. Access to water and places to wash and dry reusable pads and clothes or to dispose of used materials are often scarce. Such factors can increase their risk for exposure to violence and exploitation, particularly at nighttime when seeking out private spaces to manage sanitary needs.

Water Sanitation and Hygiene

When people flee their homes, they often struggle to safely and easily access adequate water, sanitation and hygiene facilities, endangering their health and survival.

Depression and Mood Disorders

Refugees and IDPs are subjected to mental health problems. Loosing near ones, fear of exposure to sexual violence and economic hardships make them more susceptible to depression and mood disorders. Moreover in many cases violence, rape and other hardships become a reality, leading to insecurities and depression and increasing rate of suicide.

Prostitution

IDPs and refugee women are forced to take on responsibilities of family due to economic hardships and minimal resources. Inability to get respectful job, may force them to engage in prostitution, in exchange for food, clothing and shelter.

The Impact of Refugees on Host Countries

Refugees and IDPs create a lot of financial burden including economic and social costs to host country. Developing countries that host refugees experience long-term economic, social, political, and environmental impacts. From the moment of arrival, refugees may compete with local citizens for already scarce resources such as water, food, housing, and medical services. Their presence increases the demands for education, health services, infrastructure such as water supply, sanitation, and transportation, and also in some cases, for natural resources. The impacts of the refugee presence are both positive and negative. The dynamic between positive and negative factors is complex and varies depending on several factors, including the political economy of hosting countries, urban–rural interactions, and the nature of host-refugee relations.

Looking for Solutions—Who Can Help?

65–70% of displaced persons are women and children. They are subjected to leave home country due to conflicts, disasters, terrorism and wars. Throughout their journey they are at risk of violence, rape, sexual exploitation and abuse, sexual harassment, psychological violence, trafficking, early and forced marriage, transactional sex and domestic violence. Even when they have reached the host country, they have limited access to support services, security and proper facilities. Poor and marginalized women are at increased risk of maternal mortality and morbidity. It is important to channelise resources towards poor and banished ones which can improve their health and survival. Refugee situation is very difficult for the displaced people—women and children specially, but also for the host country as it puts tremendous pressure on their resources and needs a lot of financial and administrative support. Setting up of facilities, ensuring protection and rights to the vulnerable group, ensuring daily amenities, protecting against STI, securing reproductive health services and contraception are all huge challenges. Other equally important challenges are finding shelter, education of this group, finding them jobs, overcoming the cultural constraints and helping them to integrate with the indigenous population. In long-term one has to look at rehabilitation and return of refugees and many times IDPs.

Humanitarian organizations and NGOs can play a tremendous role in this regard, by not only providing financial assistance but also by ensuring that guidelines and checklists are in place so that the handling of this issue is eased. Moreover a predesigned monitoring system would help plug in the gaps. Their presence has been an immense support in all these settings of humanitarian crisis. WHO,

UNHCR and other organisations have played an important role in this regard. IDPs must have access to basic public services, documentation, employment and income generating opportunities.

UNHCR and WHO Working for Rehabilitation of Refugee and IDPs

Their mandate is to provide, on a non-political and humanitarian basis, international protection to refugees and IDPs. There objectives are to provide a safe environment with dignity to persons of concern while durable solutions are pursued, to safeguard social rights such as adequate shelter, water and sanitation and to provide mechanisms to access services for persons with specific needs.

Ways to Improve Maternal Health in Areas of Crisis

Go Back to Basics

In area of crisis, irregular services, funding shortage and poor facilities hinder development of maternal health infrastructure. Simple paper solution can work when community and governance structure breaks down. Enabling midwives and creating awareness among pregnant ladies will be helpful.

Women Empowerment

Women and men of society should be taught about women's fundamental human rights and their right of access to health care. This can be achieved by increasing literacy rate of society and making education necessary for all.

Well-equipped Refugee Camps

Refugee camps should be fully equipped with all resources, clean and safe health facilities. Safe delivery kits and all emergencies drugs should be available with well-trained staff.

Go Mobile

Being mobile will not only helpful in collecting data but also helpful to determine security threats, creating awareness and educating peoples and giving access to family planning.

Provide Access to Contraception and Safe Abortions

In areas of conflict higher rate of maternal mortality and morbidity is due to unsafe abortions. It is important to ensure that all women must have access to full range of contraceptives and state must prioritize comprehensive sexual and reproductive health services.

Recruit Local Staff

For retention of staff, hiring should be from the local community and if recruiting people are from poor villages, they will work with more dedication and motivation.

Confront Child Marriage

Child marriages are common in crisis situations to prevent forced exploitation like rape and abuse. Preventing child marriages and giving children protection and security helps in decreasing maternal mortality rates.

Recommended Interventions for Children and Women

1. Providing safe water, sanitation and hygiene
2. Promoting equality, justice and preventing discriminating behavior of society
3. Special initiatives to protect women and girls from any type of violence
4. Efforts in helping women and girls to be empowered and confident
5. Efforts to make them self-organized and use their skills in earning livelihood.
6. Ensuring schooling and affordable education to children
7. Giving vocational and skill training to adolescents to make them self sufficient
8. Protection of girl child from child marriages and abuse
9. Safe and secure places from girls

10. Promoting women and adolescent participation in decision making

Key Health Matters to be Tackled

1. Ensuring that good health facilities services are easily available, accessible without discrimination at affordable rates and culturally acceptable and sensitive to gender.
2. Treating like early pregnancy, STDs and HIV, unsafe abortion, menstrual hygiene and nutritional deficiencies.
3. Preventive care: Providing condoms, emergency contraceptive pills, prevention of sexual and gender-based violence.
4. Treatment: For accidents and emergencies, facility for orthopedic surgery, availability of emergency obstetrics and neonatal care services, ensuring presence of skilled birth attendants, post-natal care, rehabilitation and care for survivors of sexual violence, provision of family planning and safe abortion services, treatment of STDs and antiretroviral therapy should be available.
5. Ensuring availability of kits: Menstrual hygiene kit, post-rape kit, contraception kit, sexually transmitted infection kits.
6. Ensuring availability of medical devices: Manual vacuum aspiration, vacuum extractor, sonic aid and ultrasound.

Resettlement and Reintegration of Refugees

Refugees require restoration, relocation and rehabilitation. An integrated approach is required and close cooperation of countries of origin, host states, humanitarian and developmental agencies, as well as the refugees themselves, and usually offers the best chances for success. It is important to stop trafficking and racism and government stop blaming refugees for economic burden and social problems rather work for their welfare.

Ensuring Voluntariness of Return

IDPs are citizen of their countries, enjoy all rights of citizen and liberty to move. They should voluntarily decide whether they want to go to their area of origin or want to resettle at new place. In safeguarding return, it has to be ensured that they do not suffer from any insecurities, harassment, bullying upon return to their land. IDPs must have access to property restoration and funds for reconstruction and help to settle down.

Conclusion and Recommendations

As a result of wars and conflicts women are dying two types of death—a physical and an emotional death. The physical death is when you are no longer alive and the emotional death is when you no longer see signs of hope and are dead inside. When women are exposed to sexual violence and rape, they are emotionally dead. No matter how hopeless a situation is, change is always possible, and good leadership makes that possible. This leadership is not one person, it is a collective effort. Empowering women with knowledge about their rights will bring the change. Providing and supporting reproductive, maternal, newborn, child and adolescent health is essential to human dignity. Educating women and girls is solution of all problems.

There is limited data available on the obstacles encountered during provision of service to the refugees and IDPs an important step would be to collect and analyze data with full participation of stakeholders. Governments should strengthen their existing partnership with donors and human right agencies and different supporting organizations for generating sufficient resources. The resources can be used to make them self-organized, help in developing skills, improve camp facilities and start vocational training for adults and schooling for children.

Rules and regulations must be amended to prevent sex crime amongst refugees and IDPs by introducing adequate control and accountability mechanisms. There is need for gender diversification in police and peace keeping troops responsible for refugee camps.

Additional staff and training of precious staff is required on prevention and response to violence and assaults. There should be a proper framework for rapid and timely access to justice and legal remedies. Host countries should focus on legal system regarding this matter.

In addition to country laws local camps rules can be developed with contribution of camp residents as they consist of mixture of refugees customs and are adopted top camp setting.

Emergency management committee can be formulated holding representatives from the refugees/IDPs to register their issues and funding solutions. They can develop connections with NGOs, human right associations and donor agencies. Laws about women trafficking, violence and prostitution of host country must be applied to refugees. Governments should also take action and prevent early forced marriages in the camps.

To conclude, there is no one solution but a host of solutions to deal with the issues. Developing a universal template to put basic structure in place to help the situation would be beneficial. Every country can make amendments to this universal template of dealing with the refugees or IDPs. A lot of hard work is required before systems can be in place to deal with this essential human rights issue.

BIBLIOGRAPHY

1. "Bangladesh PM asks Myanmar to take back Rohingya refugees". Channel NewsAsia. Retrieved 20 March 2017.
2. 11 ideas to improve maternal health in areas of conflict and extre… poverty | Global Development Professionals Network | The Guardian
3. 2005 Kashmir earthquake From Wikipedia, the free encyclopedia.
4. 2010 Pakistan flood From Wikipedia, the free encyclopedia
5. 32Parker A, Smith JA, Verdemato T, Cooke J, Webster J, Carter RC. Menstrual management: a neglected aspect of hygiene interventions. Disaster Prev Manag. 2014;23(4):437–54.
6. 8 ways to solve the world refugee crisis, https://www.amnesty.org/en/latest/campaigns/2015/10/eight-solutionsworld- refugee-crisis/
7. C. Palmer, Reproductive Health for Displaced Populations, Relief and Rehabilitation Network (RRN) Paper no. 24 (London: Overseas Development Institute, 1998).
8. Challenges faced by women & girl refugees, https://medium.com/@chayn/challenges-faced-by-women-girl-refugee
9. Conflict and development Ejaz Ghani, Lakshmi Iyer 23 March 2010 https://voxeu.org/article/conflict-and development-lessons-south-asia
10. Conflicts in South Asia: Causes, Consequences, Prospects S D Muni ISAS Working Paper No. 170, 26 March 2013
11. DAWN https://www.dawn.com/wps/wcm/connect/dawn-contentlibrary/ dawn/news/pakistan
12. Donatella Lorch, ed. (August 1, 2001). "Afghan Refugees in Pakistan at Risk". UNHCR. Retrieved June 3, 2012.
13. Durable Solutions for Internally Displaced Persons: An Essential Dimension of Peacebuilding
14. Hayden T. Menstrual hygiene management in emergencies: Taking stock of support from UNICEF and partners. New York City: UNICEF; 2012.
15. https://www.cordaid.org/en/news/stop-sexual-violence-idp-camps/ sexual violence in IDPs camps
16. Humanitarian Responses in Pakistan Humanitarian forum.
17. Internal Displacement in South Asia Wednesday, March, 06, 2019 | 28, Jumadi ul Sani, 1440 | 32nd Year of publication, Greater Kashmir.
18. Nawaz J, Lal S, Raza S, House S. Screened toilet, bathing and menstruation units for the earthquake response in NWFP, Pakistan. Colombo: 32nd WEDC International Conference; 2006.
19. Pakistan observer Women worst victims of Kshmir conflict: Naseem Shafai January 22, 2017.
20. Refugee or IDP-What's the difference? https://preemptivelove.org/blog/refug ee_or_idp_what_s_the_difference/
21. Refugees and Internally Displaced Persons https://pesd.princeton.edu/? q=node/262
22. Refugees in South Asia https://www. every-culture.com/South- Asia/Refugees-in-South-Asia.html
23. Saleem, Farukh (14 October 2014). "India disappointed by Zarb-e-Azb's success". The News

International, editorial. The News International. Retrieved 17 December 2014.

24. Sexual and reproductive health, https://www. unfpa.org/sexualreproductive-health

25. Sherrill Hayes, Brandon D. Lundy & Maia Carter Hallward Conflict-Induced Migration and the Refugee Crisis: Global and Local Perspectives from Peacebuilding and Development Pages 1–7 | Published online: 08 Dec 20

26. Sohail Khattak, ed. (August 15, 2011). "Independence Day: We are Pakistanis now, say Afghans". The Express Tribune. Retrieved March 23, 2012.

27. Sommer M, Ferron S, Cavill S, House S. Violence, gender and WASH: spurring action on a complex, under-documented and sensitive topic. Environ Urban. 2014;27(1):105–16.

28. The 10-Point Plan Solutions for refugees Chapter 7 https://www.unhcr.org

29. The express tribune by APP Published April 16 2018.

30. The Impacts of Refugees on Neighboring Countries: A Development Challenge1 July 29, 2010 World Development Report 2011.

31. The Social, Political and Economic Effects of the War on Terror: Pakistan 2009 To 2011 Mr. Tariq Khan1.

32. The Status of Refugees in India by Nafees Ahmad September 12, 2017.

33. The UN Refugee agency Water, Sanitation and hygiene

34. The UN refugee agency, https://www.unhcr. org/aboutus/background/4ec262df9/1951-convention-relating-status-refugeesits-1967-protocol. html

35. UN refugee agency Nepal https://www.unhcr. org/nepal.html

36. UNFPA, Working to Empower Women: Women and Armed Conflict, accessed online at www. unfpa.org/modules/intercenter/beijing/armed. htm, on May 17, 2002.

37. UNHCR welcomes new government policy for Afghans in Pakistan (UNHCR Feb. 7, 2017)

38. UNHCR. Trends at a glance: forced displacement in 2015. Geneva: UNHCR; 2016.

39. UNHCRs global strategic objectives https:// www.unhcr.org

40. United Nations high commissioners for refugee, https://www.unhcr.org/figures-at-a-glance. html

41. United Nations, AIDS as a Security Issue (United Nations Special Session on HIV/AIDS, June 2001).

42. Walter KälinThursday, March 13, 2008

43. Yvette Collymore, Uprooted People and HIV/ AIDS in Africa: Responding to the Risks, accessed online at www.prb.org/uprootedpeople, on May 20, 2002.

11

Adolescent Issues

Noreen Zafar, Asifa Naureen, Kiren Khurshid

PREAMBLE

Adolescent is a transformation from childhood to adulthood which is characterized by physical, psychological and social transformation. WHO defines adolescence as the time period between 10 and 19 years in Sustainable Development Goals. Young section of a country's population is the backbone for development and future progress. The health of adolescents is one of the major determinants for the success of a country. There are an estimated 1.2 billion adolescents globally, which accounts for almost 16 percent of the world population. Over 50 percent of the world's adolescents, nearly 340 million, live in South Asia. Adolescents form a significant proportion of the population in SAFOG countries too. In Pakistan, the recent census reveals the significant youth bulge, 64 percent of the total population is below the age of 30 while 29 percent is between the ages of 15.

Whereas the youth is an asset to a country, this is true only when their health, education and personal development is well taken care of. The tragedy we are facing is that the health, well-being, personal development and hence the success of this, important section of population especially in developing countries is severely compromised. The youth and more so adolescent girls as deprived of their basic human rights for health, education and their talents go un-nurtured.

The Sustainable Development Goals are the roadmap created to help the developing nations achieve a better and more sustainable future for all. Adolescents have a crucial role to play in helping their nations achieve the Sustainable Development Goals. SDG specifically dealing with adolescent health are number 3 and 5. SDG 3.7 and 5.6.

a. Percentage of women of reproductive age (15–49) who have their need for family planning satisfied with modern methods **(3.7.1)**

b. Adolescent birth rate (10–14, 15–19) per 1,000 women in that age group **(3.7.2)**

c. Proportion of women aged 15–49 who make their own informed decisions regarding sexual relations, contraceptive use and reproductive health care **(5.6.1)**

d. Number of countries with laws and regulations that guarantee women aged 15–49 access to sexual and reproductive health care, information, and education **(5.6.2)**

For the SDGs to materialize, the young people's health, education and developmental opportunities have to be optimized. The 8 SDGs, number 1, 2, 3, 4, 5, 8, 10 and 16 that cannot be achieved without ensuring optimal opportunities for health, education and ensuring well-being of adolescents.

According to WHO 1 in 6 persons of the world population are from 10 to 19 years of age. They form a very volunerable group in terms of exposure to social and environmental hazards.WHO reports in 2017 that 3000 of

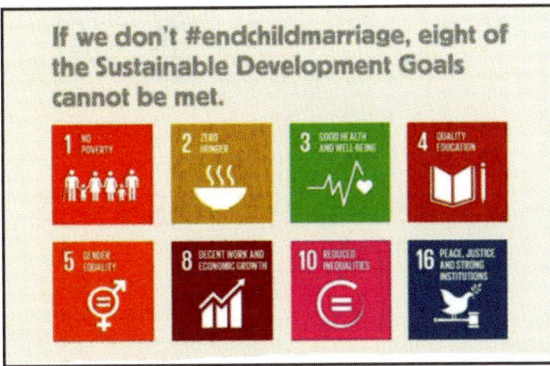

If we don't #endchildmarriage, eight of the Sustainable Development Goals cannot be met.

adolescents die per day globally and most of them by preventable causes. The leading causes are road traffic accidents, pneumonia, suicide and diarrhoea ultimately represent lesser safety and awareness in this age group.

ADOLESCENT PROBLEMS

Common adolescent issues in south Asia can be broadly put in different categories, though they have a great degree of overlap and underlying causes are interlinked:

- General issues
- Reproductive rights and sexual health issues
- Gender-based violence
- Mental issues

There is a multiple array of reasons responsible for adolescent problems and major contribution is from socio-cultural environment of South Asia and harmful traditional practices in this region.

REPRODUCTIVE RIGHTS AND SEXUAL HEALTH ISSUES

Adolescent Pregnancies

Approximately 16 million girls aged 15 to 19 years and 2.5 million girls under age 16 years give birth in developing regions.

Teenage or adolescent pregnancies are defined as pregnancies occurring in young girls aged 15–19 years of age. Most of these pregnancies are unplanned and are associated with significant social and medical consequences. Teenage pregnancies are a significant contributor to maternal and neonatal mortality.

The risk of death associated with pregnancy is about a third higher among 15 to 19 years old than among 20 to 24 years old. It appears that young adolescents are also more likely to experience obstructed labor, fistula, and premature delivery and to give birth to low birth weight babies than older women.

In Pakistan PDHS 8% of women age 15–19 had begun childbearing: 6% had a live birth, and 2% were pregnant at the time of the interview. The proportion of teenagers who had begun childbearing rises rapidly with age, from 1% at age 15 to 19% at age 19.

This group also contributes to the unsafe abortion numbers. Terrible long-term psychological and physical sequelae are common in those who survive. The babies born to these young mothers are also adversely affected due to high risk of low birth weight, risk of pre-term delivery and neonatal morbidity. Babies born to girls younger than 15 are more likely to die before their 5th birthday suffer from malnutrition and experience stunting. This initiates the cascade of a repeat pregnancy soon after, which further adversely affects the health and well-being of the mother.

There are severe socio-economic consequences. Violence is much more common in this situation. As the girls are forced to leave the school, their education and hence personal development and opportunities for a successful life are reduced.

Key Facts

- Approximately 16 million girls aged 15 to 19 years and 2.5 million girls under 16 years give birth each year in developing regions.
- Complications during pregnancy and childbirth, such as hemorrhage, sepsis, obstructed labor and complications from

unsafe abortions are the leading cause of death for 15 to 19 years old girls globally.

- Adolescent mothers (ages 10 to 19 years) face higher risks of eclampsia, puerperal endometritis, and systemic infections than women aged 20 to 24 years, and every year, some 3.9 million girls aged 15 to 19 years undergo unsafe abortions.
- More than 1.1 million adolescents aged 10–19 years died in 2016, over 3000 every day, mostly from preventable or treatable causes.
- Globally, nearly one in three adolescent girls aged 15–19 years (84 million) has been a victim of emotional, physical and/or sexual violence perpetrated by their husband or partner.
- Every year an estimated 21 million girls aged 15 to 19 years and 2 million girls aged under 15 years become pregnant in developing regions.
- The global adolescent birth rate has declined from 65 births per 1000 women in 1990 to 47 births per 1000 women in 2015.
- According to the United Nations Population Fund (UNFPA), "Pregnancies among girls less than 18 years of age have irreparable consequences. It violates the rights of girls, with life-threatening consequences in terms of sexual and reproductive health, and poses high development costs for communities, particularly in perpetuating the cycle of poverty".
- The UN Population Division puts the global adolescent birth rate in 2018 at 44 births per 1000 girls this age—country rates range from 1 to over 200 births per 1000 girls.

TRADITIONAL PRACTICES AND EFFECTS ON SEXUAL RIGHTS

Selective sex selection and female infanticide: Gender discrimination works to the disadvantage of girls, even prior to birth. Female infanticide refers to deliberate termination of a pregnancy, following the diagnosis of a female foetus on board. This tragedy is prevalent in many SAFOG countries. India has one of the highest female infanticide numbers in the world and selective abortions based on the diagnosis of a female foetus. During the period 1991–2011, the child sex ratio (0–6 years) declined from 945 to 914.

Child Brides

Getting married as a teenager or young girl imposes serious threats to the health and safety. These girls are immature physically and emotionally. They often have poor or no education and are totally not ready for the great responsibility that entails being a wife. Most of them are from poor families and with poor nutritional status and are often married at a young age, one less mouth to feed. These girls are often undernourished and anaemic and getting married young, further perpetuates the cycle of poverty and ill health.

These young girls have almost no decision-making powers and are poorly informed. Getting married practically eliminates their chances of any personal development or pursuing education. They form poor relationships and are vulnerable to depression and abuse. Even if they ever start work, being unskilled means poor pay. In 2018, the global adolescent birth rate is 44 births per 1,000 women aged 15 to 19, compared to 56 in 2000.

Teenage Marriage

Marriage prior to 18 years of age is a sheer violation of human rights. A girl getting married to such a young age is almost inevitably denied of her right to study, empower herself and achieve her true potential in life. An estimated 5% to 33% of girl's ages 15 to 24 years who drop out of school in some countries do so because of early pregnancy or marriage.

This is further complicated by her poor nutritional status and lack of knowledge and choices about reproductive health, self-care and use of contraception.

The vicious cycle of adolescent pregnancy starts which often results in significant morbidity and even mortality. This initiates a cascade of poor maternal health replicating into poor obstetric outcomes. There is clear evidence that young married girls are often subjected to violence. It is also known that girls with no or poor education are more likely to be married young. Each year, about 15 million girls are married before the age of 18 years, and 90% of births to girls aged 15 to 19 years occur within marriage.

One of the specific targets of the health Sustainable Development Goal (SDG 3) is that by 2030, the world should ensure universal access to sexual and reproductive health care services, including family planning, information and education, and the integration of reproductive health into national strategies and programs. Better access to contraceptive information and services can reduce the number of girls becoming pregnant and giving birth at too young age. Laws that are enforced that specify a minimum age of marriage at 18 can help.

Vani

This custom is practiced in different parts of the country especially Pakistan under different names. It is called vani in Punjab. Different names are used in other areas like sawra and bada. This involves giving a girl away in marriage in order to settle a feud. Since the two families are adversaries, these poor girls are never really accepted as a family member and face severe hostility at the hands of their in-laws.

Dowry Violence

Dowry refers to the stuff the girl's families give as a gift to their daughter at the time of the wedding. Supposed to be a voluntary sending of gift, this has become a brutal compulsion. The groom's family often set their own terms and the girl's family has to comply. Even worse, if the groom's family is not happy with the dowry, the girl is often tortured and forced to ask her family to give more. Failing this many brides are killed mercilessly. This tragedy also affects the younger brides more frequently.

SAFOG countries continue to suffer from the menace of dowry deaths. In one year alone, dowry related violence claimed the lives of 325 women and contributed to 66.7 per cent of the violent incidents against women in Bangladesh, insufficient dowry claims have been punished by throwing acid at the brides. It is estimated that there are over 200 acid mutilations per year (Heise et al., 1994).

MARRIAGE WITH HOLY BOOKS AND OBJECTS

Women and girl children are deprived of their property rights by symbolically marrying them to the Holy Quran in some areas in Pakistan. This ensures that the girl child or woman will not bear children in the future and will not demand her rightful share in the family property. Sometimes poor parents who cannot afford to marry their daughters resort to this symbolic arrangement. This practice of marriage of girls with holy and spiritual value objects as some trees is also seen in India.

Watta Satta

It refers to a double marriage within two families. A son and a daughter of one family are married to the son and daughter of the other. So, a brother and sister are married to a brother and sister. Many times, these marriages are arranged so as to compensate for a weaker partner. The dual arrangement puts unnecessary and constant pressure on the wives in both marriages. The situation is worse for the younger bride.

Role of a gynecologist for adolescent reproductive Health: Young girls and not small women, they are unique individuals with their own specific set of clinical problems. Dealing with them requires an entirely different set of skills and expertise. Clinical history and examination techniques are different. The investigations and treatment are entirely different from the adult counterparts of prime importance is the first visit of a teenager to the gynaecologist this is actually set the tone of how she is going to relate to reproductive health seeking behavior.

This is the one opportunity for the young girl to establish a bond of comfort and trust with her doctor. If this visit goes well, she will develop a positive relationship with her physician and will be able to go back and discuss any future concerns. This is an extremely important landmark of the girl. The attending doctor must be kind and well-versed in dealing with the problems.

It is of prime importance that this visit is conducted in a relaxed and yet confidential environment. The young girl must be made comfortable and reassured that physical examination is not a part of this visit.

The American College of Obstetrics and Gynecologists recommends that the adolescents should visit the doctor around the age of 13 to 15 years. The main purpose of this visit is to get the young girl to have her first interaction with the gynaecologist and an opportunity for her to discuss any general issues like body image, weight, skin and any period issues. Vaccination including MMR and HPV may be offered too. This is also an opportunity to discuss the contraceptive needs should that be the case and also protection against sexually transmitted diseases, contraception, and prevention of sexually transmitted infections (STIs).

Violence and Abuse

Violence against women and specially adolescents is a growing menace in the SAFOG countries. As a human rights issue the Sustainable Development Goal No 5 stands for eliminating all harmful practices and all discrimination and violence against women and girls (SDG 5.2 and 5.3).

Percentage of women aged 20–24 years who were married or in a union before age 15 and before age 18 (**5.3.1**).

Proportion of ever-partnered women and girls aged 15 years and older subjected to physical, sexual or psychological violence by a current or former intimate partner in the previous 12 months, by form of violence and by age (**5.2.1**) 1 in 10 girl reports sexual violence under the age of 20 globally. Proportion of women and girls aged 15–49 who have undergone female genital mutilation (**5.3.2**).

Whether or not legal frameworks are in place to promote, enforce, and monitor equality and non-discrimination on the basis of sex (**5.1.1**).

Rape and sexual violence are on a rise especially in India. According to the Indian National Crime Records Bureau, one woman is subjected to sexual violence every 22 minutes. A 2009 report, the Maternal Mortality and Morbidity Study 2008-09 by the Family Health Division of the Department of Health Services in Nepal and circulated by IRIN, the United Nations news and information service, reveals the high suicide rate among young women and states the causes are family issues, including domestic mental and physical abuse. The study also revealed that 21 per cent of the suicides were committed by women under 18.

General Issues

Adolescents have developmental needs in social context, problems with body image and weight management. Poor nutrition (anemia), stunted growth and inadequate physical activity in the countries of this region share as common problems in adolescents.

Anemia

In South Asia poor dietary practices, poverty, bad hygiene, worm infestations, menorrhagia and gender-based food disparities are common causes for anemia in adolescent girls. This is further aggravated by lack of priority for girls nutrition. In many household, even the affluent ones, it is a custom to feed the boys and men first. More meat and rich foods are considered to the necessity of the males. This is in paradox to the naturally increased requirement of better iron stores for the young girls, who loose blood in menstruation

Poor Hygiene

No information about menstruation and self-care during this time is available to young girls. In the poor household specially, the purchase of hygienic protection and its safe disposal is also a problem. It is not uncommon for these girls to use old, redundant pieces of clothes, which are often unclean. Prolonged use forms a basis for possible ascending infections.

There are multiple myths and taboos surrounding daily life activities during menstruation too. For example, in many families, the girls are forbidden to take a shower or bathe during menstruation. Others impose dietary restrictions like not eating eggs or meat, etc. On account of the socio-cultural taboos, many families are still reluctant to bring the young girls to a gynaecology clinic. However, in the past decade or so things have changing, for a better and many more adolescents are reporting to health care facilities with their issues.

Weight Problems

Globally, in 2016, over one in six adolescents aged 10–19 years was overweight. There are different sets of weight issues seen amongst the adolescents in different socioeconomic strata. There is the affluent group with girls with unhealthy diets consisting of fast foods with high carbohydrate and fats. This is compounded by sedentary lifestyle with laptops, iPads, video games and chatting on the phones resulting in weight gain. Obesity results not only in health issues like a tendency towards developing diabetes, heart disease and joint problems but also significant psychological issues, poor self-esteem, body image problems and depression. Low mood further hampers an active lifestyle and exercise. This a vicious cycle begins which adversely affects the health. Polycystic ovarian syndrome is the commonest hormonal problem in young girls, with a raising incidence. The adolescence is a time of physical and psychological changes and body image is an important concern. The phenotypic manifestations of polycystic ovarian disease, cause a significant distress to the adolescents and results in poor self-esteem and depression. Weight gain leads to appearance of the problem. The other and slightly smaller group often has weight by the lowest centimes, often due to poor dietary intake due to anorexia. In the poor strata of the population, the rampant problem is that of malnutrition and stunted growth. This not only affects their physical health but also the cognitive behaviors and hence their output as individual.

Dysmenorrhoea

It is a common problem among the adolescents seen in the gynecology clinics. Unfortunately, this significant cause of distress to the young girls is often not dealt with properly within the family. Mothers are commonly reluctant to share this with their husbands and mostly tell the girls not to use any analgesia, as per the common belief that pain killers will stop the menstruation. It is important to counsel the mother and the girls in a factual but reassuring way. It is important for the health care provider to help remove myths and misconceptions.

ACOG recommends proceeding with laparoscopy in adolescents with persistent dysmenorrheal who do not respond to oral contraceptive pills (OCP) and non-steroidal anti-inflammatory drug therapy, so that diagnosis of endometriosis is not missed.

However, in the socio-cultural atmosphere of South Asia, this is difficult to practice. There is reluctance of the family for the unmarried young girl to go through any surgical procedures. So often the clinicians have to rely on ultrasounds and resort to medical management.

HIV

South Asia accounts for 4% of adolescents living with HIV. Globally adolescent girls are more at risk of contracting and developing AIDS.

Smoking

Globally, at least 1 in 10 adolescents aged 13 to 15 years uses tobacco. Cigarette smoking is rising in our part of the world, whereas this trend is declining among younger adolescents in some high-income countries. The adolescents have therefore no real information about high risk behaviors like smoking and sheesha. They often find these things attractive and many of the teenagers from affluent backgrounds use these under peer pressure, just for the fun of it.

Mental Health

Self-harm is the third leading cause of death for adolescents and depression is among the leading causes of disability.

Psychological problems often arise due to patterns of behavioral or psychological symptoms that impact multiple areas of life. Another important reason for depression among young girls is the plight of their mothers in the household.

Suicide and accidental death from self-harm were the third cause of adolescent mortality in 2015, resulting in an estimated 67,000 deaths. Self-harm largely occurs among older adolescents, and globally it is the second leading cause of death for older adolescent girls. It is the leading or second cause of adolescent death in Europe and South-East Asia.

ROOT CAUSES OF COMMON ADOLESCENT PROBLEMS

Lack of Information and Awareness

Adolescence is the most formative and vital part of a young girl's life and yet most of the girls pass through it being minimally or completely uninformed. Not only this a body of myths and misconceptions surrounds this important phase of life. Although menstruation is a hallmark of successful stepping into womanhood, it is surrounded by myths and taboos.

While being deprived of the factual information, the youngsters are exposed to multiple sources of unclassified and often incorrect information about reproductive health issues. These further taints their perception and understanding of their personal issues and makes healthy choices more distant target. The mothers or teachers in school often do not communicate with the adolescents about issues like onset of menstruation, menstrual hygiene, self-protection and abuse.

Social and Cultural Norms

Nutritional deprivation, increased demand of adolescent's body, and excessive menstrual loss, all aggravate and exacerbate anemia and its effects. Menstrual disturbances are not uncommon and may add further disruption during this difficult phase for adolescents and their families. The social norms often demand that the boys are fed better than the girls. Many adolescents with menstrual disturbances never present to their family doctor or gynecologist. Embarrassment about discussing menstruation, fear of disease, and ignorance about available services may lead to delayed presentation.

Lack of Education

Financial difficulties are a common reason for families to discourage girl's education. Socio-cultural barriers and patriarchal mind-set, not allowing the girls to travel distances for the school are common. Daughters are often used as home helps for the overburdened mothers and to look after their younger siblings, an eventually intended role for them. The expenditure on boys' education is thought of being a worthwhile investment, while the families think it would be waste to spend on the girls' education, as they will go their new homes after getting married.

The SDGs address this important issue and ensure that all girls and boys complete free, equitable and good quality primary and secondary education (SDG 4.1).

Patriarchal Practices

Adolescent is a crucial time for both parents and boys, specifically in the girls as menstruation, as the initiation of menstruation imposes extra demand on the youngster's body. Paradoxically there in the several regions boys have a preference not only in education, opportunities, but also for health facilities. This disparity forms the foundation for poor personal development and ill health for adolescent girls. Lack of a priority for girls education and personal development creates imbalance in the dynamics for the society and also for the country.

Lack of Recreational Activities

WHO recommends for adolescents to accumulate at least 60 minutes of moderate-to-vigorous-intensity physical activity daily, which may include play, games, sports, but also activity for transportation (such as cycling and walking), or physical education. A big problem facing the adolescents especially those belonging to poor socioeconomic group is the total absence of any recreational activities. No designated safe places exist for their physical exercise or creative work. The facilities and centers for vocational trainings are a rarity and those who are not able to attend schools are just stuck in their houses, doing household chores, often waiting to be married off. This causes frustration and unhealthy habits are formed. This also results in aggravating the low mood, frustration and psychological problems.

The poor household often have one or two rooms for the whole family and many generations live together. The 2030 Agenda for Sustainable Development, specifically Goal 11, emphasizes the need for the provision of space towards inclusive and sustainable urbanization.

Poor Family Units

Where the family unit is not cohesive, especially in poor strata of population, contributes to immense psychological up heavily and often results in disturbed behaviours and poor personal development. Such adolescents have problems not only in education but also issues later in developing relationships when they grow up.

HUMAN RIGHTS PERSPECTIVE ON ADOLESCENT HEALTH

The WHO Constitution (1946) states, "Health is a state of complete physical, mental and social well-being and not merely the absence of disease or infirmity. The enjoyment of the highest attainable standard of health is one of the fundamental rights of every human being without distinction of race, religion, and political belief, economic or social condition", Universal declaration of Human Rights, 1948 further states, "Everyone has the right to a standard of living adequate for the health of himself and of his family, including food, clothing, housing and medical care and necessary social services".

As signatories to the Convention on the Elimination of all Forms of Discrimination against Women, bound to ensure that girls and women are free from all discrimination and be entitled to all human rights. The ten basic human rights are listed below.

The right to
Life
Health
Benefitting from science

Confidentiality
Privacy
Access to information
Non-discrimination
Autonomy in decision-making
Be able to limit their family size
Be free from inhumane treatment

All SAFOG countries are signatories to the Human Rights and yet the most basic things like the right to knowledge and access to health care are often denied or poorly executed.

There is a great and urgent need for integrating the following basic human rights in adolescent healthcare. This will translate into healthy, empowered and successful adolescents, who will be able to contribute to their nations development and lead happy and prosperous lives.

CONCLUSION

Global Evidence (GAGE) is a nine-year (2015–2024) study to explore the gendered experiences of adolescents as they progress through the second decade of their lives and into early adulthood. GAGE is undertaking research with 18,000 adolescents in six low-and middle-income countries in Africa (Ethiopia, Rwanda), Asia (Bangladesh, Nepal) and the Middle East (Jordan, Lebanon). However, the evidence available on Adolescent Health clearly conveys that in order to combat the issues related to this age group, needs to address the stakeholders and barriers in the social and cultural context. The governments in South Asian countries need to consider adolescent rights at the priority list and formulate laws and legislation for protecting their rights. To overcome barriers, school education and self awareness of youth is urgently required. Equal opportunities for healthy development of adolescents must be universal. As pregnancy and childbirth is one of the leading causes of death, focus should be on enhancement of awareness, reducing child early and forced marriages. Provision of comprehensive contraceptive and sexual education is necessary for adolescents.

Countries in South Asia are putting in efforts for improvement in quality of life of their youth as these efforts are fruitful and wise investment for future of their nations.

BIBLIOGRAPHY

1. Acta Obstet Gynecol Scand 2012; 91:1114-18. Every Woman Every Child. The Global Strategy for Women's, Children's and Adolescents' Health (2016-2030). Geneva: Every Woman Every Child, 2015.
2. American College of Obstetricians and Gynaecologists. ACOG Committee Opinion. Number 310, April 2005. Endometriosis in adolescents. Obstet Gynecol 2005 Apr; 105(4):921–7.
3. Committee on the Elimination of Discrimination against Women (1992) Violence against women (CEDAW) General Recommendation No. 19 (Eleventh session) New York, NY, United Nations
4. Darroch J, Woog V, Bankole A, Ashford LS. Adding it up: Costs and benefits of meeting the contraceptive needs of adolescents. New York: Guttmacher Institute; 2016.
5. Darroch J, Woog V, Bankole A, Ashford LS. Adding it up: Costs and benefits of meeting the contraceptive needs of adolescents. New York: Guttmacher Institute; 2016
6. Global strategy for women's, children's and adolescents' health is the adolescent birth rate.
7. Heise L, Pitanguy J, Germain A (1994) Violence against women: the hidden health burden. World Bank Discussion Paper 255. The World Bank, Washington, DC
8. http://www.sparcpk.org/2015/Other-Publications/HTP-1.pdf
9. http://www.unfpa.org/adolescent-pregnancy
10. https://data.unicef.org/topic/adolescents/demographics/
11. https://data.unicef.org/topic/adolescents/mental-health/#_ednref1
12. https://en.unesco.org/education 20 30-sdg4/targets
13. https://en.wikipedia.org/wiki/Honour_killing_in_Pakistan
14. https://en.wikipedia.org/wiki/Watta _satta

15. https://ro.uow.edu.au/cgi/viewcont ent.cgi?referer=https://www.googl e.com/&httpsredir=1&article=2532 &context=lhapapers

16. https://sustainabledevelopment.un .org/sdg3

17. https://sustainabledevelopment.un.org/sdg5

18. https://unstats.un.org/sdgs/indicators/data base/?indicator=3.7.2

19. https://www.gage.odi.org/research/our-approach/(www.gage.odi.org/research/ourapproach, n.d.)

20. https://www.girlsnotbrides.org/the mes/sustainable-development-goals-sdgs/

21. https://www.peertechz.com/article s/.pdf

22. https://www.smh.com.au/world/nepalese-women-suffering- 20110820-1j3f4.html

23. https://www.un.org/sustainabledevelopment/sustainable-development-goals/

24. https://www.who.int/news-room/fact-sheets/detail/adolescent-pregnancy

25. India loses 3 million girls in infanticide. The Hindu, 9 October 2012, http://www.thehindu.com/news/national/ india-loses-3-million-girls-in-infanticide/article3981575.ece

26. Neal S, Matthews Z, Frost M, et al. Childbearing in adolescents aged 12–15 years in low resource countries: A neglected issue. New estimates from demographic and household surveys in 42 countries.

27. Nove A, Matthews Z, Neal S, et al. Maternal mortality in adolescents compared with women of other ages: Evidence from 144 countries. The Lancet Glob Health. 2012; 2: e155–e164.

28. Pakistan Demographic and Health Survey 2017-2018 Key Indicators.

29. PDHS 2017-2018

30. UN DESA, Population Division. World Population Prospects: The 2017 Revision, DVD Edition. New York: UN DESA; 2017. UNDESA, Population Division. World Population Prospects, the 2015 Revision (DVD edition). New York: UNDESA, Population Division, 2015

31. UNFPA. Girlhood, not motherhood: Preventing adolescent pregnancy. New York: UNFPA; 2015.

32. UNFPA. Girlhood, not motherhood: Preventing adolescent pregnancy. New York: UNFPA; 2015.

33. UNFPA. Motherhood in childhood: Facing the challenge of adolescent pregnancy: The State of World Population 2013. United Nations Population Fund, New York; 2013:163–196.

34. UNICEF analysis of DHS, MICS, and other national household surveys, 2013–2017.

35. UNICEF. Ending child marriage: Progress and prospects. New York: UNICEF, 2013

36. WHO and partners (2017) Global Accelerated Action for the Health of Adolescents (AA-HA!). Geneva 2017.

37. WHO and partners (2017) Global Accelerated Action for the Health of Adolescents (AA-HA!). Geneva 2017 (WHO and Partners)

38. WHO. Global health estimates 2015: deaths by cause, age, sex, by country and by region, 2000–2015. Geneva: WHO; 2016.

39. World Bank. Economic impacts of child marriage: Global synthesis report. Washington, DC: World Bank; 2017.

12

Violence Against Women

Ferdousi Begum, Rowshan Ara Khanom, Yeasmin Jahan

BURDEN OF DISEASE

Violence against women and girls is major health and human rights issue.

At least one in five of the world's female population has been physically or sexually abused by a man or men at some time in their life. (WHO, 1997) Many, including pregnant women and young girls, are subject to severe, sustained or repeated attacks. What is done to a woman in her house is accepted, whereas the same act done elsewhere is recognized as a crime. The abuse of women is effectively condoned in almost every society in the world. Prosecution and conviction of men is rare when compared to the number of assaults. Violence and/or the threat of violence are a means to maintain and reinforce women's subordination. Rape is used as a weapon in a conflict, further reinforcing the idea of the woman as a possession.

By 1990s all gender-based violence was recognized as an abuse of human rights. In late 1993, the General Assembly of the United Nations adopted a declaration against violence against women.

Violence against women is defined as: Any act of gender-based violence that results in or is likely to result in physical, sexual or psychological harm or suffering to women including threats of such acts, coercion or arbitrary deprivations of liberty whether occurring in public or in private life.

TYPES OF VIOLENCE

This definition encompasses, but is not limited to violence occurring in the family, including battering, sexual abuse of female children in the household, dowry related violence, marital rape on spousal violence and violence related to exploitation, female genital mutilation and other traditional practices harmful to women. Violence occurs within the general community, rape, sexual abuse, sexual harassment and intimidation at work, in educational institutes, trafficking in women and forced prostitution, violence perpetrated or condoned by the state.

Effects on Health and Society

- Violence against women has important effects on health and development.
- Effect on socio-economic development
- Socio-economic development is slowed because gender violence reduces women's ability to contribute fully.
- Fear of stranger-perpetrated violence similarly limits women's participation in public life by restricting themselves, not going out or not going to certain places, or not moving out at certain times or in certain dress.
- As a result of abuse, women and girls do not attain the educational and income level for which they have ability. They see the outside world is dangerous and limit

themselves in what they do. This attitude continues and affects their children as well.

- To avoid violence, women learn to restrict their behaviour to what they think will be acceptable to their husbands and partners. Threats or fear of violence control women's minds as much as do acts of violence, making women their own jailers.
- The restriction and the underlying fear may even exacerbate under nutrition.
- Distrust and hatred of men affects the normal working relationship with male colleagues.

Effects on Maternal Health

- Surveys show that pregnant women are prime targets of abuse.
- Violence is also responsible for a sizable but often unrecognized share of maternal mortality.

Effects on Family Planning

- Many women limit their use of contraception out of fear of abuse.
- Sexual victimization may be directly and indirectly related to unwanted pregnancy.
- Effect on STD and HIV/AIDS prevention
- **Violence can increase a woman's risk of STD and HIV/AIDS**
- Through non-consensual sex or
- By limiting her willingness or her ability to get her partner to use a barrier contraceptive.

Effects on Children

- Children who witness wife abuse are at risk of being assaulted themselves.
- Children who witness violence and abused children may experience emotional and behavioural problems.
- Abuse has an effect on children's sense of security and their developing personalities.
- Violence may affect child survival in a more subtle way: Being less self-confident and have less power, They cannot pay proper attention to the children.

- Low birth weight babies are more prevalent if the mother is abused.
- Female children who see their mothers as powerless often have low self-esteem and so are at risk of being sexually exploited.
- Male children are more likely to grow up and become batterers. Children from abusive homes are 1,000 times more likely to abuse their spouse or batter their own children.
- Research in South Asia has shown that:
  - Children of abused women are at a higher risk of stunting and wasting
  - Domestic violence is estimated to account for about 60% of runaways

Health Care Costs

- Violence against women burdens an already over-burdened health care system.
- Costs a lot for treating serious physical injury and psychological problems.
- Involves other direct costs for police, courts and legal services. Incurs costs for social services including child protection.

Violence Related to Women's Reproductive Health

Pregnancy is a physiological process. Proper care during pregnancy, delivery and puerperium is the right of a woman. Family and society often ignores this resulting in many acute and chronic complications, many a times resulting in death or disability. Women of our society are not aware of their rights and or not empowered to obtain that right. Family and society due to lack of awareness, in correct cultural norms and traditions. Lack of culture of caring during pregnancy often do not give due importance to pregnant women. Deprivation of this human right of pregnant women is a form of violence. The result of which is far reaching, two-thirds of the babies whose mothers dire, dies within one year of life. The children who survive are brought up with lack of care, no or less education, less nutrition, early marriage, etc. This results in delinquent behavior of society and for female children to enter into the vicious cycled of early marriage, early child bearing and its sequel.

1. **Induced abortion:** Most of the husbands in Bangladesh are unwilling to use any contraceptives by themselves. They think this is the responsibility of women to safe herself from unwanted pregnancy. Few women can't tolerate hormonal contra-ceptives, few do not want permanent method and few are not suitable for IUD. So they become pregnant repeatedly and their husbands send them for induced abortion.

2. **Secondary to sexual abuse:** Married women may become pregnant due to contraceptive failure or non-use of contra-ceptive by the male partner. Unwanted pregnancy leads to induced abortion. Unmarried girls, separated or widows may become pregnant due to sexual abuse. Careful history taking, not judgmental attitude and empathy may give her the opportunity to break her silence on her abuse. This group of women may seek induced abortion, which may endanger their lives.

3. **Septic abortion: Violence in silence:** Results for an anthropological study Published by Bangladesh Association for Prevention of Septic Abortion reports that most patients suffered for several days and even weeks before they sought admission. By the time they reached hospital they were in a critical condition and required emergency care. Within marriages abor-tion is sometimes a husband's sole decision. Though the husband has an equal share in the pregnancy, many a times the husband did not come to visit her or did not bear the expenses of her treatment. Over 50% (27 out of 53) respondents had been using some contraceptive methods at the time they got pregnant and most are process failure.

Where the doctor has been in attendance before death, she/he may be able to give information as a result of examination, including:

i. Relevant details obtained from the woman, even including an admission of induced abortion. The admissibility of such hearsay evidence is a matter for the court.

ii. Signs of interference such as scratches or bruises on thighs and vaginal walls, cervix, etc. Several places of local damage often tend to confirm that the abortion was self-induced.

iii. Presence of foreign material such as disinfectants or other agents exuding from the vagina or cervix

iv. Presence of other complications such as perforation, infection.

4. **Infertility:** It is known that in 30% cases female only, 30% male only and in 40% both male and female factors is the cause of infertility. Whether the cause of infertility lies with the female or not, usually she is the one to bear the blame. The concept that both male and female are involved in the conception of a child is ignored, many a times the husband's disease may cause wife's infertility. The female is the partner who mostly has to use the contraceptive (which may result in infertility), has to be the victim of STI which her promiscuous husband transmits to her and which results in her getting pelvic inflammatory. Disease and as a result her fallopian tubes are blocked or cannot work properly.

Sometimes the husbands are too confident to be investigated themselves. But the wife is blamed and brushed. The female of an infertile couple is frequently the victim of violence even if the cause of infertility lies in the male.

5. **Fistula: Vesico-vaginal, recto-vaginal:** Often the VVF or most fistulae are the results of neglect during pregnancy and

delivery. Lack of proper care during pregnancy and delivery prevents the screening of high risk cases and appropriate management. Prolonged and obstructed labour are the two important causes of VVF and women in labour are often neglected as a result of poor status of women, less importance being given to the suffering, lack of empowerment and access to money, power and different sociocultural reasons.

Once they develop a VVF, which is through no fault of their own, their husbands and family often abandon them. They often become social outcasts subject to taunts, physical violence and neglect. The BIRPERHT study of maternal morbidity found 2% of women had VVF and 18.9% of them reported a deteriorated relationship with their husband. 77.7% of these women did not seek care for their condition. The violence of neglect produces their condition and their condition leads to greater neglect and violence.

6. **Eclampsia:** Early marriage and early child bearing is the social norm on our society especially in rural setting. Eclampsia usually occurs in pregnant women who are primigravida of teenage or grand multipara. Pre-eclampsia is not preventable but eclampsia is preventable through antenatal care and timely intervention.

How is it related with violence against women?

Due to neglect and poor status of women in the family as well as in the society, lack of power to utilize money the women cannot get timely treatment. Getting antenatal, intranatal and postnatal care is a human right, therefore, women right, so it is the isolation of human and women's right and became a violence against women.

7. **Pelvic inflammatory disease (PID):** Repeated MR or induced abortion may lead to PID. If husband is infected with STIs and not treated completely, the married women become a sufferer of chronic PID. Dysparunia and lower abdominal pain are the leading presentation in case of OI which leads to familial disharmony and more abuse. A rape victim may be infected with STIs and often does not seek care during acute phase. So they suffer of chronic PID and this may be a source of abuse as the husband blames the wife for it. PID in unmarried girls may be due to sexual abuse by the infected person.

8. **Delayed treatment:** When a woman seeks treatment for an injury or illness after quite some delay, then this may be a sign of violence as the cause of the injury or a type of violence related to the value placed on the women's life. Delay in seeking treatment may be a sign of violence.

Since she may have to recover sufficiently to be able to get herself to treatment, since she may have to wait for the perpetrator to leave before she can seek assistance.

Since the victim may go first to the police and this causes a long delay, since she may wait for the injury to be less disfiguring before going out in public.

Delay in providing treatment may be a form of violence as it involves deprivation of the liberty of movement, of access to health care.

It can be a violation of a woman's human rights. It may involve delay in taking the decision to seek care. Delay caused by the method used to reach care. Delay in the time taken to provide care at the facility.

The tendency to blame the victim contributes to these delays and this tendency is found at every level, the family, the community, the police, the social workers and the hospital staff.

9. **Undernutrition:** Discriminatory practices against women begin in early childhood. The girl child is given less food and is the last to be fed. The consequences of this may be a delayed menarche, delayed and poor skeletal growth leading to a small pelvis and increased risks of obstructed labor. Various social taboos restrict the foods given to pregnant and lactating women. Nutritional anemia also affects a woman's health. Pregnant women also rely on their iron stores to produce sufficient blood but these often do not exist. Women are socialized to continue this by depriving themselves of food so that the rest of the family has sufficient food. This is a form of violence, which has serious health effects for the woman, and for the children she bears.

10. **Psychological distress:** Another form of violence is psychological distress. It may be a manifestation of other types of violences against women. This may result in the woman's loss of appetite. This may be the only symptom for which she seeks treatment. She may be unaware of the connection between the violence and her loss of appetite. On examination, she may show other signs and symptoms of depression. Another presentation is the woman who requests medicine to make her fat. This may be particularly true in those with recently acquired wealth, as the husband is demanding that she be fat as a sign of his prosperity. In this situation, undernutrition is a sign of violence especially of mental torture.

11. **Chronic pain:** One of the most frequent presenting complaints of women is that their whole body is aching. This may be due to a number of factors such as nutritional deficiency. As already mentioned lack of sufficient caloric intake. Deficiency in micronutrients, and insufficient fluid intake make a generalized weakness, anemia and poor muscular tone.

12. **Exhaustion:** Excessive physical work for long hours done by already malnourished women puts strain on the joints and results in the early onset of osteoarthirits and in generalized muscular pain.

13. **Tension:** There is much reason for tension within a family. A few may be named. Women are the ones who bear the brunt of actually getting food on the plates for the family and for economic reasons have inadequate resources but hungry children asking for food.

14. **Psychological problems:** Psychological problems may be:

    Primary resulting in violence being used against the woman.

    Secondary as the result of violence.

    For many women, the psychological effects of abuse are more debilitating than the physical effects. Fear, anxiety, fatigue, post-traumatic stress disorder and sleeping and eating disturbances are common long-term reactions to violence. Abused women may become dependent and suggestible and they may find it difficult to make decisions alone. They frequently become isolated and withdrawn as they try to hide the evidence of their abuse. In Dhaka a study of psychosocial stressors in depression, it was found that mental discord and recurrent abuse by husband or family members were significantly more common in depressed patients than in a control group. Rape survivors suffer severe and prolonged psychological effects. A study in the United States found that rape victims were nine times more likely than nonvictims to have attempted suicide and twice as likely to experience a major depression. Follow-up studies of rape victims have shown that rape survivors have higher rates of post-traumatic stress disorder than victims of other traumas.

15. **Attempted suicide, suicide:** In all the countries except Bangladesh, a greater

number of men committed suicide compared to women, the pattern was reversed in Bangladesh with 58% women committing suicides compared with 42% of men. Bangladesh perspective: In Bangladesh an average of 600 suicides per month during 1972–1988. The numbers of committing suicides are increasing day-by-day. In 1992–93 it was 984 per month. The overall national rates are estimated to be 10 per 100000 during 1992–93, based on secondary sources. A recent study in Jhenaidah revealed that torture by family members, quarrels with relatives, extreme poverty and acute scarcity of food, loss of agricultural land, suffering from incurable disease and lack of money for health care were the major causes for suicide. A study by Fauveau and Blanchet in Matlab, Bangladesh found that there were 13.8% more deaths from injury (suicide, homicide, assault and complications from induced abortion) among unmarried than among married teenage girls. This reinforced their pregnant outside of marriage. Murder may be disguised by presenting the appearance of suicide and this call for good forensic examination to make the distinction.

CIRCUMSTANCES SUGGESTING HIGH SUICIDAL INTENT

Planning in advance precaution to avoid discovery, no attempts to obtain help afterwards, dangerous method, final acts—suicide note or making a will.

GENDER ISSUES AND VIOLENCE

Gender is an old word which has taken on a new meaning. It is a portmanteau word, containing a set of interrelated ideas. Because this use of the word is new, a kind of shorthand, it is difficult to translate. The friend of an Oxfam warder in Ethiopia was both curious and amazed that Oxfam appeared to be spending three days discussing sex. In fact, the workshop in Addis Ababa examined the distinction between sex and gender.

Understanding this difference, and the concept of gender, is essential to our understanding of how development processes affect men and women, girls and boys, in different ways.

Sex is a fact of human biology, we are born male or female, it is men who impregnate, and women who conceive, give birth and breastfeed the human baby. On this biological difference, we construct an edifice of social attitudes and assumptions.

Behaviours and activities: These are our gender roles and identities. Questioning them may feel threatening, attacking the very foundations of our understanding of ourselves, our personal and social relations, our culture and traditions.

Gender analysis and inequalities: Gender analysis reveals the roles and relationships of women and men in society and the inequalities in those relationships. The much quoted UN statistics remain as true today as they were when they were first formulated over a decade age:

- Women perform two-thirds of the world's work
- Women earn one-tenth of the world's income
- Women own less than one hundredth of the world's property

One Stop Crisis Center (OCC) Bangladesh

One stop crisis center, a multispectral program on violence against women, started its activities on 19th August 2001 at Dhaka Medical College Hospital to provide all the sorts of services to the survivors (victim) from a common center without any cost lane, it is named One Stop Crisis Center (OCC). In Rajshahi Medical College Hospital another OCC center already started its activities. OCC is a multi-sectoral Program on VAW under Ministry of Women and Children affairs (lead Ministry) and funded by Royal Denmark Government (DANIDS). Other implementing ministries are Ministry of Health and Family Welfare, Home Affairs, Social Welfare, Information and Ministry of Law and Justice, and Parliamentary Affairs.

Pakistan's Violence Against Woman Center (VAWC) was established in 2004 in Karachi. The VAWC has been set up in an agricultural belt which is particularly dangerous for the Pakistani woman, who is treated worse than cattle. The Punjab Protection of Women against Violence Act (VAWA) passed in 2016 covers sexual, domestic, physical, economic, cyber, or psychological abuse.

Objectives of the Program

General: Prevent and reduce of violence against women in Bangladesh improved through coordinated multi-sectoral Integrated Ministerial approach.

Specific:

- Improved handling of violence cases by the health services
- Improved handling and investigation of violence cases by the police
- Improved women's access especially for poor women to the justice
- Increased public awareness, condemnation and resistance to type of violence against women. OCC deals with the violence of:
  1. Sexual assault
  2. Physical assault
  3. Burn

Services:

1. Medical treatment.
2. Medicolegal examination of the victim at OCC by the forensic department
3. Psychological counseling
4. Legal counseling and support by lawyer.
5. Security and counseling by OCC police

6. Social welfare service by the social welfare office
7. Temporary shelter.
8. Research and training (academic activity)
9. OCC hotline services

OCC working Group

- OCC working group is formed with the Director of MCH as
- Chairperson and OCC Coordinator as member secretary
- Other member's are:
  - Head of the department of casualty
  - Head of the department of gynae and obstetrics
  - Head of the department of forensic medicine
  - Head of the department of radiology
  - Head of the department of burn and plastic surgery
  - Representative from project implementation unit
  - Nursing Superintendent
  - Social Welfare Officer
  - Representative from nongovernmental organization working with the OCC

Besides this OCC working group can co-opt any official as member. But total number of the working people should not be more than twenty. The extension of OCC activities in other MCH situated at divisional level will start soon.

CONCLUSION

Gender-based violence against women and girls is multi-dimensional, deeply rooted in inequitable societal norms, and persists throughout the life cycle. Excess child mortality rates and a deep-rooted bias against girls often begins in the womb. Although it is widely recognized that domestic violence can include physical, sexual, psychological, and economic violence, half of the countries that have domestic violence laws do not include protections against economic violence. While domestic violence laws in South Asia include protection against sexual and economic abuse, 74 percent of women (age 15+) in the EAP are not protected from sexual violence and 76 percent of women are not protected from economic violence. There is also variation in who is protected by such laws.

Limited awareness, capacity, and lack of political will hinder women's legal protection. Laws against domestic violence and other forms of gender-based violence are just the starting point. There is no shortage of legislation, and most laws have been accompanied by awareness raising campaigns. Human rights lawyers and activist organizations have been on the frontlines, bringing these measures into place and lobbying for justice.

Difficulties in implementation these laws hindered due to limited awareness among the general public about the content or even existence of such laws; archaic legal systems and courts that are insensitive to the needs of victims, or the alternative of the controversial and patriarchal jirga systems; and weak administration and local government capacity.

Need of time is implementation of a multi-sectoral response to urgently address gender-based violence against women and girls across this diverse region.

A collaborative and coordinated response is needed in every country, concrete guidance for services that should be available to every survivor, no matter where she lives or who she is. It builds on existing standards and applies to the health, social services, police, and justice sectors, as well as to overall governance and coordination.

RECOMMENDATIONS

- Survivor-centered care
- Need to develop a Code of Conduct
- A coordinated approach
- Leaving no one behind
- Economic support
- Analytical work on violence against women and girls
- Conducting workshops and building evidence on what works to prevent GBV
- Develop GBV risk assessment tool
- Incorporating GBV issues in infrastructure projects in recent years.
- To employ women in the industry.
- Introduction of an implementation framework.

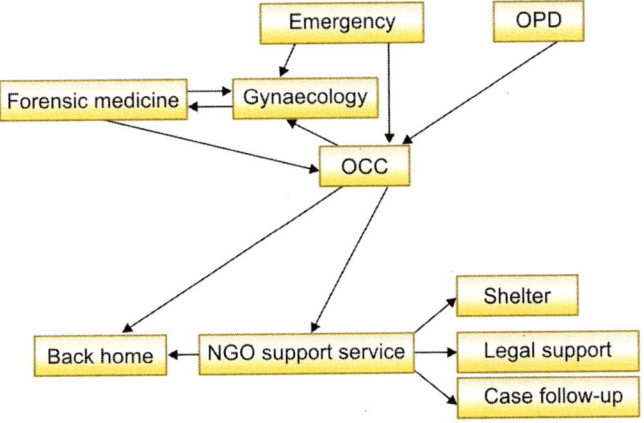

Fig. 12.1: Protocol for sexual assault

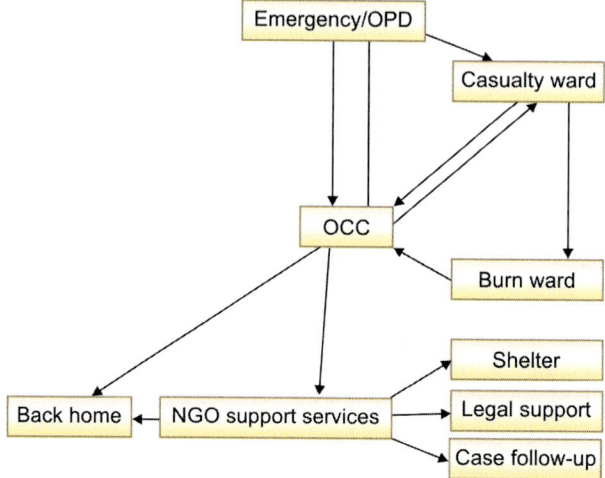

Fig. 12.2: Protocol for burn (VAW)

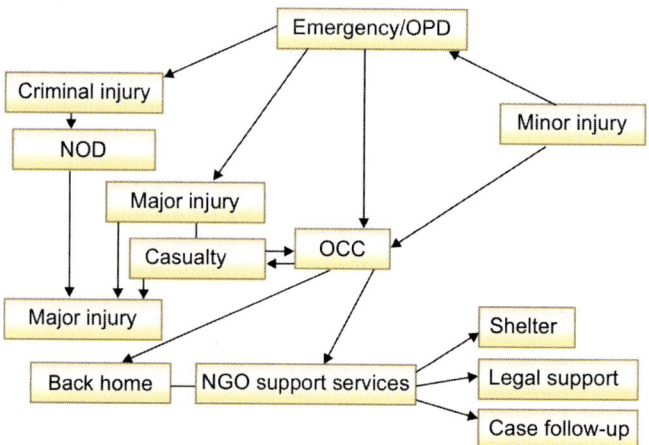

Fig. 12.3: Protocol for domestic violence

BIBLIOGRAPHY

1. Bano S, Balzani M, Siddiqui H, Sharma K, Wilson A, Mitra T, Patel P, Kelly L. Violence against women in South Asian communities: Issues for policy and practice. Jessica Kingsley Publishers; 2009.
2. Bunch C. The intolerable status quo: Violence against women and girls. The progress of nations. 1997;1:41–5.
3. Ellsberg M, Arango DJ, Morton M, Gennari F, Kiplesund S, Contreras M, Watts C. Prevention of violence against women and girls: what does the evidence say? The Lancet. 2015;385(9977):1555–66.
4. Fulu E, Miedema S. Violence against women: globalizing the integrated ecological model. Violence against women. 2015;21(12):1431–55. Bhanot S, Senn CY. Attitudes towards violence against women in men of south Asian ancestry: are acculturation and gender role attitudes important factors? Journal of Family Violence. 2007;22(1):25.
5. García-Moreno C, Riecher-Rössler A. Violence against women and mental health. In violence against women and mental health 2013 (Vol. 178, pp. 167–174). Karger Publishers.
6. Hester M. Future trends and developments: Violence against women in Europe and East

Asia. Violence against women. 2004; 10(12): 1431–48.

7. Ina R, Thomas LS. Health consequences of sexual violence against women. Best Practice & Research Clinical Obstetrics and Gynaecology. 2013;27(1): 15–26.

8. Jejeebhoy SJ, Santhya KG, Acharya R. Violence against women in South Asia: the need for the active engagement of the health sector. Global public health. 2014;9(6):678–90.

9. Khan ME, Townsend JW, Pelto PJ. Sexuality, gender roles, and domestic violence in South Asia. New York: Population Council; 2014.

10. Mehta M. Towards ending violence against women in South Asia. Oxfam International, 2004.

11. Niaz U. Violence against women in South Asia. InViolence against women and mental health 2013 (Vol. 178, pp. 38–53). Karger Publishers.

12. Palermo T, Bleck J, Peterman A. Tip of the iceberg: reporting and gender-based violence in developing countries. American Journal of Epidemiology. 2013;179(5):602–12.

13. Piper N. Feminization of labor migration as violence against women: International, regional, and local nongovernmental organization responses in Asia. Violence Against Women. 2003; 9(6):723–45.

14. Silverman JG, Decker MR, Kapur NA, Gupta J, Raj A. Violence against wives, sexual risk and sexually transmitted infection among Bangladeshi men. Sexually transmitted infections. 2007; 83(3):211–5.

15. Solotaroff JL, Pande RP. Violence against women and girls: Lessons from South Asia. The World Bank; 2014 Sep 4.

16. Terry G. Poverty reduction and violence against women:Exploring links, assessing impact. Development in Practice. 2004;14(4):469–80.

13

Special Situations Violating Women's Rights

Uma Pandey, Ruchika Garg, Neharika Malhotra Bora

INTRODUCTION

South Asia is the most populated and one of the poorest regions of the world. It faces huge socioeconomic and health challenges. One of the most important challenges is gender inequality and violence against women which is pervasive in the region and is associated with the region's cultural incorporation of patriarchal norms.

The current situation is still influenced by the old cultural norms which have prevailed since the longest of times and which perpetuate the secondary position of women in the society. In the region women have to suffer serious consequence both physical and mental due to the aggressive behavior of men. Practices which depreciate and endanger the life and health of the women include son preference, dowry deaths, honor killings, female circumcision, sati and marriage to Quran.

Traditionally there is emphasis on male dominance with a male member being a head of the family. Then women are financially dependent on men and female autonomy is not encouraged. Even in the present day and age, women are deprived of their legal rights. They have to bow to discriminatory laws and social injustice. The scenario is changing but at a snail's pace.

In this chapter some practices prevalent in the region are discussed such as *sati*, rape, honor killing, dowry and female genital mutilation.

SATI

Sati means the burning or burying alive of any widow along with the body of her deceased husband or any other relative or with anything or article associated with husband or such relative, or any woman along with the body of any of her relatives. Such burning or burying may either be voluntary or otherwise.

In this age of ascending feminism and focus on equality and human rights, it is difficult to assimilate the Hindu practice of *sati*, the burning to death of a widow on her husband's funeral pyre, into our modern world. Indeed, the practice is outlawed and illegal in today's India, yet it occurs up to the present day and is still regarded by some Hindus as the ultimate form of womanly devotion and sacrifice. *Sati* (also called suttee) is the practice among some Hindu communities by which a recently widowed woman either voluntarily or by use of force or coercion commits suicide as a result of her husband's death. The best known form of *sati* is when a woman burns to death on her husband's funeral pyre. However other forms of sati exist, including being buried alive with the husband's corpse and drowning.

The term *sati* is derived from goddess Sati, also known as Dakshayani, who self-immolated because she was unable to bear her father Daksha's humiliation of her (living) husband Shiva. *Sati* as practice is first mentioned in 510 CCE, when a stele commemorating such an incident was erected at Eran, an ancient city in the modern state of Madhya Pradesh. The custom began to grow in popularity as evidenced by the number of stones placed to commemorate satis, particularly in southern India and amongst the higher castes of Indian society, despite the fact that the Brahmins originally condemned the practice.

Over the centuries the custom died out in the south only to become prevalent in the north, particularly in the states of Rajasthan and Bengal. While comprehensive data are lacking across India and through the ages, the British East India Company recorded that the total figure of known occurrences for the period 1813–1828 was 8,135; another source gives the number of 7,941 from 1815–1828, an average of 618 documented incidents per year. However, these numbers are likely to grossly underestimate the real number of *satis*.

A few rulers of India tried to ban this custom. The Mughals tried to ban it. The British, due to the efforts of Hindu reformers like Raja Ram Mohan Roy outlawed this custom in 1829.

There are not exact figures about the number of *Sati* incidences. In general, before this custom was outlawed in 1829, there were a few hundred officially recorded incidences each year. Even after the custom was outlawed, this custom did not vanish completely. It took few decades before this custom almost vanished. But still there are rare incidences in which the widow demands to voluntary commit *sati*. In 1987 an eighteen years old widow committed Sati in a village of Rajasthan with the blessing of her family members. In this incidence the villagers took part in the ceremony, praising and supporting the widow for her act. In October 1999 a woman hysterically jumped on her husband's pyre surprising everyone. But this incidence was declared suicide and not *sati*, because this woman was not compelled, forced or praised to commit this act.

In different communities of India, *sati* was performed for different reasons and different

manners. In communities where the man was married to one wife, the wife put an end to her life on the pyre. But even in these communities not all widows committed *Sati*. Those women who committed *Sati* were highly honored and their families were given a lot of respect. It was believed that the woman who committed *Sati* blessed her family for seven generations after her. Temples or other religious shrines were built to honor the *Sati*.

In communities where the ruler was married to more than one wife; in some cases only one wife was allowed to commit *Sati*. This wife was normally the preferred wife of the husband. This was some kind of honor for the chosen wife and some kind of disgrace for the other wives. In other communities some or all of the wives and mistresses were immolated with the husband. And in some cases even male servants were immolated with the kings. This kind of *Sati* in which the wives and servants were treated as the ruler's property.

In some very rare incidences mothers committed *sati* on their son's pyre and in even more rare cases husbands committed *sati* on their wives pyres.

Sati is a malpractice which is still prevalent in a few regions. We cannot turn a blind eye to it. The idea of *sati* should be curbed and never praised. In modern societies like ours even a single victim of *sati* pratha brings a huge shame to society.

FEMALE GENITAL MUTILATION

Female genital mutilation (FGM) is internationally recognized as a violation of the human rights of girls and women, reflecting deep-rooted inequality between the sexes. FGM is mostly carried out on minors, it is also a violation of the rights of children. It involves partial or total removal of the external female genitalia, or other injury to the female genital organs like piercing.

A major reason is believed to ensure the girl conforms to key social norms, such as those related to sexual restraint, femininity, respectability and maturity.

Fertility enhancement, social acceptance and preservation of virginity are some of the reasons for its conduct. In India such operations usually take place in the Mullanis house, and those who practice it are given permission from the clergy of Dwoodi Bohra sect. Bohra community in Pakistan also practices it. This is taught to young girls as a normal process of growing up. The women are made to believe that FGM is necessary to ensure acceptance by their community and are unaware that FGM is not practiced in most of the world. Family honour, increasing sexual pleasure for the male are attributed as the reasons for conducting it.

Women are either too afraid or too embarrassed to raise their voice against such oppression. The girl's circumcision has been kept an absolute secret not only from outsides but also from the men of the community.

Many health complications like severe bleeding, tetanus, infections and some cases of frigidity as it is performed with a razor are some of its consequences and the perpetrators often used abeer or kapurkanchi powder mixed with silk thread ashes to put over the clitoris after cutting takes place for its cooling effect and for its adhesive value which is totally unhygienic. The other health hazards include severe pain and shock, complications in pregnancy and childbirth, sexual dysfunction, difficulties in menstruation and psychological damages among many consequences. In addition to these there are considerable psychosexual, psychological and social consequences of FGM. Women undergone this barbaric practice of FGM faced a significantly greater risk of requiring a Cesarean section, an episiotomy and an extended hospital stay, and also of suffering postpartum hemorrhage. Women who have undergone infibulation suffer from prolonged and obstructed labor, sometimes resulting in fetal death and obstetric fistula. The infants of mothers who have undergone more extensive forms of FGM are at an increased risk of dying at birth.

There is also a high risk of HIV transmission in the women undergone the process. Because the procedure is coupled with blood loss, and because one instrument is often used for a number of operations, FGM increases the risk of HIV transmission. This is particularly the case in communities where a large group of girls are cut the same day as part of a socio-cultural rite.

Legal sanctions against FGM are the most common type of intervention at the national and international levels but there is strong evidence that laws alone are not enough. Nevertheless, legislation creates an enabling environment for interventions at the local.

Reducing gender discrimination, improving social justice and supporting human rights, community development, and empowerment and literacy among women and girls might see fall in the brutal practice.

Rape

"Our society is one not of spectacle but of surveillance."

Under sexual assault comes molestation, eve-teasing, child sex abuse, rape, marital rape, domestic violence of all these crimes, rape is the most heinous crime which is committed against women. Rape means an unlawful intercourse done by a man with a woman without her valid consent. Rape outrages a woman's modesty. After a rape incident, a woman lives a pathetic life which includes fear, depression, guilt complex, suicidal action and social stigma. It appears that the rapists are not scared of laws. Also, cases are being reported where minors and elderly women are being raped. Stigmatizing the victim and encouraging the victim to compromise gives a further impetus to this horrendous crime. They are encouraged to marry their rapist by telling them that nobody will marry them now and it will bring shame to her family. There may be several multitude sexual offences unreported. In majority incidents, the aggrieved women and parents do not want to publish such news and do not want to complain to the police with a fear that the reporting to the police and publishing in newspapers would further cause low-degradation and shame in the society.

Rape is not only physical but also psychological. The victim is mentally and emotionally scarred for life. It causes permanent aversion to sexual behavior and social awkwardness. Victims may feel numb and disorganized. They often feel detachment from their life and people leading to poor social, academic and occupational functioning. Victim also experience post-traumatic stress disorder. Rape victim may hide the incidence from her society and/or from her family to avoid social and marital rejection. Shock, denial, confusion, anger, irritability, mood swings, fear, guilt, anxiety, shame, self-blame or suicidal thoughts may follow rape. Rape victim is physically, emotionally and socially challenged. Therefore, while treating a rape victim it should always be addressed.

GENDER-BASED UNSAFE ABORTION

Gender discrimination works to the disadvantage of girls, even prior to birth. Female infanticide refers to deliberate termination of a pregnancy, following the diagnosis of a female fetus on board. This tragedy is prevalent in many SAFOG countries. India has one of the highest female infanticide numbers in the world and selective abortions based on the diagnosis of a female fetus. During the period 1991–2011, the child sex ratio (0–6 years) declined from 945 to 914. Maternal mortality is a key indicator of women's health and social status. A 2014 systematic analysis of worldwide data estimates that approximately 8% of all maternal deaths are attributable to unsafe abortion and related complications. Unsafe abortion is defined by WHO as "a procedure for terminating an unwanted pregnancy either by persons lacking the necessary skills or in an environment lacking minimal medical standards or both." While maternal mortality rates have declined, the proportion of maternal deaths attributable to these complications has remained relatively constant over the past decade. Unsafe abortion is commonly carried out by women self-administering unapproved and typically ineffective drugs or taking approved drugs incorrectly; these types of abortion attempts often result in incomplete abortion and further complications. Providers who have medical training but lack specific training in abortion procedures are another source of unsafe abortions. Additionally, traditional providers without any medical training may use sticks, roots, herbal medicines or other unsafe and ineffective means for terminating a pregnancy, but the prevalence of these methods seems to have declined considerably in recent years. D&C remains a common abortion method, although there has been an encouraging transition to EVA, MVA and medical methods in recent years. Especially if performed by an untrained person or under unhygienic conditions, D&C is more likely to result in post-abortion complications than these less invasive methods. It is important to note that safety of abortion does not correspond directly with its legal status: While most legal abortions (those performed by certified providers at approved facilities) are likely safe, illegal abortions may be either safe or unsafe, depending largely upon the provider's training and where the abortion is done.

KARO-KARI

Karo-Kari is a type of premeditated honor killing, practiced in rural and tribal areas of Sindh, Pakistan. These are primarily committed against women who according to them have brought dishonor to their family by engaging in illicit pre-marital or extra-marital relations. To restore this honor, a male family member kills her. Although legally proscribed, socio-cultural factors and gender role expectations have given legitimacy to Karo-Kari within some tribal communities. In addition to its persistence in areas of Pakistan, there is evidence that Karo-Kari may be practiced in other parts of the world due to migration. Moreover, perpetrators of honor killings often have motives outside of female adultery. Analysis of the socio-cultural and psycho-pathological factors associated with the practice of Karo-Kari can guide the development of prevention strategies.

DOWRY

One of the worst social crimes thriving in our country and in South Asia is "Dowry System". It is badly influencing most of the parents who have given birth to a girl child. And this crime has also become the reason of another cruel crime of "Female Feticide". The system of dowry takes place where groom's family are greedy and want to do a business deal with bride's family and demands cash, vehicle, clothes, gold, furniture, appliances, utensils or other things on the cost of their son and they name it "wedding ceremony". They have forgotten the pure and sacred feelings of wedding and just have made it as a business deal.

Results of Dowry System

It is quite obvious that result of Dowry system has been always very bad for all and further it will be more dangerous.

1. Till now several baby girls are killed before birth as their parents don't want to have burden of a girl child, because at the time of their daughter's wedding they have to give dowry to the groom side.
2. Bride's parents are forced to sale their house, agriculture fields or other expensive properties to get rid of the debt which they had taken at the time of their daughters

wedding to fulfil the demands of groom side.
3. Accidental incidents like suicide or burning happens with the bride when her parents could not be able to fulfil the unlimited demands by her husband's parents or relatives.

Solutions to this Problem

Solutions for this unacceptable problem are:
1. Firstly the law against this crime should be strict and rigid with no concession.
2. Women education and empowerment is must for preventing this crime.
3. Awareness by advertisements and campaigns should be spread all over country to tell people about the hazardous effects of this crime.
4. Women should take stand against this illogical demand by groom side.

One of the worst crimes that is arising its head in most of the communities during wedding is "dowry system", that is completely nonacceptable for all. One side we say that boys and girls are equal in all matter and girls are not less than boys; on the other side, we make such a huge difference between them at the time of their marriage when boy's parents have right to demand dowry from bride side and bride side is forced to fulfil their demand at any cost. If we want to be called successful and developed, then dowry system should be completely abolished.

BIBLIOGRAPHY

1. Abortion Law Reform in Nepal: Women's Right to Life and Health. G Shakya, S Kishore, C Bird, Jr Barak. An intl J on sexual and reprod health and rights. 2004;12 (Issue sup 24):75–84.
2. Achievements of the FIGO Initiative for the Prevention of Unsafe Abortion and its Consequences in South-Southeast Asia. S Zaidi, F Begum, J Tank, P Chaudhary, H Yasmeen, M Dissanayake. Int J of Gynae Obs. 2014. 126(1). 520–23.

3. Challenging assumptions about women's empowerment: Social and economic resources and domestic violence among young married women in urban South India. CH Rocca, S Rathod, T Falle, RP Pande, S Krishnan. Int J of Epidemiology. 2009;38(2);577–85, https://doi.org/10.1093/ije/dyn226

4. Conflict in the Indian Kashmir Valley I: exposure to violence. Kd Jong, N Ford, S Kam, K Lokuge, S Fromm, R Galen, B Reilley, R Kleber. Confl Health. 2008;2:10. PMCID: PMC257518

5. Current global status of female genital mutilation: A review. GAO Magoha, OB Magoha. East Afric Med J. 2000;77(5):268–72.

6. Dowry in 21st-Century India: The Sociocultural Face of Exploitation. PR Banerjee. Trauma, Violence, and Abuse. J 2013 https://doi.org/10.1177/15248380134 96334

7. Dowry in Bangladesh: A Search from an International Perspective for an Effective Legal Approach to Mitigate. A Begum. J of Int Women's Studies. 2014;15(2):249–67. http://vc.bridgew.edu/jiws/vol15/iss2/1

8. Female genital mutilation in Pakistan, and beyond. A Chohan. August 18, 2011. https://blogs.tribune.com.pk/story/752 3/female-genital-mutilation-inpakistan- and-beyond/

9. Female Genital Mutilation: Many Pakistani women's painful secret. F Zahidi. February 6, 2013. https://blogs.tribune.com.pk/story/159 79/female-genital-mutilation-manypakistani-womens-painful-secret/

10. Female Genital Mutilation: Secret Practice in India. S Nazeer. Int J Scientific and Research Publications. 2017;7(7):341. ISSN 2250–3153.

11. Honour Killing in Pakistan. A Malik Am J of Criminal Law. 20 Mar 2014. https://papers.ssrn.com/sol3/pa pers.cfm?abstract_id=2411680

12. https://en.qantara.de/content/rape-in-india-and-pakistan-endemic-misogyny

13. Karo Kari: The murder of honour in Sindh Pakistan: An ethnographic study. Bhanbhro, Sadiq, Wassan, MR Shah, Muhbat, Talpur, Ashfaq A, A Ali. http://shura.shu.ac.uk/7287/

14. Karo-Kari: A Form of Honour Killing in Pakistan. S Patel, AM Gadit. Transcult Psychiatry 2008; 45(4):683–94.

15. Menstrual regulation, unsafe abortion, and maternal health in Bangladesh. A Hossain, I Maddow-Zimet, S Singh, L Remez. Europe PMC. 2012(3):1–8.

16. Rape in Rural Bangladesh. N Ali, S Akhter, N Hossain, N Khan. Delta Med College J. 2015;3(1):31–5.

17. Ray of hope: Opportunities for reducing unsafe abortions! SS Khowaja, A Pasha, S Begum, MN Mustafa. JPMA. 2013.Vol. 63(1).

18. Sati Problem: Past and present. SK Pachauri. Journal of Indian Law Institute. Vol.45(2) (April-June 2003):253–61.

19. Sati Tradition - Widow Burning In India: A Socio-Legal Examination. January 2009. www.researchgate.net/publication/23 7707719_Sati_Tradition_-_Widow_Burning_In_India_A_Socio-Legal_Examination

20. Sati: A review article. W Menskt. Bulletin of the School of Oriental and African Studies/Volume 61/Issue 01/February 1998.p 74–81 DOI:10.1017/S0041977X00015767, Published online: 05 February 2009 Link to this article: http://journals.cambridge.org/abstract_S0041977X 00015767

21. Social change and the family: Comparative perspectives from the west, China, and South Asia. AT Thomas, E Fricke. Sociological Forum. 1987;2(4);746–79.

22. Violence against women in Pakistan: A framework for analysis. PA Ali. MIC Bustamante. JPMA 2008;58(4):198–203.

23. Women's mental health in Pakistan. U Niaz. World Psychiatry 2004;3(1):60–62.

14

Unsafe Abortion—Where Do We Stand?

Mriganka Mouli Saha, Asma Mushtaq

BACKGROUND

An unsafe abortion is the termination of a pregnancy by people lacking the necessary skills, or in an environment lacking minimal medical standards, or both. For example, an unsafe abortion may be an extremely dangerous life-threatening procedure that is self-induced in unhygienic conditions, or it may be a much safer abortion performed by a medical practitioner who does not provide appropriate post-abortion attention.

South Asia (Bangladesh, India, Nepal, Pakistan, and Sri Lanka) is home to 28% of the world's people and accounts for about a third (30%) of the world's maternal deaths. Thirteen percent of all maternal deaths in South Asia are attributed to complications of unsafe abortion and are almost entirely preventable.

Restrictive laws hamper safe abortion in most of the region, but even where laws are more liberal, limited awareness of the law has been a barrier to access. Such health system barriers as an insufficient number of trained providers, inequitable distribution of services, and excessive costs have contributed to death from unsafe abortion.

Disease burden in South-Asian countries and situation analysis: During 2010–2014, an estimated 35.5 million induced abortions occurred each year in Asia. The annual rate of abortion for the region is an estimated 36 per 1,000 women of reproductive age (15–44), which is down slightly from 41 per 1,000 in 1990–1994. The regional abortion rate is roughly 36 per 1,000 for married women and 24 per 1,000 for unmarried women. Abortion rates in four of Asia's five subregions (Eastern, Southern, Southeastern and Western) are close to the overall regional rate; the rate in Central Asia is higher (42 per 1,000 women). The proportion of all pregnancies in Asia ending in abortion each year, estimated at 27% in 2010–2014, has remained roughly the same since 1990–1994; by subregion, the proportion ranges from 22% in Western Asia to 33% in Eastern Asia.

It is estimated that around 6 million abortions occur annually in India out of which two million are spontaneous and the rest are induced. Only 15 % of those are legal and rest are performed illegally. Unsafe abortions account for 8% of all maternal deaths in India. 60% of these are in the age group of 15–24 years.

ABORTION LAWS AND CURRENT SITUATION

In an attempt to safeguard against indiscriminate abortion, different laws have been implemented in different south Asian countries. After introduction of Medical Termination Act (MTP) in 1972 in India, reported cases of MTP have been raised significantly. Authorized MTP centers have increased from 1877 in 1976 to 7121 in 1991. Similarly the number of MTP cases have been raised from 25 reported cases in the year 1972–73 to 15.6 million cases in 2015–16 in India.

Till 1997 abortion was permitted only to save the life of the mother in Pakistan. The situation changed when Commission of Inquiry for Women was appointed by the government of Pakistan, which recommended that " women's right to obtain an abortion by her own choice within the first 120 days of pregnancy be unambiguously declared an absolute right "Past time, the unmet need for family planning in Pakistan was quiet high and use of contraceptive methods was not so much popular. Data retrieved from a 2012 national study focusing on abortion-care with related complications estimated that there were 2.2 million abortions in Pakistan in 2012, an annual rate of 50 per 1,000 women. Earlier study demonstrated an abortion rate of 27 per 1,000 women in 2002.

Unfortunately, the abortion rate has likely increased substantially between 2002 and 2012. Contraceptive-use patterns and abortion rates varies among the provinces, with higher rates in Baluchistan and Sindh than in Khyber Pakhtunkhwa and Punjab. Actually strategies for coping with uniformly high unintended pregnancy rates will differ among provinces.

Previously Bangladesh law has allowed abortion only to save the life of the mother.

The government has recognized the role of comprehensive abortion care in the eve of rapid population growth. Data from the Bangladesh Fertility Survey provides a unique framework for discussion of current attitude towards and prevalence of abortion in Bangladesh. The Bangladesh Fertility Survey (BFS) was conducted on a nationally representative sample survey where 88% of Bangladeshi women approved of abortion if the woman had conceived as a result of rape and premarital sex. Danger to mother's life is a more acceptable basis for abortion in 53% cases, followed by malformed child (30%). Abortion due to economic reasons was acceptable to only 17% of women.

Educated couples were more liberal found to be more approving of abortion than the less educated. Around 646,600 induced abortions were conducted in Bangladesh in 2010, which indicates an annual rate of 18 abortions per 1,000 women in reproductive age. The abortion rate is comparable with the national average in Dhaka and Sylhet, whereas higher than average in Rajshahi and Khulna, lower than average in Chittagong and very low in Barisal. The abortion rate in Bangladesh is higher than the estimated ratio for South-central Asia in 2008 (26 per 100).

Before 2002, the law to perform abortion in Nepal was highly reserved only for saving the life of a woman. Unsafe form of abortion was more common, and maternal mortality from abortion-complications was accountable for most of maternal deaths in major hospitals. Honorable Supreme Court of Nepal legalized the right of women to terminate a pregnancy at up to 12 weeks of gestation on demand and up to 18 weeks of gestation where it resulted from rape or incest. In the year of 2014, Nepal had 323,100 abortions out of which 137,000 were only legal, and 63,200 women were treated for abortion complications.

Overall the abortion rate in Nepal is 42 per 1,000 women aged 15–49 years, and the ratio is 56 per 100 live births currently. The abortion rate in the central Nepal is relatively higher which is 59 per 1,000 live birth than the national average.

In spite of nation-wide freely available contraception is in Sri Lanka, the absolute number of illegal abortions is growing on the top. In a report by Health Ministry stated that, daily over 500 abortions are being performed in Colombo. Sri Lanka is restrictive on abortion law and strict enforcement which resulting avoidance in giving information by the women for abortions. It is also difficult to determine the actual prevalence rate for illegal abortions. It has been estimated a decade ago that 125,000 to 175,000 abortions among which mostly are illegal, performed in a year. Recently it has been reported that much higher rate of induced abortions per day amounting to

240,170 per year, contributing an abortion ratio of 741 per 1000 live births. Unfortunately illegal abortion contributes to 12.5% of all maternal deaths which is the third most common cause of maternal death in Sri Lanka.

Afghanistan is leading with the highest birth rate in Asia. On an average, an Afghan woman has approximately six children throughout the course of their reproductive lives. Most of the women lack the necessary education to find out about the various methods of birth control. According to UNICEF, approximately 79 % of women in Afghanistan do not use birth control. Unsafe abortions in the Maldives was evaluated in 2008 by International Planned Parenthood Federation (IPPF), which found that abortion is commonly seen amongst unmarried youth than married couples. It has been also intercepted that abortion is "a risk-free procedure" which is viewed as a "safe alternative to contraception". It is evident that abortion is frequently sought by young unmarried Maldivian women as a solution. Penal Code of Bhutan does not legalize abortion unless it is caused due to rape, mother critically ill and mentally challenged. In the year 1999, Ministry of Health and Education regularized the "Medical Termination of Pregnancy" (MTP) as law where opinion of two medical practitioners is required. The number of abortion for medical termination is reported very low as per hospital data. Strong adherence to social beliefs and women's acceptance of children born out of wedlock is an important issue. Recently increasing number of Bhutanese women are seeking unsafe abortion in the neighboring areas of India.

CONSEQUENCES OF UNSAFE ABORTION

Induced abortion is medically *safe* when WHO-recommended methods are used by trained persons, *less safe* when only one of those two criteria is met and *least safe* when neither is met.

In 2012, approximately eight per 1,000 women of reproductive age in Asia (excluding Eastern Asia) were treated for complications from unsafe abortion. In all, about 4.6 million women in the region are treated for such complications each year. In 2014, at least 6% of all maternal deaths (or 5,400 deaths) in Asia were from unsafe abortion. The majority of women with an unwanted pregnancy usually contact close friends or go to traditional healers. They may otherwise find and take the non-recommended, abortifacient such as castor oil or some forms of herbs. This may either prove to be successful or result in disastrous situations such as hemorrhage, shock, infections, sepsis, perforations, organ failure, chronic pelvic inflammatory disease, infertility, or even death. The unethical and unlawful practice by health care providers or traditional untrained and unskilled healers, supplemented by poor hygiene standards and lack of expertise, have caused major complications.

Unsafe abortion has negative consequences beyond its immediate effects on individual women's health. Treating complications from unsafe abortion increases the economic burden on poor families and incurs considerable costs to already struggling public health systems. The extent to which medication abortion is used to induce abortions in Asia is not known; however, evidence indicates that sales of these drugs have increased in the region in the past decade.

The most common complications from unsafe abortion are incomplete abortion, excessive blood loss and infection. Uterine perforation with or without intestinal involvement is also well-known complication.

Most of the abortions occur in the first trimester, during which the uterus is placed in the pelvis in proximity to the sigmoid colon and rectum, making them more susceptible to injury. With the increasing size of the uterus, the small bowel becomes more prone to injury during unsafe abortion.

Some women with untreated complications experience long-term health consequences, such as chronic pain, inflammation of the reproductive tract, pelvic inflammatory disease and infertility. Poor and rural women are the most likely to experience an unsafe abortion and severe complications thereof.

SIGNS AND SYMPTOMS REQUIRING IMMEDIATE TREATMENT

Initial assessment of patient is mandatory for appropriate treatment and referral to proper health facility so that complications should be managed accurately. Following sign and symptoms need immediate attention and management:

- Pain in abdomen
- Excessive or abnormal vaginal bleeding
- Fever
- Foul smelling purulent vaginal discharge
- Shock (collapse of the circulatory system)

Sometimes difficulty in diagnosing complications occurs as a woman with ectopic pregnancy may present history of unsafe abortion and symptoms of incomplete abortion. So health care provider should be prepared to refer such patients to health facility where a definitive diagnosis can be made and patient can be managed with standard and quick care.

Treatment

In case of hemorrhage treatment of heavy blood loss should be on emergency basis with replacement of blood and blood products. Delay at this step can lead to DIC and multiple organ failure.

Infection should be treated with broad spectrum antibiotics and if there possibility of retained product of conception manual vacuum aspiration (MVA) should be done under antibiotic cover as soon as possible.

If injury to genital tract is observed repair should be considered. Appropriate level of health care involvement is needed if injury to internal organ such as intestine urinary system is suspected. Responsibility of health care providers regarding treatment for abortion complications.

Regardless the legal status for abortion, its obligation of health care providers to provide life-saving medical care to any woman who suffers abortion-related complications, includes treatment of complications from unsafe abortion. The practice of extracting confessions from women emergency medical care as a result of illegal abortion puts women's lives at risk. The legal requirement for doctors and other health care personnel to report cases of women who have undergone abortion, delays care and increases the risks to women's health and lives. UN human rights standards call on countries to provide immediate and unconditional treatment to anyone seeking emergency medical care.

Reasons to Choose Unsafe Abortion?

There are certain reasons why female have to choose for unsafe abortions.

Strict Laws

Before 1997, abortion was only allowed to save the life of the woman, but in 1997, the law was amended to allow abortion in early pregnancy not only to save the life of the woman but also to provide necessary treatment.

Personal Believes of Health Professionals

Health professionals are known to refuse termination on the basis of their own personal beliefs (either ethically or religiously driven). It has been suggested that doctors who feel ambivalence about providing abortion services undergo a values clarification and attitude transformation exercise; hence, they should be able to separate their personal beliefs from their professional responsibilities of saving women's lives. According to the Federation of International of Gynecologists and Obstetricians (FIGO) Resolution 2006, doctors who refuse termination on the basis of conscientious objection are still under ethical obligation to refer women to safe services and provide the service themselves in case of an emergency.

OVERBURDENED HEALTH FACILITIES

In 2012, almost 6.2 million women have been treated for post-abortion complications in both the public and private sectors. This rate is quite high when compared with other neighboring third-world countries. The poor state of public health facilities in Pakistan, apart from the rapidly increasing population, has exerted pressure on state institutions. This has allowed the private sector to step in and provide health care to the majority of the population of these mismanaged cases were treated by unskilled individuals, such as midwives who are not even licensed to handle such cases.

LOW SOCIOECONOMIC CONDITIONS

The low socioeconomic status of people has urged them to seek cheap medical services, which has contributed to the increased frequency of complications related to abortion. The workload on the public sector and the cost-related issues of good quality in the private sector has also encouraged people to look for alternate options. Even if treated by professionals, one cannot be sure about the standard of facilities that the private sector offers, particularly in rural areas.

UNINTENDED PREGNANCY AND UNMET NEED

By 2017 almost 132 million women of re-productive age in Asia have an unmet need for modern contraception, that is, they want to avoid pregnancy but are either not practicing contraception or are using traditional methods, which are less effective than modern methods.

Most women who have an abortion do so because they become pregnant when they do not intend to. As of 2010–2014, the rate of unintended pregnancies in Asia is 54 per 1,000 women aged 15–44. An estimated 53.8 million unintended pregnancies occur each year in Asia. Of these, nearly two-thirds (65%) end in abortion.

Lacking Women Empowerment

Right of male relatives to make reproductive decisions, the strong social stigma against extramarital pregnancy also put women at risk of unsafe abortion. Women either have no knowledge of family planning services or they cannot opt any method of contraception independently without asking their husbands.

PREVENTION AND CONTROL

Prevention of unintended pregnancies must always be given the highest priority and every attempt should be made to eliminate the need for abortion. Women who have unintended pregnancies should have ready access to reliable information and counseling. Any measures or changes related to abortion within the health system can only be determined at the national or local level according to the national legislative process. In circumstances where abortion is not against the law, such abortion should be safe.

All women should have access to quality services for management of post-abortion complications. Post-abortion counseling, education and family-planning services should be offered promptly, which will also help to avoid repeat abortions. Unsafe abortion can be prevented through:

- Use of effective contraception, including emergency contraception
- Comprehensive sexuality education
- Prevention of unintended pregnancy through
- Provision of safe, legal abortion.

According to WHO, use of pharmacological measures and manual vacuum aspiration

(MVA) to terminate pregnancy should be promoted.

Mortality and morbidity from unsafe abortion can be reduced through the timely provision of emergency treatment of complications.

The positive attitude of health providers is very important to reduce the impact of unsafe abortion. Provision of contraceptive methods should be readily available at the same site where post-abortion care of termination of pregnancy is provided. This will help to prevent repetition of abortion.

RECOMMENDATIONS

Policies that improve knowledge, access and use of contraceptive methods must be implemented to reduce unintended pregnancies, abortions or unplanned births.

The provision and quality of post-abortion care should be improved and expanded to reduce illness and death from unsafe abortion. Need for increasing provider training along with improving availability of PAC equipment and medicines. Public facilities in particular lack essential components for providing PAC services, such as MVA kits, disinfection equipment, and trained providers available around the clock.

The grounds for legal abortion should be broadened and access to safe abortion services should be improved to reduce the number of clandestine procedures and the negative consequences.

Standard service provision guidelines must be adopted. Health care providers must be trained and governments must be committed to ensure that safe abortion services are available.

Safe abortion must be provided or supported by a trained person using WHO recommended methods appropriate for the pregnancy duration.

Almost every abortion death and disability can be prevented through sexuality education, use of effective contraception, provision of safe legal induced abortion, and timely care for post-abortion complications.

BIBLIOGRAPHY

1. Ahmad R. Attitude towards induced abortion in Bangladesh. Bangladesh Dev Stud. 1979;7(4): 97–108.
2. Augustin G, Majerovic' M, Luetic' T: Uterine perforation as a complication of surgical abortion causing small bowel obstruction: a review. Arch Gynecol Obstet. 2013,288:311-323.10.1007/s00404-013-2749-4
3. Badakali MA, Kalburgi EB, Goudar BV, Pujari LL: Entero-uterine fistula: a rare complication of an unsafe abortion. J Clin Diagn Res. 2012;6:1301–2.
4. Bulletin of the World Health Organization. Infant and under-five mortality in Afghanistan: current estimates and limitations. https://www.who.int/bulletin/volumes/88/8/09-068957/en/ (accessed on Feb 22, 2019).
5. Chavkin W: Conscientious objection to the provision of reproductive healthcare. Int J Gynaecol Obstet. 2013,123:39–40. 10.1016/S0020- 7292(13) 00601-2.
6. Choden J, Pem R, Pathak A. Prevalence, determinants and outcomes of unplanned pregnancy and perspectives on termination of pregnancy among women in Nganglam, Bhutan. Bhutan Health Journal 2015;1:30–37.
7. Darroch JE and Ashford LS, Adding It Up: The Costs and Benefits of Investing in Sexual and Reproductive Health 2014, New York: Guttmacher Institute, 2014.
8. De Silva IW. The Practice of Induced Abortion in Sri Lanka. Harword School of Public Health, 1997. Rajapakshe LC. Estimates of Induced Abortion using RRT Technique. Colombo, 2000.
9. Godakanda S. Regional Workshop on FIGO initiative on unsafe abortion. International Federation of Gynecology and Obstetrics (FIGO). Mumbai, 2016.
10. Government of Pakistan. The First Ordinance of the Qisas and Diyat Law. Islamabad, Pakistan: Ministry of Law, Justice and Parliamentary Affairs (Law and Justice Division); 1990.

11. Guttmacher Institute, Adding it up: investing in contraception and maternal and newborn health, 2017, Fact Sheet, New York: Guttmacher Institute, 2017.

12. Henderson JT, et al. Effects of abortion legalization in Nepal, 2001-2010. PLoS One. 2013;8(5): e64775. doi:10.1371/journal.pone. 0064775.

13. http://www1.umn.edu/humanrts/research/ srilanka/statutes/Penal_Code.pdf (accessed on Feb 22, 2019).

14. Huda F et al., Strengthening Health System Capacity to Monitor and Evaluate Programmes Targeted at Reducing Abortion-Related Maternal Mortality, Dhaka: International Centre for Diarrhoeal Disease Research, Bangladesh, 2010.

15. Imoedemhe DA, Ezimokhai M, Okpere EE: Intestinal injuries following induced abortion. Int J Gynaecol Obstet. 1984,22:303–306. 10.1016/0020-7292(84)90087-0

16. Khan A. Induced abortion in Pakistan: Community-based research.J Pak MedAssoc. 2013 Apr; 63(4 Suppl 3):S27–32.

17. Mbele AM, Snyman L, Pattinson RC: Impact of the choice on termination of pregnancy act on maternal morbidity and mortality in the west of Pretoria. S Afr Med J. 2006,96:1196–8.

18. Ministry of Health 2008. Adolescent Health and Development, A country profile. Ministry of Health, Thimphu, Bhutan. MoH (2011) Annual Health Bulletin 2010. Thimphu: Minstry of Health, Royal Goverment of Bhutan.

19. Ministry of Health and Population, New ERA and ICF International. Nepal Demographic and Health Survey 2011. Kathmandu, Nepal: Ministry of Health and Population and New ERA; Calverton, MD, USA: ICF International; 2012.

20. Nasratullah A, et al. Assessing Post-Abortion Care in Health Facilities in Afghanistan: A Cross Sectional Study. BMC Pregnancy and Childbirth 2015;15 (1):1–9.

21. Nepal Ministry of Health. National Safe Abortion Policy. Kathmandu, Nepal: Ministry of Health; 2002.http://www.mohp.gov.np/images/pdf/ policy/National%20abortion%2, accessed on 22.2.19.

22. NIPORT, Bangladesh Maternal Mortality and Health Care Survey 2010.

23. NIPORT, Mitra and Associates, and ORC Macro, Bangladesh Demographic and Health Survey, 1999–2000, Dhaka, Bangladesh: NIPORT and Mitra and Associates; and Calverton, MD, USA: ORC Macro, 2001.

24. Oludran OO, Okonofua FE: Mortality and morbidity from bowel injury secondary to induced abortion. Afr J Reprod Health. 2003,7:65–8.

25. Paul M, Danielsson KG, Essén B, Allvin MK. The importance of considering the evidence in the MTP 2014 Amendment debate in India-unsubstantiated arguments should not impede improved access to safe abortion. Glob Health Action. 2015 Mar 30;8:27512.

26. Peldon S. Should abortion be legalized? Bhutan Observer 2011.

27. Rahman A, Katzive L, Henshaw SK: A global review of laws on induced abortion, 1985-1997. Int Fam Plann Persp. 1998,24:56–64.

28. Safe Abortion: Technical and Policy Guidance for Health Systems, page 12 (World Health Organization 2003): "a procedure for terminating an unwanted pregnancy either by persons lacking the necessary skill or in an environment lacking the minimum medical standards, or both."

29. Saleem S, Fikree FF. The quest for small family size among Pakistani women-is voluntary termination of pregnancy a matter of choice or necessity? J Pak Med Assoc. 2005 Jul;55(7):288–91.

30. Samandari G, et al. Implementation of legal abortion in Nepal: A model for rapid scale-up of high-quality care. Reproductive Health. 2012;9:7. doi: 10.1186/1742-4755-9-7.

31. Sample registration bulletin, maternal mortality in India: 1997–2003. Trends, causes and risk factors. Registrar general India.

32. Sathar Z, Singh S, Rashida G, Shah Z, Niazi R: Induced abortions and unintended pregnancies in Pakistan. Stud Fam Plann. 2014, 45:471–91. 10.1111/j.1728-4465.2014.00004.x

33. Sedgh G, Guttmacher Institute, New York, personal communication, Apr. 26, 2012.

34. Senanayake L, Willatgamuwa S, Moonasinghe L, Tissera S. Unwanted/Unplanned pregnancies and their aftermath. Colombo: The Family Planning Association of Sri Lanka in collaboration with the College of General Practitioners of Sri Lanka, 2012.

35. Serour GI: Ethical guidelines on conscientious objection. FIGO Committee for the Ethical Aspects of Human Reproduction and Women's Health. Int J Gynaecol Obstet. 2006, 92:333-334. 10.1016/j.ijgo. 2005.12.020

36. Siddique S, Hafeez M. Demographic and clinical profile of patients with complicated unsafe abortion. J Coll Physicians Surg Pak. 2007 Apr; 17(4):203–6.

37. Singh S and Maddow-Zimet I, Facility-based treatment for medical complications resulting from unsafe pregnancy termination in the developing world, 2012: A review of evidence from 26 countries, BJOG, 2015, doi:10.1111/1471-0528.13552.

38. Singh S et al. Estimating the level of abortion in the Philippines and Bangladesh, International Family Planning Perspectives, 1997, 23(3):100–7;144.

39. Special tabulations of updated data from Sedge G et al. Abortion incidence between 1990 and 2014: global, regional, and subregional levels and trends, Lancet, 2016,388(10041):258–67.

40. Sri Lanka Penal Code Section 303. University of Menesota,1883.

41. Summary of Key Findings and Implications, Dhaka, Bangladesh: NIPORT, 2011.

42. Thapa PJ, Thapa S, Shrestha N. A hospital-based study of abortion in Nepal. Studies in Family Planning. 1992;23(5):311–8.

43. Thapa S, Sharma SK, Khatiwada N. Women's knowledge of abortion law and availability of services in Nepal. Journal of Biosocial Science. 2014;46(2):266–77.

44. The Maldives Study on Women's Health and Life Experiences, 2007, Ministry of Gender and Family, Maldives/UNFPA/UNICEF/WHO.

45. The Reproductive Health Baseline Survey, Ministry of Health, Maldives/UNFPA, 1999.

46. Unpublished data from Bangladesh Association for Prevention of Septic Abortion (BAPSA), Dhaka, Bangladesh, 2012. Bangladesh Bureau of Statistics (BBS), Report of the Household Income and Expenditure Survey, 2010, Dhaka: BBS, 2012.

47. Unpublished data from Singh S.

48. "Unsafe abortion: Global and regional estimates of the incidence of unsafe abortion and associated mortality in 2003" (PDF). World Health Organization. 2007. Retrieved March 7, 2011. The estimates given in this document are intended to reflect induced abortions that carry greater risk than those carried out officially for reasons accepted in the laws of a country.

49. Winikoff B, Sheldon W. Use of medicines changing the face of abortion, International Perspectives on Sexual and Reproductive Health, 2012, 38(3):164–6.

15

STDs and HIV/AIDS

Ruchika Garg, Narendra Malhotra, Shahlla Kanwal, BB Rewari

Sexually transmitted diseases/infections (STIs) and HIV/AIDS are a major public health concern in South Asia not only because of their high prevalence worldwide but also because of their permanent sequale in untreated patients. After subsaharan Africa this region has the largest burden of disease. There are more than 30 different types of sexually transmitted bacteria, viruses and parasites. Among all these infections, gonorrhea, chlamydia and HIV are most common.

BACKGROUND

The exact data of sexually transmitted infection in South Asia is sparse. WHO estimated that South Asian countries accounted for major proportion of all new STI infections globally in the mid-1990. The incidence and prevalence of curable STIs, particularly ulcerative chancroid and syphilis, were extremely high and closely linked to rapid early spread of HIV in and urban areas and along well-traveled migrant and trucking networks. However, interventions to improve those conditions and increase condom use in sex work led to large STI declines and slowing of HIV epidemics during the 1990s and early 2000s.

Progress in India, which accounts for over two-thirds of the region's population, has likely had the greatest overall impact on regional STI epidemiology over the last 15 years. During this period, large scale interventions to reduce HIV/STI transmission among key and bridging populations documented large STI declines in several populous and highly affected states.

The Epidemiology of STIs in the South Asia Region

Most published STI prevalence data cannot be directly extrapolated to inform general population estimates. While overall global estimates have changed little over twenty years.

The STIs have declined in Sri Lanka. STIs have not been controlled elsewhere, and the situation remains largely unknown, due to insufficient data, in several countries. Evidence of increasing rates of syphilis and other STIs is emerging from a number of Asian countries. Syphilis has declined and eliminating mother to child transmission (MTCT) in some countries, supports feasibility of regional elimination of syphilis.

Syphilis among men having sex with men (MSM) has increased. Combinations of syndromic and etiologic reporting have proven useful in guiding control efforts in several countries. In Sri Lanka and Maldive, microscopy with Gram stain has helped to distinguish gonococcal from non-gonococcal infections.

BRIEF COUNTRY PROFILES OF STIs

Sri Lanka

STIs have been in decline in Sri Lanka. STI, gonorrhea have declined since 2003 and syphilis in 2012, were detected by surveillance, and largely brought back under control.

UNAIDS

According to UNAIDS estimates, about 97,000 people were living with HIV in Pakistan at the end of 2009. Officially reported cases are, however, much lower. As in many countries, underreporting is due mainly to the social stigma attached to HIV, limited surveillance and voluntary counseling and testing systems, and the lack of knowledge among the general population.

Inadequate Blood Transfusion Screening and High Level of Professional Donors

It is estimated that 40 percent of the 1.5 million annual blood transfusions in Pakistan are not screened for HIV. About 20 percent of the blood transfused comes from professional donors.

Large Numbers of Migrants and Refugees and Commercial Sex Workers

World Bank response: The World Bank was the largest financer of HIV/AIDS programs in Pakistan. It assisted the government's HIV/AIDS efforts through funding the second Social Action Program (1998–2003). In addition, the World Bank worked with the government and other development partners (CIDA, DFID, USAID, and UN agencies) to support the government's program through the HIV/AIDS Prevention Project. The Bank provided US$37.1 million, 75 percent of which was a nointerest credit and 25 percent of which was grant money. The project which closed in December 2009 supported HIV prevention services to most at risk groups, mass media campaigns aimed at raising awareness and reducing stigma, promoting safe blood transfusion and building management and institutional capacity.

India

India is accounting for over two-thirds of the population. STI transmission, and the early AIDS epidemic, followed migrant pathways to metro cities. Early efforts focused on the large metropolitan areas. From about 2004 onwards, large-scale efforts were made, first in high-prevalence states (Avahan), then nationwide (NACO). STI prevention, screening and treatment were major program components. Evidence of significant declines of several common curable STIs is there by many surveys.

STI services and reporting also improved considerably during this period. During the FY 2016-17, 8.6 million patients were managed for STI/RTI following national protocols, nearly 95% of NACO target. STI reporting increased from about 65% in 2008-09, to 95% of STI clinics (DSRC) and 85% of KP TI Projects in recent years, but trends are difficult to interpret due to the increased reporting.

Significant declines in syphilis prevalence has been documented from 2005-06 and 2016-17 among DSRC attendees, ANC attendees, KPs and blood donors (Fig. 15.1). HSS 2014-15 reported 0.14% syphilis prevalence among ANC attendees. Yet, syphilis prevalence reported from NHM, based on partial ANC testing coverage (17% of 30 million ANC attendees) is significantly higher (1.5%).

Bangladesh

Patients usually seek care in the private sector or at health facilities run by non-governmental organizations, such as CARE, BRAC Action, Poricharja, and also by Bangladesh Medical Association, Bangladesh Private Medical Practitioners Association. Sex with a sex worker is the main culprit.

Bangladesh acted early to improve HIV/STI prevention among sex workers and clients— to mobilise sex workers. Syphilis prevalence was very high but has declined greatly since the early 2000s (Fig. 15.2).

Nepal

In Nepal, interventions with sex workers started slowly from the mid-1990s with education and condom promotion.

More recent IBBS data (2011) (Fig. 15.3) support apparent stabilisation of HIV among

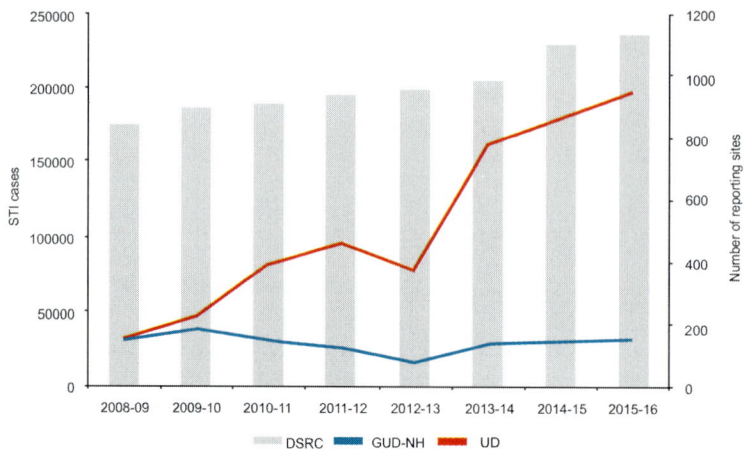

(a) Rising UD and falling GUD as DSRC attendance and reporting picked up

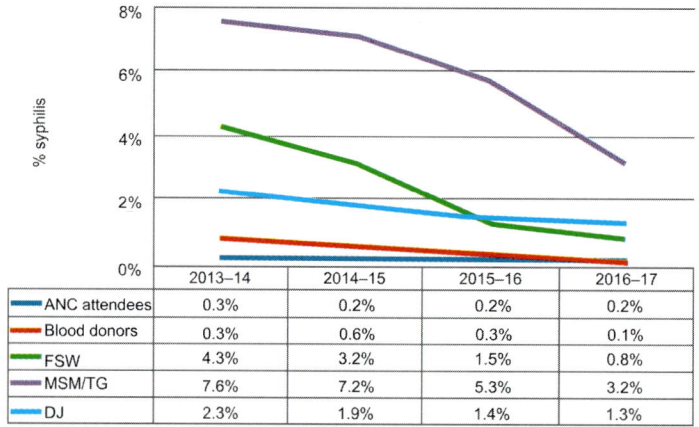

(b) Declining syphilis prevalence KPs among general population

Fig. 15.1: India: Increased STI reporting (DSRC) and declining syphilis prevalence

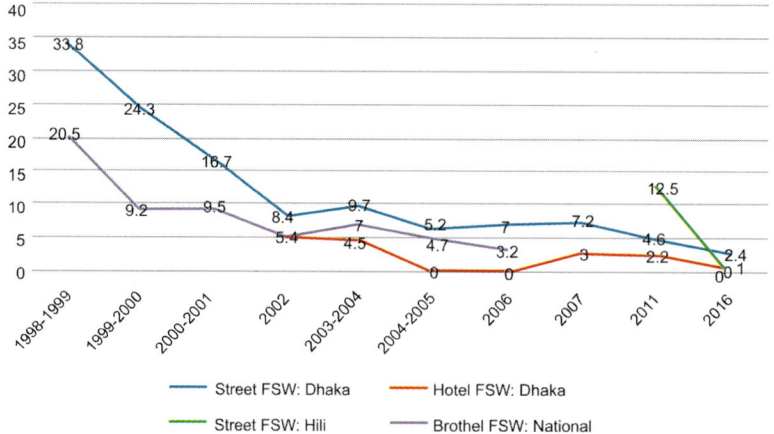

Fig. 15.2: Declining prevalence of active syphilis among sex workers in Bangladesh

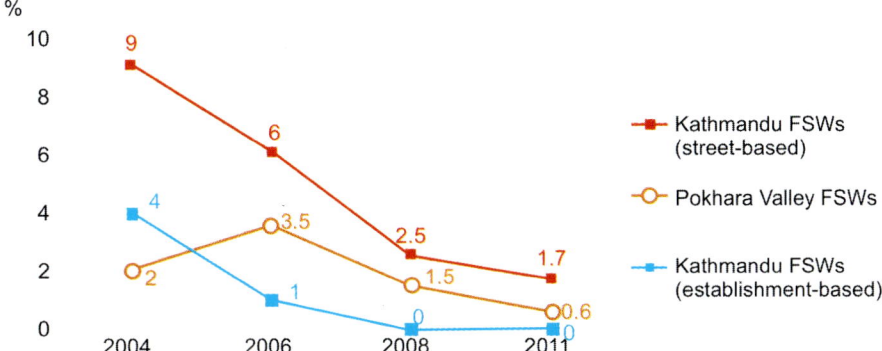

Fig. 15.3: Active syphilis prevalence among female sex workers in Kathmandu and Pokhara Valley, 2004–2011 (*Source; S/C p. 209*)

sex workers at around 2% in the same regions as reported condom use has risen and syphilis continues to decline. Large reductions in gonorrhea have been documented.

Maldives

The HIV and STI epidemics in the Maldives are very low level. The country does not have a separate programme for STI. STI control is incorporated in the National HIV/AIDS Programme. Syndromic management approach is applied in all health care facilities except a few where laboratory facilities are available. (Fig. 15.4).

Bhutan

Although exact magnitude of STIs in Bhutan is not known. Gonnorrehea is most common

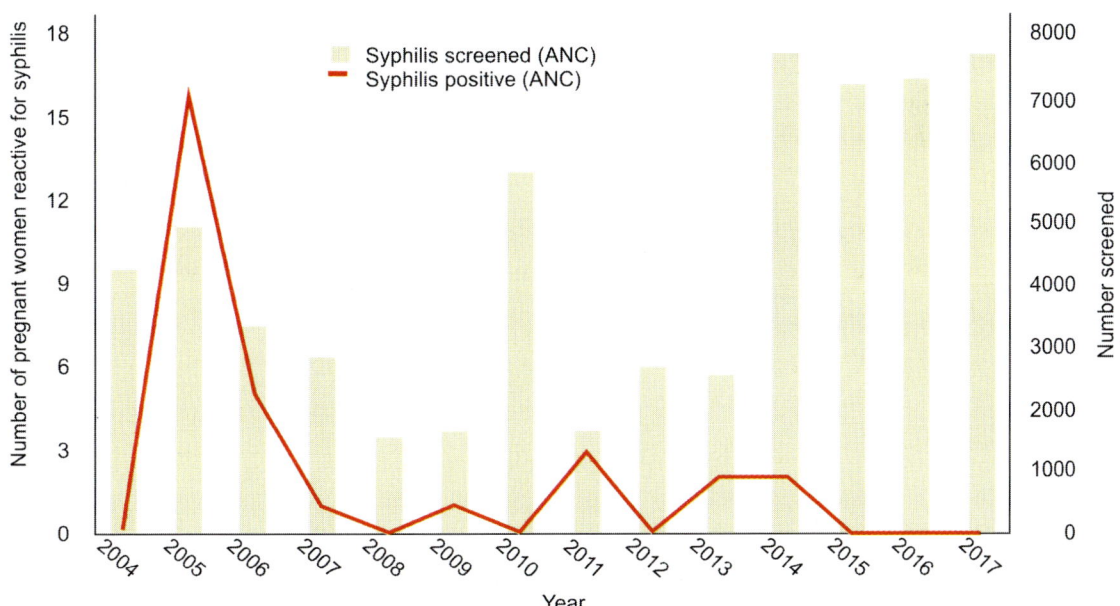

Source: Health Protection Agency, Ministry of Health and Family

Fig. 15.4: Antenatal clinic (ANC) syphilis screening trends

infection which has estimated annual incidence of about 2%. Syphilis for which blood donors and pregnant woman are screened showing slightly small data. STI symptoms found about 5–6% of men and 8% of woman. According to UNAIDS less than 1000 people have HIV/AIDS at the end of 2009. Most of whom are unaware of their infection. The Royal Government of Bhutan initiated National HIV/AIDS and STD control program (NACP). Despite of national program, there are is a project of HIV/AIDS and STI prevention along with World Bank.

Afghanistan

Reliable data on STDs prevalence in Afghanistan is sparse. UNAIDS and WHO estimate that there could be between 2000 and 3000 Afghan living with HIV. In order to maintain low prevalence <0.5% and to reduce morbidity and mortality related to HIV, Ministry of Health developed strategic framework into program operational plan (POP). Funding of these program is by national and international NGOS UNICEF, UNFPA, WHO, Asian Development Bank, USAID and UNODC.

The Program Response to STI

STI prevention and control have widespread public health benefits and contribute to progress towards SDGs. In 2016, WHO released its Global Health Sector strategy on sexually transmitted infection 2016–2021 with the goal of ending STI epidemics. To measure progress against the strategy's goal, key targets have been identified are by 2030: ≤50 cases of congenital syphilis per 100 000 live births in 80% of countries:

- 90% reduction in *T. pallidum* incidence globally (2018 global baseline);
- 90% reduction in *N. gonorrhoeae* incidence globally (2018 global baseline);
- 90% national vaccination coverage and at least 80% district coverage in countries with HPV vaccine in their national immunization program, prevention maternal to child transmission… defined three priority areas: (1) reducing STI incidence in high transmission networks; (2) improving STI case management for all; and (3) ensuring reliable data to guide the response. Basic clinical services, maintain stocks of effective STI treatments, conduct basic STI surveillance and monitor antibiotic resistance are required.

Sri Lanka have documented high levels of control. Human resources are required for HIV testing, ART, PrEP. Little or no funding or personnel were left for STI diagnostics, treatment and related control activities such as contact tracing and surveillance. Table 15.1 summaries the key STI activities in countries

Table 15.1: STI guidelines

	STI guidelines (last revision)	Reliable STI surveillance (>80% sites reporting)	ANC syphilis screening (>90% pregnancies)	STI contact tracing (actively supported)	KP routine STI screening and/or PPT
Bangladesh	2006				
Bhutan	2006		Yes		
India	2014	Partial	Yes (to verify)		Yes
Pakistan		No	No	No	
Maldives	2013		Yes		
Nepal	2014				
Sri Lanka	2013 updated, now revising	Yes	Yes	Yes	Yes

Table 15.2: Gaps in STI programs by programmatic area

Programmatic area	Status	Gaps/constraints
Strategic planning	National strategic plans (NSP) for HIV/STI program increasingly oriented towards HIV-specific targets, little attention to STI control.	STI generally low priority, may include some provision for STI treatment services. Recent attention to triple elimination may be opportunity to improve ANC syphilis screening.
Resources	Resource allocation aligned to NSP, including GFATM and other donors, few resources for STI activities.	Lacking separate line items for core STI control activities.
Commodities	Condom promotion and distribution for HIV also works for STIs. STI drugs and diagnostics often overlooked.	Gaps include reliable supply of STI diagnostics and treatment, logistics and supply management to avoid stockouts.
Outreach	Outreach to KP and bridge groups works for both HIV and other STIs.	Outreach with single focus (i.e. HTC only) misses opportunities for broader STI prevention and risks alienating KP.
Clinical service delivery	Variable attention across countries.	Monitoring of quality, supervision, refresher training, etc.
Contact tracing	Neglected in most countries.	Lacking dedicated staff to follow-up contacts of index cases.
Guidelines development, training and supervision	Many countries in region have not updated STI case management guidelines in last 5 years.	Guidelines updates, training and supervision required to maintain effective STI case management.
STI surveillance	Neglected in most countries.	Requires dedicated staff to ensure complete, accurate and timely reporting, analyse and disseminate data, etc.
Anti-microbial resistance (AMR) monitoring	Neglected in most countries.	Requires planning, funding and technical assistance for periodic AMR surveys.

in South Asian STI services for key populations (MSM IDUs, TG, FSW)—including quarterly medical checkups, presumptive treatment for asymptomatic infections and regular syphilis screening—have resulted in rapid STI control, including virtual elimination of common STIs in two Indian districts, Kolkata and Mysore.

HIV/AIDS

More than 70 million people have been infected globally of whom 35 million people have already died because of HIV/AIDS. Decline in AIDS related deaths and new HIV infections over the years is well known. ART has changed HIV from a virtual death sentence to a chronic manageable disease.

Global Scenario of HIV Estimates

Africa, global epicenter, is the region with the largest epidemic. Next largest number of HIV infected people live in Asia and Pacific. While rates remain low relative to some other regions, well over 5.2 million are living with HIV in this region as on Dec 2017.

Global summary of the AIDS epidemic 2017
Number of people living with HIV
Total   36.9 million [31.1–43.9 million]
Adults   35.1 million [29.6–41.7 million]
Women (15+ years) 18.2 million [15.6–21.4 million]
Children (<15 years) 1.8 million [1.3–2.4 million]
People newly infected with HIV in 2017
Total   1.8 million [1.4–2.4 million]
Adults   1.6 million [1.3–2.1 million]
Children (<15 years) 180 000 [110 000–260 000]
AIDS-related deaths in 2017
Total   940 000 [670 000–1.3 million]
Adults   830 000 [590 000–1.2 million]
Children (<15 years) 110 000 [63 000–160 000]

Antiretroviral therapy (ART) has reduced HIV-related mortality and morbidity, and HIV transmission. In 2016 UN General Assembly adopted a resolution to move towards 90-90-90 by 2020 and end AIDS as general health issue to public by 2030. India accounts for 60% of HIV burden. India has a prevalence of 0.26% but reports a higher HIV prevalence in southern and north-eastern states of India* and in Papua.

Adolescents and young adult PLHIV (15–24 years old), account for 44% of all new HIV infections. But epidemic modeling suggests that their numbers have declined in Nepal. New group of less than 15-year-old will shift into sexually active adults greatly increasing risk of resurgence of new infections.** There are 1.3 million (39%) women, 15 years and above, living with HIV out of 3.5 million PLHIV living in South Asia Infections amongst women considered to be at low risk because they are intimate partners of key populations (partners with clients of sex workers and people who inject drugs). Migrants also serve as bridge population introducing new infections back home.

THE HIV RESPONSE IN SOUTH ASIA

Focus on adolescent's girls and young people will need to be enhanced.

Prevention responses vary across countries. Opioid substitution therapy and needle syringe exchange sites for PWID, and only India, have reached the global standard of >200 needles distributed per person per year in 2016. Condoms reported usage varies across populations. Reported condom use is high (>80%) in India, Nepal but less than 50% in Bangladesh and Sri Lanka in MSM Population.[1] Pre-exposure prophylaxis (PrEP) for those at substantial risk of HIV is now recommended by WHO as part of the prevention-combination package, but currently India offers PrEP as a prevention intervention in pilot projects for sex workers and men who have sex with men.

The coverage for prevention of mother-to-child transmission (PMTCT), is low. Estimated 43% pregnant women living with HIV receiving ART compared with the global average of 76%. Sri Lanka is on verge of elimination of mother to child elimination of HIV as is Maldives. ART is recommended irrespective of CD4 count for all PLHIV, the remaining have agreed to 'test and treat' in principle. Viral load testing as a routine component of patient care in most countries is lacking. Punitive laws, stigma and discrimination against key populations potentially serve as barriers.

Adequate funded program with a rights based people centered approach will be required urgently.

PPTCT and ART in Pregnant Women

HIV transmission is preventable with appropriate intervention, by providing anti-retroviral therapy (ART) to mothers and anti-

---

*NACO (2015). India HIV estimation 2015 Technical Report. NACO. New Delhi. Available at: http://www. naco.gov.in/sites/default/files/India%20HIV%20 Estimations%202015.pdf
**The countries in SEAR started the demographic transition, a situation where countries experience transformation of their age structure and face a phenomenon known as youth bulge, in 2000. WHO. Health situation and trends assessment: regional health observatory. Available at: http://www.searo.who.int/entity/health_situation_ trends/data/chi/age-structure/en/

retroviral (ARV) prophylaxis to infants. All these HIV infected pregnant women have to be detected and provided with timely ART in order to reduce mother to child transmission and ultimately to eliminate pediatric HIV.

Table 15.3: Risk of HIV transmission from mother to child with ARV interventions

ARV intervention	Risk of HIV transmission from mother to child
No ARV, breastfeeding	30–45%
No ARV, no breastfeeding	20–25%
Short course with **one ARV**, breastfeeding	15–25%
Short course with **one ARV**, no breastfeeding	5–15%
Short course with **two ARVs**, breastfeeding	5%
3 ARVs (ART) with breastfeeding	2%
3 ARVs (ART) with no breastfeeding	1%

PPTCT Services

The National PPTCT programme recognizes the 4 elements to prevent HIV transmission among women and children.

PPTCT: Interventions During Pregnancy

- Primary prevention of HIV in childbearing women
- Provide HIV information to all pregnant women
- Antenatal visits are opportunity for PPTCT
- Prevention of unwanted pregnancies in HIV-positive women
- Prevention of PTCT through ART
- Safe obstetric practices

How HIV affects Women's Health

Weight loss, comorbid psychiatric illness, psychotropic medications, illicit substance use, thrombocytopenia, renal dysfunction may cause secondary amenorrhoea more often than menstrual disorders. Acute HIV infection initially leads to flu-like illness. Dedicated approach to treat HIV infection has positive impact on life expectancy. Motivation of patient is important in this regard.

Screening

All pregnant women are counseled to have screening for HIV at booking antenatal visit.

Rapid HIV tests are recommended who present **in labour with unknown HIV status**.

- Screening HIV, *syphilis, hepatitis B,* early in pregnancy
- At initial screening if female is HIV negative but still have risk factors, test should be repeated.

  Treatment might be delayed until after first trimester.

  If no breastfeeding, the risk of MTCT in women taking HAART less than 1%.

Antiretroviral Therapy

- All pregnant HIV positive woman have same first line regimen of ART as non-pregnant woman.
- Every effort should be made that all pregnant HIV positive woman should have access to it.
- In resource poor countries criteria for initiating ART should be based on CD4 count and WHO clinical staging.
- Most of pregnant HIV positive woman booked late in antenatal clinic and not willing to take HRT alternative option should be discussed.

Mode of Delivery

The safest way deliver of HIV positive pregnant woman depends upon viral load during pregnancy. In general vaginal delivery is preferred for safety of mother and fetus if the risk of transmission is low.

Scheduled cesarean section at 38 weeks to minimize perinatal transmission of HIV.

Woman diagnosed positive > 32 weeks may still have planned vaginal delivery if she commences HAART and achieves a viral load <50 copies/ml by 36 weeks.

- For viral load >50 copies/ml at 36 weeks elective cesarean section—38 weeks,
- Should continue her HAART
- Intravenous ZDV at delivery.

Management of Delivery

PPTCT: Interventions during labour and delivery:

- Minimise vaginal examinations
- Avoid prolonged labour, consider oxytocin to shorten labour
- Avoid artificial rupture of membranes
- Early cord clamping after it stops pulsating and after giving the mother oxytocin
- Use non-invasive fetal monitoring
  - Avoid invasive procedures
  - Avoid routine episiotomy/support perineum
  - Minimise the use of forceps or vacuum extractors

Considerations in Mode of Delivery

1. In India, normal vaginal delivery is recommended unless the woman has obstetric reasons (like foetal distress, obstructed labour) for a caesarean section
2. Use of ART can reduce risk of PTCT better and with less risk than a C-section. Intravenous ZDV is started four hour before start of c-section and continued until cord is clamped.

Forceps is preferable to ventouse.

Postpartum Care

- Breast milk suppression is recommended within 24 hours of delivery.
- Contraceptive advice should be given in the postpartum pre-pregnancy management.
- Pre-conception counseling is essential for all HIV-positive woman who are planning pregnancy. This conversation should be non-judgmental and concerning their reproductive desires.

- Ideally this counseling should be initiated shortly after the diagnosis of HIV in reproductive age.
- Counsellor should address individual needs of woman.
- Encourage sexual partner for HIV testing.
- Assess safe sexual practices and contraceptive method (condom). If female partner is HIV negative, assisted conception with donor insemination or sperm washing is recommended.
- Yearly cervical cytology should be done
- They can use all available contraceptive methods, including hormonal contraception and emergency contraception.
- Labour room nurse informs the ICTC counsellor and lab technician for further confirmation of HIV test as per guidelines.

ARV Prophylaxis for Infant

The infant should be started on nevirapine. The duration of NVP prophylaxis will depend on duration of ART that has been given to mother during her ante-natal period.

- Infant should be stared on daily NVP prophylaxis at their first encounter with health services.
- Daily infant NVP prophylaxis can be started even if more than 72 hours have passed since birth and should continue by which time the mother should be linked to appropriate ART services.

Duration of daily infant NVP prophylaxis will depend on "how long the mother was on life-long ART [for a minimum of 24 weeks (6 months) or not]".

- The duration of NVP to infant is minimum of 6 weeks, regardless of whether exclusively breastfed or exclusive replacement fed
- Six weeks nevirapine prophylaxis should be increased to 12 weeks, if ART to mother was started in late pregnancy, during or after delivery and has not been on adequate period of ART as to be effective to achieve optimal viral suppression (which is at least 24 weeks–6 months)

- The recommendation on extended nevirapine duration (12 weeks) applies to infants of breastfeeding women only and not those on exclusive replacement feeding.
- Infants of women with prior exposure to NVP to get syrup zidovudine (AZT) in place of syrup nevirapine
- If syrup zidovudine is not available, syrup nevirapine may be used as per weight band.

Care of the Neonate

All neonates should be treated with anti-retroviral therapy within 4 hours of birth.

> Choice of breastfeeding should be the decision of woman under proper information; Counseling on breastfeeding should begin during ante-natal period itself.

Sexually Transmitted Diseases

Our aims of treatment are to cure the infection as rapidly as possible, and to eliminate contagiousness to interrupt transmission and to prevent reinfection and recurrent infection.

Trichomonas Parasitic Infection

The NAAT, APTIMA has a sensitivity of 95.3–100% and specificity of 95.2–100%. Specimens can be sent from urine, vagina, endocervix, or urethra. Cultures and wet preparations are decreasing in popularity because of lower sensitivities.

Viral STDs

Amongst viral STDs, some viral infections have local manifestations like herpes, genital warts and molluscum contagiosum, whereas HIV/AIDS, hepatitis B, C and D have systemic manifestations.

Human Papillomavirus (HPV)

The high burden of cervical cancer in South Asia is due to high prevalence and lack of screening. Genital warts and benign cervical lesion are caused by 11 low risk type of HPV.

As this infection leads to cancerous lesion so universal screening, early detection and simple timely interventions are key factors for prevention of cancer. Woman should have access to screening and vaccination. The management of genital warts is difficult. Sometimes after topical treatments surgery is required. HPV is not only causative agent for cervical cancer (99%), anal cancer (90%), vaginal, vulval and penile cancer (70%). Anal cancer is more common among HIV-positive homosexual men 70–100 per 100000.

Herpes Simplex Virus (HSV) Infection

The prevalence of HSV is low in South Asian countries as compared to worldwide. It is most common cause of painful genital ulcers. High risk sexual behaviour and perinatal transmission contribute to its high prevalence. It also increases risk of HIV infection. Educate the patient to explain nature and purpose of treatment to avoid false expectation from cure.

Haemophilus ducreyi

These infections are less common nowadays. It is transmitted through skin to skin contact. Painful ulcerative lesions appear within 4 to 10 days on external genitalia, cervix and anus.

Syphilis

Syphilis in clinical stage I, II, or III is called "early syphilis" for the first year after the date of infection and "late syphilis" at later times.

Painless ulcer with an indurated edge (ulcus durum) is seen in half of the patients. Mode of transmission is same like other STIs. It has long-term implications on female health.

Hepatitis B

The prevalence of this infection in South Asia is around 15–20%. Serological diagnostic modalities are available. In low middle income countries like Pakistan, India and Afghanistan females have limited access to screening services. Only chance of screening is during antenatal periods. There are social and financial barriers. There is need to address these issues as every female has right to be treated.

Hepatitis C

It is increasingly becoming a public health problem. Homosexuality and multiple sexual partners contributing to its high prevalence. Important aspect of this infection includes.

- Targeted screening
- Preconception and pregnancy care
- HIV-positive woman should have annual screening of HCV.

Cure rate is More Than 90%

Chlamydia and Gonorrhea

- Chlamydia is a silent killer of woman and it is neglected STI in South Asia.
- The prevalence in South Asia is 6.5%.
- Untreated chlamydia infection results in 40% PID which leads to infertility
- Gonorrhea leads to 15% infertility.
- Nucleic acid amplification tests (NAATs), are sensitive diagnostic tool for both infections.
- Safe sexual practices like use of condom, limited number of sexual partners and annual screening of chlamydia and gonorrhea will help to prevent chlamydia and gonorrhea.

The WHO STI guideline recommends that local resistance data should determine the choice of therapy. In settings where local resistance data are not available, it is recommended to use dual therapy over single therapy for people with genital or anorectal gonorrhoea. In people with gonococcal infections who have failed treatment, if reinfection is suspected, re-treat with a WHO-recommended regimen, reinforce sexual abstinence or condom use, and provide partner treatment. If treatment failure occurred after treatment with a regimen not recommended by WHO, re-treat with a WHO-recommended regimen in double dose. If treatment failure occurred and resistance data are available, re-treat according to susceptibility.

Genital Ulcer Disease

The common causes of genital ulcer are syphilis and herpes simplex. *T vaginalis, candidiasis and BV are the three common pathological causes of an abnormal vaginal discharge.* T. vaginalis is sexually transmitted and causes an offensive malodorous discharge with vulval soreness and irritation. It may also present no symptoms at all.

Candida albicans is uncommon in adolescents prior to puberty. If present, the adolescent may have a discharge, vulval itching, dyspareunia, a peri-anal soreness or a fissuring at the introitus. Attacks of candida vulvitis may be cyclical in nature and correspond to menstruation. Bacterial vaginosis does not produce a vulvitis and the adolescent will not complain of itching or soreness.

Pelvic Inflammatory Disease

Women presenting with lower abdominal or pelvic pain and at least one of the following on pelvic examination should be treated presumptively for PID.

- Uterine tenderness, or
- Cervical motion tenderness, or adnexal tenderness.

STIs in Adolescents

Adolescent acquires half of all new STDs. The most common STD is caused by chlamydia and HPV. These young adults are at risk of STDs due to behavioral biological and cultural reasons. This increased susceptibility to infection is due to cervical ectopy. The main factor in increase of adolescent STDs is multiple barriers in access to screening and prevention programs. These barriers include:

- Inability to pay
- Lack of transportation
- Long waiting times

- Conflict between clinic hour and work schedules
- Embarrassment attached to seeking STD services
- Concern about confidentiality

There is risk of a child acquiring STI as a result of sexual abuse. Interventions only address individual level factors which do not address high level factors like peer norms and media influence. The intervention for risk adolescent and young adults should address underlying social and cultural aspects that sexual behaviour. In designing STDs program, more attention should be paid toward extending times, taking care of privacy and cost. These early infections can lead to PID and its complication in later life. It is mandatory to screen and treat these young adults.

Criteria for STI Drugs

Drugs for treating STI should meet the following criteria:
- High efficacy
- Low cost
- Acceptable side effects
- Resistance unlikely to develop
- Single dose oral route
- Not contraindicated for pregnant or lactating women

Violation of sexual and reproductive rights of female. An integrated approach to health and human rights lies at the heart of ensuring dignity and well-being of female around the world and is linked to improvements in the uptake of services and incidence of positive outcomes. Through the roll of treatment, advances in overcoming stigma and discrimination, and response have given hope for a healthy life for many around the world. However, for those who remain the most vulnerable, there is not nearly enough progress. Women and girls, for instance, remain especially vulnerable to STIs because of a host of biological, social, cultural and economic reasons, including women's entrenched social and economic inequality within sexual relationships and marriage.

Sometimes female rights are violated as she does not know the HIV/STIs status of her husband. So without use of safety measures female gets that infection and bears all consequences including social, medical, pschycological. HIV is not only driven by gender inequality, but it also entrenches gender inequality, leaving women more vulnerable to its impact. Moreover, women and girls at risk of, or living with, STIs have additional challenges linked to sexual and reproductive health that includes risk of unintended pregnancy, complications arising from unsafe abortions and a host of other sexual and reproductive health morbidities.

Social Stigma

Violence, whether it be physical, sexual and/or emotional, or fear of violence can prevent women from negotiating safer sex and from learning and/or sharing their HIV status if the results turn out positive. In addition, women living with HIV are sometimes blamed for bringing HIV into the family and for being immoral and breaking sexual norms. Many women living with HIV can achieve safe and satisfying sex lives, but there is still a long way to go for this to be a reality for the most vulnerable amongst them who face repeated violations of their rights.

Solutions

- Placing human rights and gender equality at the centre of a comprehensive approach to health programming, in particular, in relation to sexuality and sexual health.
- Ensuring health systems responsiveness to inequalities in access to health care and quality of care that often do not meet the needs of women living with HIV.
- Engaging and empowering women living with HIV in the development of policies and programs that affect them.

- Strengthening monitoring, evaluation and accountability procedures to provide good quality data and ensuring remedial action against violations of health and human rights of women living with HIV.

  In India and other countries of South Asia, there is no fully functional STI surveillance system. The consensus is that syphilis and gonorrhea is declining. Genital herpes, human papillomavirus and Chlamydial infections are increasing. The bacterial STDs are decreasing because of the syndromic treatment at peripheral centers, reducing the need for tertiary centres.

- STIs are a major cause of serious gynecological and psychological consequences. There is correlation between sex behaviour and infection. Safe sex behaviour includes use of condoms, limiting sexual partners, limited use of alcohol and illicit drugs.

- Presentation varies from acute illness, infertility even long-term disability and death. Sexually transmitted infections are asymptomatic in up to 90% patients. Type 2 herpes simplex virus (HSV-2) infection is also asymptomatic in up to one-third pregnant women.

- Our aims of treatment are to cure the infection and to interrupt transmission and to prevent re-infection and recurrent infection.

Handling the Situation

This is public health issue, which needs prompt identification and treatment to avoid long-term consequences. Ideally there should be sexual health clinic on 24/7 services. In low middle income countries like Pakistan, Bangladesh and other countries of south Asia where these issues were highly ignorant.

Psychological Support

- Management of STIs requires members of staff to be respectful to patients and not to be judgmental. Clinical examination must take place in appropriate surroundings where privacy can be ensured and confidentiality guaranteed. The sexual partner(s) of patients should also be examined for STIs and promptly treated as the index patient.

- Counseling of targeted groups regarding compliance of medication, desensitization and safe sexual practices. This should be done by pschycologist or some trained personnel.

- Another important component of pschycological support is peer group formation, it will enhance self-confidence and motivation.

Role of Family

Role of family is of utmost importance especially in case

- Sex education to teenager
- Parents feel uncomfortable talking about this issue to their children. There is an evidence that parents involvement is effective and important component of sexual behaviour of teenagers.
- Positive role of spouse to provide moral, financial and social support.

Rehabilitation

This sector is most neglected although it needs prime importance in South Asia. There are a few NGOs working off and on in this regard but there should be a sincere effort at Government level.

NGOs

There are different NGOs in different countries of South Asia like *NAIE ZINDGI* in Pakistan working for social, pschycological and financial support. All these NGOs in countries of South Asia are funded by UNAIDS, UNICEF and global funds. The intermittent availability of these funds effect the performance of these NGOs.

Helplines

- Most of countries have their helplines. In Pakistan there is 24/7 helpline 0800-22209

- Provide basic information regarding HIV/HCV
- Telephonic counseling
- Referral services
- Receiving complaints, suggestion, and feedback about provision and quality of services These information are available in Urdue, Sindhi, Balouchi and Pashto language. Anonymity, confidentiality and neutrality are major principles for functioning of helpline.

BIBLIOGRAPHY

1. Available at: https://www.cdc.gov/std/stats15/adolescents.htm. Accessed Feb. 27, 2017.
2. BHIVA Guidelines for the management of HIV infection in pregnant women 2012, HIV Medicine 2014;15(4):1–77.
3. Branson BM, Handsfield HH, Lampe MA, et al. Revised Recommendations for HIV Testing of Adults, Adolescents, and Pregnant Women in Health-Care Settings.
4. Centers for Disease Control and Prevention. 2015 Sexually Transmitted Disease Surveillance: STIs in Young Adolescents and Adults. (2016, Oct. 18).
5. Centers for Disease Control and Prevention. Syphilis-CDC Fact Sheet (Detailed). Feb. 13, 2017. Available at: https://www.cdc.gov/std/syphilis/stdfact-syphilis-detailed.htm. Accessed Feb. 23, 2017.
6. Dixit R, Bhavsar C, Marfatia YS. Laboratory diagnosis of human papillomavirus infection in female genital tract. Indian J Sex Transm Dis 2011;32:50–2.
7. Guidelines for the management of sexually transmitted infections. Expert Consultation on Improving the Management of Sexually Transmitted Infections (2001: Geneva, Switzerland) ISBN 92-4-154626-3 World Health Organization 2003.
8. Jayanna K, Washington RG, Moses S, Kudur P, Issac S, Balu PS, et al. Assessment of attitudes and practices of providers of services for individuals at high risk of HIV and sexually transmitted infections in Karnataka, South India. Sex Transm Infect. 2010;86:131–5.
9. Meyers D, Wolff T, Gregory K, et al. USPSTF Recommendations for STI Screening American Sexual Health Association. STDs/STIs. Available at: http://www.ashasexualhealth.org/stdsstis. Accessed Feb. 21, 2017.
10. Mignone J, Washington R, Ramesh BM, Blanchard JF, Rajaretnam T, Moses S. Discrepancies between the self-reporting of STI preventive care and the actual care provided by male doctors to male patients in Karnataka, India. Sex Transm Infect. 2010;86:391–2.
11. Mishra S, Naik B, Venugopal B, Kudur P, Washington R, Becker M, et al. Syphilis screening among female sex workers in Bangalore, India: comparison of point-of-care testing and traditional serological approaches. Sex Transm Infect. 2010;86:193–8.
12. Mogasale V, Wi TC, Das A, Kane S, Singh AK, George B, Steen R. Quality assurance and quality improvement using supportive supervision in a large-scale STI intervention with sex workers, men who have sex with men/transgenders and injecting drug users in India. Sex Transm Infect. 2010;86 Suppl 1:i83–8.
13. Ramakrishnan L, Gautam A, Goswami P, Kallam S, Adhikary R, Mainkar MK, et al. Programme coverage, condom use and STI treatment among FSWs in a large-scale HIV prevention programme: results from cross-sectional surveys in 22 districts in southern India. Sex Transm Infect. 2010;86 Suppl 1:i62–8.
14. Sexually Transmitted Diseases Treatment Guidelines. (2017, January 25). Available at: https://www.cdc.gov/std/tg2015/default.htm.
15. The Presentation, Diagnosis, and Treatment of Sexually Transmitted Infections Florian ME Wagenlehner, Prof. Dr Med.1 Norbert H. Brockmeyer, Prof. Dr Med.2 Thomas Discher, Dr. Med.3 Klaus Friese. Dtsch Arztebl Int 2016;113(1-2):11–22.

Contraception—A Rights Issue

Syeda Batool Mazhar, Zeenat Nasreen, Bushra Haq

Contraception provides control over pregnancy timing and prevention of unintended pregnancy. Around 214 million women of reproductive age in developing countries who want to avoid pregnancy are not using a modern contraceptive methods (WHO 2018).

Family planning implies the ability of individuals and couples to anticipate and attain their desired number of children and spacing and timing their births using temporary contraceptive methods such as periodic abstinence, coitus interrupts, oral pills, long-acting injections, implants, placement of IUCDs, or barrier methods, i.e. using condoms, diaphragms and spermicide. Present methods of contraception include male and female sterilization. As the world experiences a population explosion during the second half of the present century, the need of fertility control extended beyond family to society levels as a means of limiting the population growth to a level within their socio-economic capabilities. In Asia, a wide number of women now use contraception, the trend which is seen as contributing towards containing the ever-expanding world population. Within the region, the highest levels of contraceptive use are found mainly in the Eastern and South Eastern regions, with an estimated high of 83.4 percent in China. In all, countries in Asia have contraceptive prevalence levels of 50 percent or more. The lowest level of contraceptive prevalence in Asia was in Pakistan at 38.5 percent in 2015.

CONTRACEPTIVE PREVALENCE RATE

This refers to the proportion of all couples of child bearing age who are currently using a particular contraceptive method. This includes modern and traditional methods.

TOTAL FERTILITY RATE

This refers to the number of live births a women would have throughout her entire reproductive life. The assessment of fertility trends indicate that no country has achieved the desired fertility rate to an ideal replacement level of 2.1 births per women without achieving a contraceptive prevalence rate of at least 50 percent.

SUSTAINABLE DEVELOPMENT GOALS

The sustainable development goals are a call to action to end poverty, protect the planet and ensure peace and prosperity everywhere.

Picking up where the Millennium Development Goals left off, the Sustainable Development Goals now seek to reduce the maternal mortality ratio to less than 70 deaths per 100,000 live births by 2030. If we are going to reach this ambitious goal, then we need to get serious about contraceptives that ever done.

Contraception reduces the need for abortion and especially unsafe abortion, thereby prevents deaths of mothers and children. Lots of barriers and challenges need to be overcome to achieve the targeted goal.

Goal 3: **Ensure healthy lives and promote well-being for all women at all ages.** Ensuring healthy lives and promoting the well-being for all at all ages is essential to sustainable development. Significant strides have been made in increasing life expectancy and reducing some of the common killers associated with child and maternal mortality.

But limiting family by contraceptive has tremendous benefit for women well-being. The global agenda emphasize on women's health for which contraceptives are the keystone.

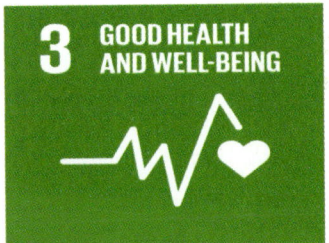

Goal 3: Good health and well-being

Goal 5: Providing women and girls with equal access to education, health care, decent work, and representation in political and economic decision-making processes will fuel sustainable economies and benefit societies and humanity at large.

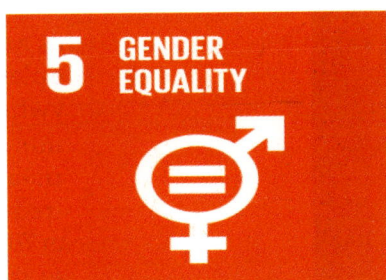

Goal 5: Achieve gender equality and empower all women and girls

CONTRACEPTION AND SOUTH ASIA

The contraceptive prevalence rates according to the last reports available from the three countries are as follows (*see* Graph 16.5).

- 23.9% in Pakistan.
- 41% in India.
- 45% in Bangladesh

Pakistan is far behind its neighbors in the transition to lower fertility. With its high annual population growth rate of 2.8 percent Pakistan is likely to become the world's third most populous country by 2050 (Ann Tinker). Although all three countries are socio-economically, culturally and religion-wise very similar, there is still a lower contraceptive prevalence rate in Pakistan as compared to the other two countries (Graphs 16.1 and 16.3). The level of literacy is almost the same for all three countries (62–76 percent). Therefore, the main issue is not only education but also there are other reasons for the comparatively lower contraceptive prevalence rate in Pakistan. More research is necessary to look into the reasons for the acceptability and the non-acceptability of contraceptives in Pakistan. A family planning programme should be geared towards the promotion and availability of methods that are more acceptable to the women of Pakistan. Health workers can play a major role in educating people about family planning methods. A large number of women are still not using contraception.

Table 16.1: Preferred method for future use of a contraceptive method (in percentages)

Method of contraception	%
Female sterilization	18%
Male sterilization	0%
Oral contraceptive pills	14.5%
Injectable contraceptives	17.5%
IUD	8.7%
Condom	10.4%
Vaginal methods	0.3%
Abstinence	2.4%
Withdrawal	1.5%
Other methods	7.9%
Don't know any method	17.9%

Pakistan DHS 1990–91

Table 16.2: Percentage of men out of 1354 interviewed revealed

Method	%
Know of one method	79%
Approved of family planning	56%
Used a contraceptive method	18%
Had used any method at all	25%
Currently using a modern method of contraception	10%
Were using any method of contraception	15%

(Pakistan DHS 1990–91).

Table 16.3: Percentage of users of various contraceptive methods in Pakistan and Bangladesh

Method of contraception	Pakistan 1996–97	Bangladesh 1993–94
Any method	23.9%	44.6%
Oral contraceptive pill	1.6%	17.4%
IUD	3.4%	2.2%
Injectable contraceptives	1.4%	4.5%
Vaginal Methods	0.1%	–
Condoms	4.2%	3.0%
Female sterilization	6.0%	8.1%
Male sterilization	0.0%	1.1%
Any traditional method	7.0%	8.4%
Abstinence	1.9%	4.8%
Withdrawal	4.6%	2.5%
Others	0.5%	1.1%
Number of women	7582	8980

(PFFPS 1996/97 and Bangladesh DHS 1993–94)

Graph 16.1: Percentage of women using any method of contraception in Pakistan and Bangladesh 1975–95

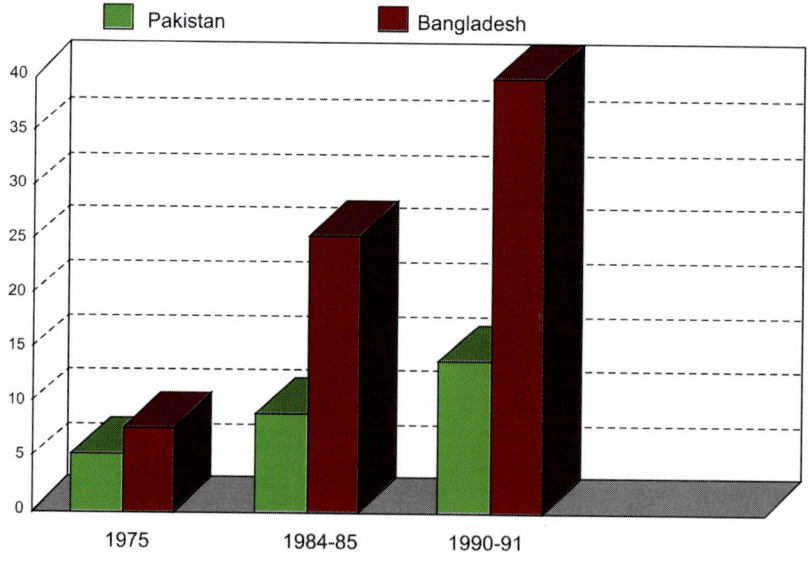

(Pak DHS 1990-91 and Bangladesh DHS 1993-94)

Graph 16.2: Contraception prevalence rates

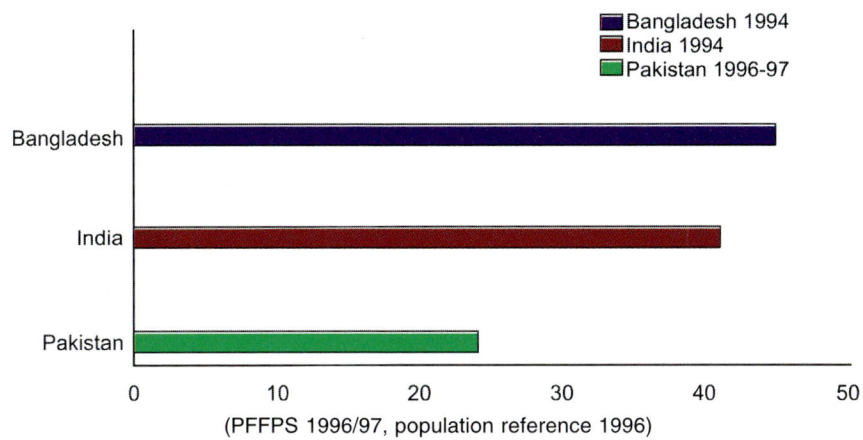

(PFFPS 1996/97, population reference 1996)

Graph 16.3: Women aged 15–50. Levels of current contraceptive use in percentages

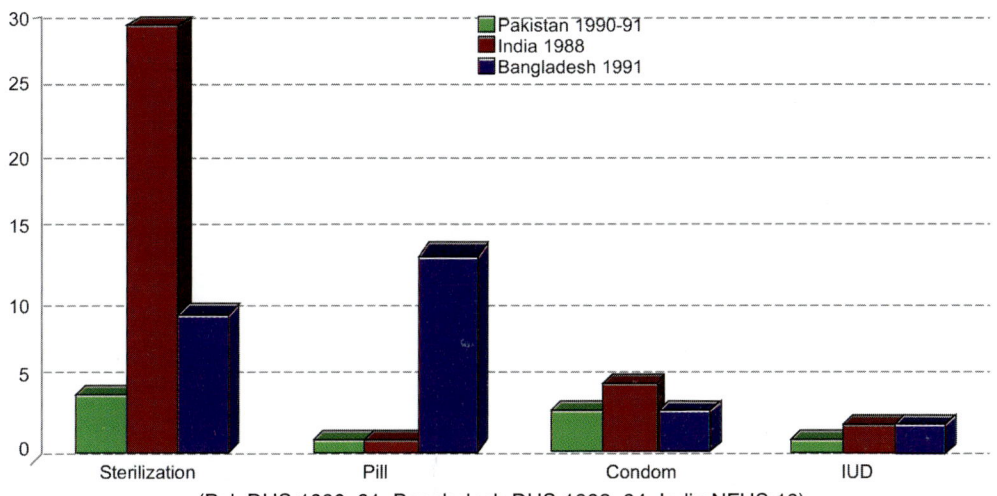

(Pak DHS 1990–91, Bangladesh DHS 1993–94, India NFHS 19)

Graph 16.4: Percentage of ever married women who have never used contraception

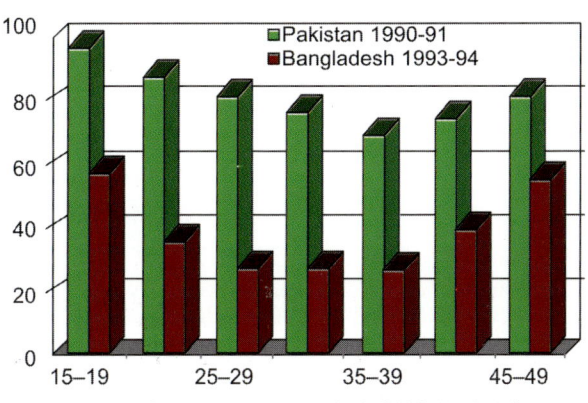

(Pak DHS 1990–91, Bangladesh DHS 1993–94)

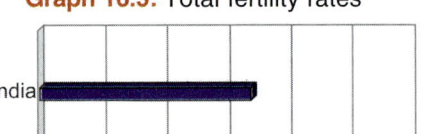

Graph 16.5: Total fertility rates

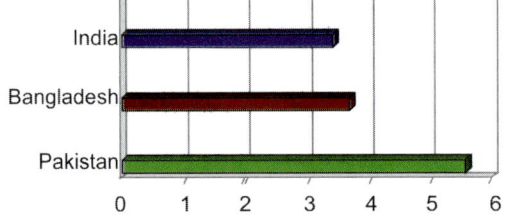

(*Source:* Improving women's health in Pakistan—Ann Tinker)

All the countries of south Asia need to give special attention. If we look around the world: In Asia, a wide number of women now use contraception, the trend which is seen as contributing towards containing the ever-expanding world population. Within the region, the highest levels of contraceptive use are found mainly in the Eastern and South Eastern regions, with an estimated high of 83.4 percent in China. In all, countries in Asia have contraceptive prevalence levels of 50 percent or more. The lowest level of contraceptive prevalence in Asia was in Pakistan at 38.5 percent in 2015.

However, data shows a stark disparity in the range of percentage of women taking recourse to contraceptive methods in South Asia.

Nepal

A meagre 1.8 percent of women were using contraceptives in 1970 in Nepal which saw an increase to 52.4 percent in 2015.

Bhutan

Only 1.8 percent of Bhutanese women used contraceptives which increased to 67.8 percent in 2015. It is estimated to reach 72.8 percent by 2030.

Pakistan

Although Pakistan has seen resistance on birth control policies, the country has updated its

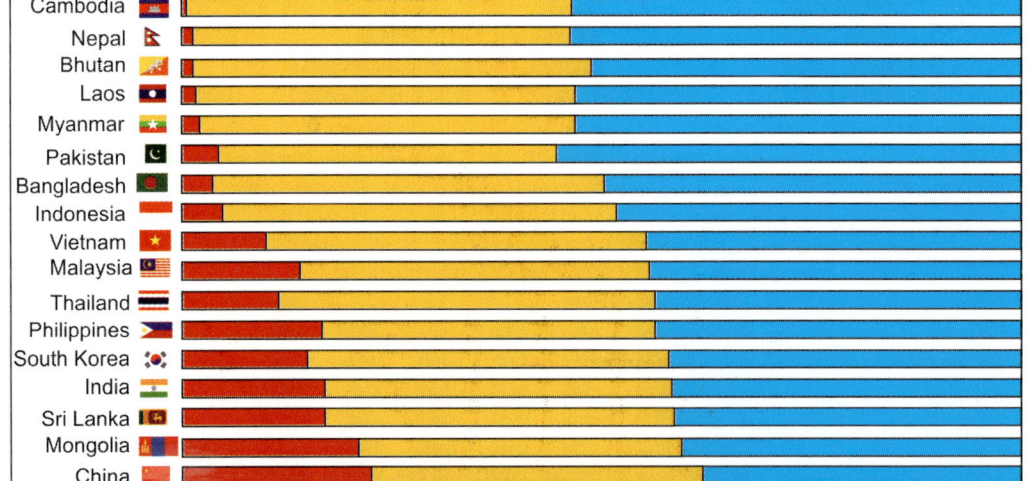

Contraception and family planning in Asia, 1970–2030

A record number of women in Asia now use contraception. But the figures show wide disparities between Asian countries.

(Figures are percentage of women using contraception)   ■1970 ▢2015 ▢2030

Compiled by: ANN/DataLEADS

Source: UN's Department of Economic and Social Affairs

Percentage of women using contraception in Asia

commitment to implement family planning methods. The percentage of women who will use contraceptives by 2030 is estimated to be 52.8.

Singapore

Singapore has been far ahead of other Asian countries in 1970 with 55.5 percent women using contraceptives in 1970. It saw an increase to 66 percent in 2015 and is expected to rise to 67.5 percent by 2030.

India

India, the first country in the world to launch a national programme for family planning, has seen a surge in number of women using contraceptives to 67.8 percent in 2015. It is estimated to rise by 1 percent by 2030.

Sri Lanka

In the South Asian region, Sri Lanka has been ahead of its neighbours at 30.3 percent in the 1970 to an increase of 71.6 percent in 2015.

Bangladesh

Fertility rate in Bangladesh is slowly declining when overpopulation remains Global concern. Sandy Walton-Elley happily mentioned that Bangladesh has been more successful than other South Asian countries (India, Pakistan, and Nepal) in reducing total fertility rate from 6.9 in 1970 to 2.2 in 2011, i.e. women have 2.1 children on average. The Government of Bangladesh updated its Family Planning 2020 commitment at the Family Planning Summit in London, UK on July 11, 2017 and pledged to take the actions for effective contraception. For this Bangladesh will mobilize USD 615 million for the family planning program over 2017, which is a 67% increase from the previous program.

Access to effective contraceptive continues to be still a challenge especially for the adolescents and for slum women. Newly married women sometimes cannot make their own decision; they need to depend on husband's decision. So they often face accidental pregnancy. OCP is popular and available, though IUD is very effective contraceptive but most Bangladeshi women are not willing to use IUD. So advocacy, round table meeting, documentary, advertisements in mass media are implemented in Bangladesh. MoHFW of Bangladesh makes the contraceptives available in all divisional hospitals. Over the counter OCP, condom, IUD are sold in subsidized rates. Emergency contraceptives are found in almost every pharmacy.

Good side, that last for few couples of years for women in Bangladesh, it has been not just life change but also empowering. No longer are women spending many years pregnant and looking after small child but rather they are able to choose to have the number of children they want.

According to the UN the region can save billions of dollars if family planning is implemented properly as it would bring down unintended pregnancies and avert unsafe abortions. Contraception use also prevents new infections in women, men and adolescents and reduces maternal mortality.

Adolescents and Contraception

Adolescents are special young adults. They are our asset, our future and for them contraception remains the real challenge.

There are an estimated 1.2 billion people aged 10–19 in the world—the largest generation of adolescents in history. They comprise 20 percent of the world's population and 18–25% of the population in member countries of South East Asia Region. In Bangladesh there are 36 million adolescents (estimated) and half of them are female.

The health and well-being of these engines of change is central to create healthier nation, so UN Secretary said "Adolescents are central to everything we want to achieve, and to the overall success of the 2030 Agenda".

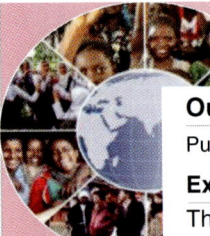

Our future: A Lancet Commission on adolescent health and well-being

Published: May 11, 2016

Executive Summary

The largest generation of adolescents and young people in human history (1.8 billion) demands more attention and action. Adolescents and young adults face unprecedented social, economic, and cultural change. *The Lancet* is dedicated to create discussion around this critical topic by publishing the best research to lead to better lives for all. Adolescence is generally thought to be the healthiest time of life and young people have therefore attracted little interest and too few resources. The 2016 *Lancet* Commission concluded that investing in adolescents will yield a triple benefit—today, into adulthood, and the next generation of children.

The latest Health Policy paper shows that investments in adolescent health and well-being are some of the best that can be made, resulting in a 10-fold economic benefit, and are vital for the progress towards achieving the UN's Sustainable Development Goals. Investments in adolescent health and well-being will not only transform the lives of girls and boys around the world, but will also generate high economic returns, especially in low income countries. The costs of inaction are too great to ignore.

About 21 million 15–19-year-old girls in developing countries become pregnant every year. Half of these pregnancies (49%) are unintended. 38 million 15–19-year-old adolescent girls are at risk of pregnancy and do not want a child in the next two years. Only 40% are using a modern method of contraception.

95% of these births occur in low middle income countries.

Abortion in Adolescents

Adolescents often resort to unsafe practices and procedures. Unsafe abortion (which is the cause of 13% of global maternal mortality) tends to be more dangerous for adolescents where it is illegal as they tend to seek abortion later in pregnancy (*International Planned Parenthood Federation, 1994*).

They usually go to unskilled providers and/or in unsafe conditions.

Among that 14% of all unsafe abortions in developing countries involve adolescent girls aged 15–19 years.

The physically devastating potential consequences of unsafe abortion include cervical tearing, perforated uterus and bowel, hemorrhage, chronic pelvic infection and abscesses, infertility, endotoxic shock, renal failure, and death. The long-term sequelae include ectopic pregnancy, chronic pelvic pain, infertility, mental health problems and also increased maternal mortality and morbidity.

High Risk Factors for Adolescent's Pregnancies

High risk factors for adolescents include low socioeconomic status, substance abuse, poor antenatal care, delayed intrapartum care and obstructed labour due to undeveloped pelvis. Again 9–86% of women with obstetric fistula develop the condition from adolescents pregnancy.

Increased risk of preterm labour and stillbirth, chance of dying in the first year of life is more than 60% higher for babies born to the under 18s than for those born to older mothers.

Social and personal consequences of pregnancy in this age group include spiral of low self-esteem, poverty and further pregnancies. (UNFPA/UNICEF/WHO, 1989).

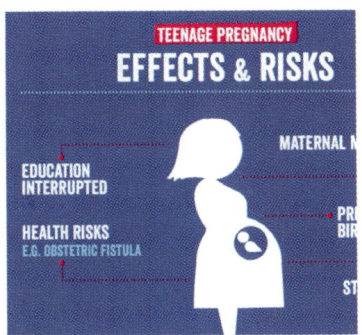

We need to stop it, need to introduce contraceptives strongly that ever done before.

In this regard Bangladesh government and NGOs have taken to provide services regarding adolescent contraceptive.

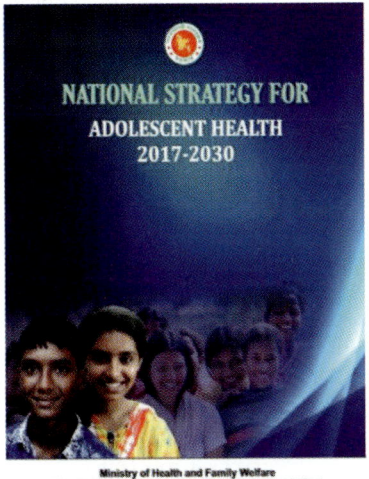

We need to stop it, need to introduce contraceptives strongly that ever done before.

The religious belief, knowledge, information level, educational status, myth, superstitions, familial pressure all guide an adolescent to decide what she might do.

So before embarking contraceptive to an adolescent, counseling is most important. Good counseling brings the high compliance.

Most important aim of counseling allow the clinician to address any knowledge deficit, misconception or exaggerated concern about the safety of contraceptive methods, to its use all of which are the barriers and also birth spacing and pregnancy care.

Adolescents contraceptive is a global challenge.

Unmet Need of Contraception

Married adolescents often do not want a pregnancy; current use of contraceptives is often lower among sexually active, married adolescents.

In Bangladesh, from 1996 to 2011 contraceptive use among women aged 10 to 49 years rose from 49% to 61%, while for married adolescents aged 15 to 19 years it rose from 33% to 47% in the same time.

Current contraceptive use prevents approximately 272 000 maternal mortalities per year, and if current family planning needs were met, another 104 000 lives would not be lost.

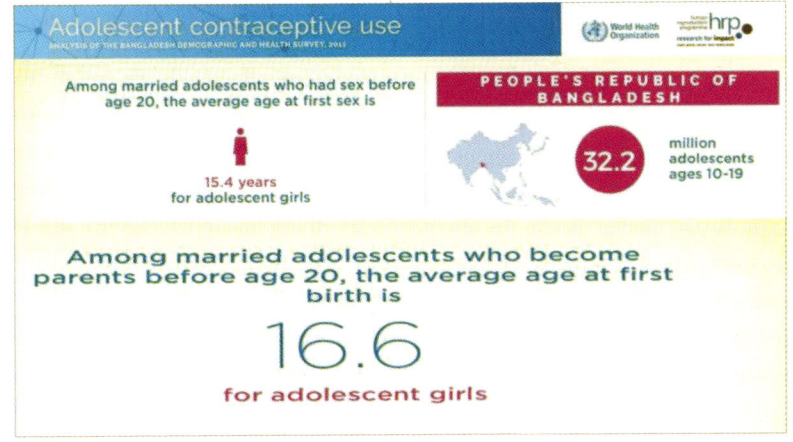

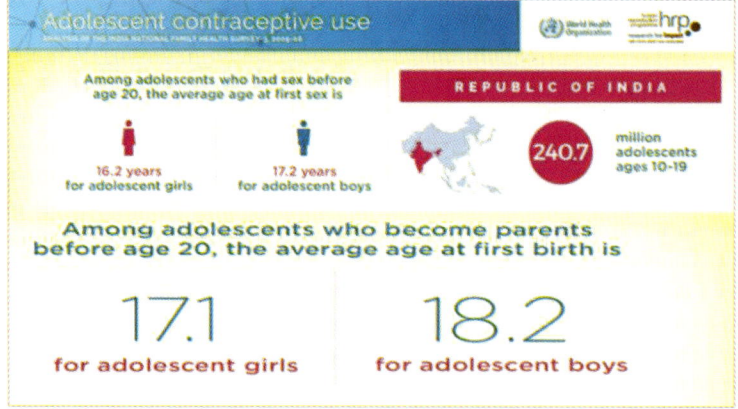

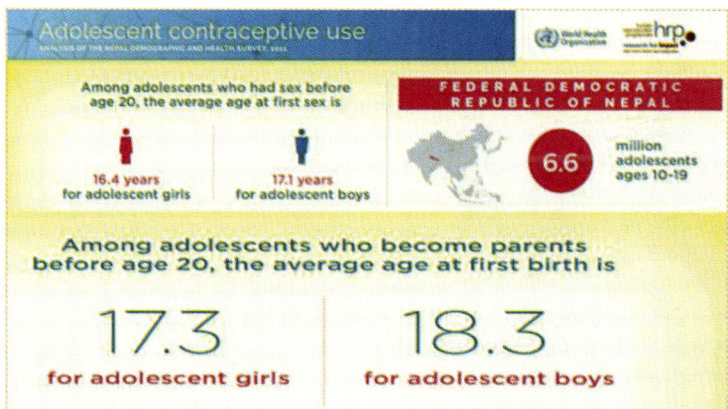

Barriers and Challenges

- Lack of laws or their enforcement to prevent early marriage, particularly for girls.
- Lack of (or no access to) safe abortion services and post-abortal care
- Lack of laws and/or their enforcement against violence including rape, sexual assault, incest, commercial sexual exploitation and sexual slavery.
- Lack of economic structures for adolescents to generate income to help protect them
- Low priority at political level

Social, cultural and Religious factors for adult women and adolescents

Various societal, cultural and religious factors create an inhibitive environment to discuss contraceptive need.

1. Unmarried adolescents are at particular risk of experiencing negative attitudes from parents, teachers and health care providers.
2. Lack of access to health information and services (services do not exist, negative staff attitudes)
3. Lack of sexual and reproductive health education within the educational system.
4. Numerous studies have demonstrated that teenagers armed with basic knowledge of reproductive biology and contraceptive methods are less likely to become sexually promiscuous, become pregnant, or contract STDs.
5. The home in which sexual behavior is discussed openly and honestly, with parents who are receptive to the special needs of the adolescent, is much less likely

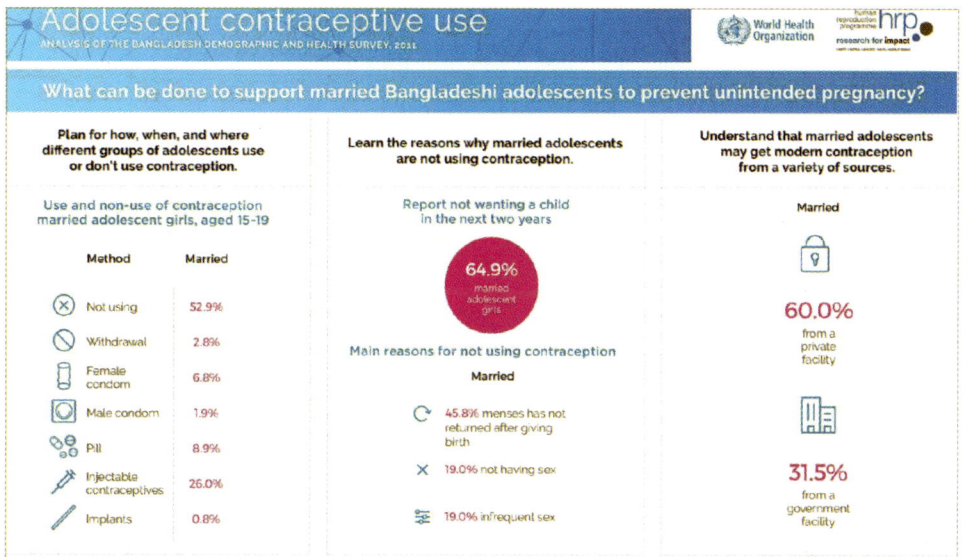

to have to endure the heartbreak of a teen's undesired, out-of-wedlock pregnancy, dropping out of school, or running away.
6. Religious believes.
7. Cultural norms and myths may prevent the women from seeking contraceptive assistance.

What we need to do?

1. Should give an opportunity to the woman to discuss their reproductive needs and contraception without the presence of the parents or guardian
2. Adolescent who discusses the issues with the parent or guardian is more likely to use contraception continuously
3. Male partner should be involved in discussions to enhance the sense of mutual responsibility
4. Need to have very strong political commitment. Women's education is one of the important factors that influence contraceptive use.

Overview of Situation

Unmet needs for contraceptive methods are considerably higher among poorer women.

There is limited political support to provide family planning services for poor people in the south Asian countries. The increasing trend of premarital sexual relationship and unintended pregnancies has created a greater need for contraceptives among young women. Sensitivities of sex-related issues in certain religious groups imposed various types of obstacles for young women's access to sexual and reproductive health information, support and practices.

In poor countries, young people's economic constraints affect their ability to buy contraceptives or seek sexual and reproductive health services.

Nepal

A study in Nepal showed that older women (35 and over), educated, living in urban, working in the business or service sectors were more likely to use modern contraceptive methods ($p < 0.05$). Ethnic disparities also affect the use of family planning services. Newars ethnicity is the highest among all ethnic groups in Nepal to use contraceptives. Analysis of Nepal Demographic and Health Survey (NDHS), indicated that despite considerable progress in meeting the Millenniumm Development Goals (MDG), different ethnic groups face many barriers for accessing family planning services, because of their illiteracy, poverty, and low social status.

In contrast, a survey of South Asian women aged 16 to 50 years, attending inner-city general practices in London, showed that unmarried women (11/13, 85%) were more likely to be using contraception than married women (54/91, [60%]) (OR = 1.4, 99% CI = 1.1 to 1.9). Thirty percent of married women at all ages and 50% (16/32) of women aged more than 30 years who said they had completed their families were not using any contraception.

Pakistan

A study among Afghan refugee women in Pakistan showed the use of contraceptive methods among women was higher in subsidized healthcare with increasing age as compared to the women in the non-health subsidy group. For example, women aged 25 years in healthcare subsidy group were 0.3 times less likely to use family planning, whereas women aged 35 years in the same group were 1.06 times more likely to use it. The potential influence of different cultures and religions on the acceptance and use of family planning methods by couples have been well documented.

India

Analysis of the National Family Health Surveys in India for Muslim and non-Muslim differentials in family planning showed that Muslim women have greater opposition to family planning. Muslims prefer to use temporary contraceptive methods while the National Family Planning Program promotes sterilization. Further, Muslims tend to utilize private-sector services due to greater privacy needs but the program rely on public-sector sources of supply of family planning. Muslim wives in comparison with non-Muslim wives usually have more children, are more likely to desire additional children, and are less likely to be using contraception when they desire no more children.

Bangladesh

Bangladesh government has given the highest priority in family planning sector. Family planning remains in the 4th health sector program (2017–2021), as a path toward achieving the sustainable goal. FWV, field workers, are knocking the doorsteps of women. All the logistics oral pills, condoms, IUCD, implants and Depo-Provera injection are widely available in upozela, sadar hospital and different satellite centers. Beside that NGOs, Marie Stops are working hard. Training is being given to doctors, nurses. Government has action plan for postpartum family planning. Also FIGO has initiated PPIUCD, which is becoming popular in Bangladesh. Though Bangladesh is doing very well but the picture in other part of Asia is not same. The use of modern contraception among other South Asian women is less than global average. In South Asia a majority of unintended pregnancies are due to using traditional contraceptive or no methods which lead to induced unsafe abortion. Cultural attitudes, lack of knowledge of methods and reproduction, socio demographic factors, and health service barriers are the main obstacles to modern contraceptive practice among South Asian women. Culturally sensitive family planning program, reforming health system, and reproductive health education through mass media to create awareness of the benefits of planned parenthood are effective strategies to improve modern contraceptive practice among South Asian women

- Challenges are lot
- Cultural factors
- Religious factors
- Fear of side effects and misconceptions

One of the most commonly cited reasons for non-use of contraception is fear of infertility.

Concerns about the side effects, health consequences and inconvenience of methods are particularly high in South and Southeast Asia. Fear of side effects and health concerns have been seen in urban areas of most countries, where barriers related to access seem to be relatively low. Method-related concerns are also common reasons for discontinuation of use among women with unmet need who had used family planning in the past.

Women's Autonomy and Decision-Making Power

The link between a woman's level of empowerment and her ability to make decision on reproduction and child bearing has been well documented.

Due to the multidimensional concept of autonomy, the factors affecting this occurrence were also varied between authors. Most of the literatures in South Asia had reported on women's participation in household decision making, control over financial resources, and. South Asian women are faced with a great disadvantage regarding to autonomy in decision making on their own health care.

A study among three Asian countries documented non-participation of women in household decision making in the majority of Nepal (72.7%) and approximately half of Bangladesh (54.3%) and Indian (48.5%) families. In all the three countries, participation of women in decision making significantly increases with age. Educated women were more likely to participate in decision making than noneducated women, OR = 1.60; 95% CI = 1.27–2.01 in Nepal, OR = 1.71; 95% CI = 1.46–1.99 in Bangladesh, and OR = 1.67; 95% CI = 1.60–1.74 in India. Urban women are always more likely to be involved in decision making than rural.

Shah in Pakistan reported that husbands in a majority (67.5%) of households decide on the desired number of children and contraceptive practice.

Limitations on women's mobility and prohibition of their accessibility to public places have been documented greatly for South Asian, Middle Eastern, and Central Asian and therefore women could not access to reproductive health services.

Researches indicate the limitation on women's mobility in Pakistan and India are connected to their limited access to contraception and abortion services.

Spouse Approval, Communication and Social Support

Husband's opposition has been reported as the main factor for not using any contraceptive method among Muslim married women. The roles of husbands as dominant member in rural areas are important in approving contraceptive practices and family size. Spousal communication about family planning has been proven to increase contraceptive use, even when other factors known to predict contraceptive practice to be controlled.

Involving males and obtaining their support and commitment to family planning is crucial for family planning service utilization. Investigation of the influence of spousal communication on the use of family planning methods in rural Nepal and Myanmar showed a strong positive impact of spousal communication on contraceptive use.

In South Asia, apart from husbands, the role of peers, mothers-in-law, and elders in contraceptive decision-making is well- documented. Urban women in Pakistan are more likely to use family planning if their mothers-in-law have discussed it with them as an option for their families.

Evidence from India showed that involving husbands and mothers-in-law in the intervention increased their support for a longer birth interval and the use of modern contraceptive methods. Moreover, the acceptance of postpartum contraception was significantly increased when the spouse discussed on reproductive issues, such as family planning, the odds ratio was 6.7 to 7.8 times greater among the couple who talked about family planning than when they did not (p<0.01).

Preference for a Son

A considerable amount of literature in South Asia, documents that the purpose of using contraception among women is to plan spacing, and number of children. The sex composition of family and the preferences for the sex of future children greatly influence women's decision making about type of contraception practice and when they use it.

The preference for sons in many East and South Asian societies have deep social, economic, and cultural roots. Son preference in India originates from the idea that economic and social benefit of sons is higher compared to daughters. In South Asia son preference is higher in urban than in rural areas, in families with more income, and more educated women. On the other hand, the picture is more mixed in Central Asia. However, son preference is similarly higher in urban than in rural areas, but higher among women with low educational status. A study among married women age 15–49 years in Ahmedabad district, India showed the son preference was more in rural areas (94%) than urban areas (81%; p<0.0001). A majority (93%) of the illiterate women preferred male child, whereas 69% of the women who completed graduation had the preference for son (p<0.01).

To Prove Fertility Soon after Marriage

Women and men face strong social pressure to prove their fertility as soon as possible after marriage. Marriage structures in many countries especially in Asia have been set up to maximize fertility and also to ensure early childbearing.

While this pattern has shifted significantly to later marriage and childbearing in East Asian countries, it is still common in South Asia. Countries such as India, Nepal, have significant high rates of early marriage and early childbearing. Strong social norms against delaying a first birth after marriage in countries like India with a high rates of adolescent childbearing make it difficult to eliminate this misconception.

Social Stigma and Embarrassment

Embarrassment and poor negotiation skills impose barriers to access sexual health information and services. Rural young people are more likely to be embarrassed than urbanites because there is a concern of stigmatization from local people in the rural areas.

Studies in Nepal and India have found that adolescents are reluctant to go to clinics and pharmacies to obtain contraceptives. They fear to be recognized by providers or people in their community and would negatively label them as sexually active. Research among Asian immigrant women had documented that they were not comfortable requesting emergency contraception from a health provider of the same ethnicity. This group of women assume that this act may result in chastise or gossip about them. They also feel uncomfortable to request emergency contraception from male doctors or pharmacists.

Health Service Factors

Running short of supply of methods and services is one of the most common cited reasons by married women for not using contraception. Non-availability of contraceptive, cost, long waiting hours at the center, shortage of the female staff and cost were reported as unsatisfactory variables in Pakistan. Studies on women's reproductive health have revealed that many health providers did not support the use of emergency contraception in Islamic countries because of concerns about promoting promiscuity. Half of the health providers thought disseminating information about emergency contraception would encourage young people to have unprotected sexual intercourse. Majority worried that increasing awareness of this method would lead to raising sexually transmitted infections because people would stop using barrier methods.

Conclusion and Recommendations

1. Contraceptive need to be the topmost priority in the national policy. In this regard Bangladesh has taken the lead by formulating and implementing the national strategy with consensus.
2. The autonomy of women was found to be a significant factor that influences contraceptive use in South Asian population. Women's autonomy in decision-making on health care should be improved in Asia particularly in South Asian region, and this could be achieved by promoting higher education and gainful employment for women. Women with higher education are more likely able to resist subjugation and to attain greater power in decision-making.
3. Confidential, personalized, adolescent's friendly service delivery need to be established.
4. Male participation in sharing the responsibility to practice and support family planning is identified as a vital strategy in increasing the contraceptive prevalence rate. In Asian countries reproductive health services are more focused on women and family planning services and information are not targeted towards men. Therefore, it is important to neutralize the stereotyping or, "feminization" of the service as a whole. Involving men in family planning program need comprehensive multilevel approach from policy to infrastructure and service delivery. Also, reproductive health educational program need to engage men to gain further support and to encourage husbands to share more responsibility in family planning.

5. Improving and implementing maternal health strategies may empower women to use effective modern contraceptive methods which in turn can help governments to achieve development goals.

BIBLIOGRAPHY

1. Ahmed S, Li Q, Liu L, Tsui AO Lancet 2012.
2. Alan Guttmacher Institute, 1994.
3. Alan Guttmacher Institute, 2002 a,b.
4. Chavada M, Bhagyalaxmi A. Effect of socio-cultural factors on the preference for the sex of children by women in Ahmedabad district. Health and population; perspectives and issues. 2009;32(4).
5. Hadley A, Chandra-Mouli V, Ingham R. Implementing the United Kingdom Government's 10-year teenage pregnancy strategy for England (1999–2010): Applicable lessons for other countries. J Adolesc
6. http://www.who.int/maternal_child_ adolescent/topics/adolescence/fram ework-accelerated-action/en/
7. http://www.who.int/reproductivehe alth/adol-contraceptive-use/en
8. https://www.researchgate.net/publication/23723565_Development_modernization_and_son_preference _in_fertility_decisions
9. https://www.researchgate.net/publication/291406934_Women's_Autonomy_and_Uptake_of_Contracepti on_in_Pakistan
10. https://www.researchgate.net/publication/305109117_Access_to_fam ily_planning_services_by_Muslim_communities_in_Nepal_- _barriers_and_evidence_gaps
11. Link CF. Spousal Communication and Contraceptive Use in Rural Nepal: An Event History Analysis. Studies in Family planning. 2011 Jun;42(2):83–92.
12. Mir AS, Malik R. Emergency contraceptive pills: Exploring the knowledge and attitudes of community health workers in a developing Muslim country. N Am J Med Sci, 2010 Aug;2(8):359–64.
13. Mishra MK. Ethnic Disparities in Contraceptive Use and its Impact on Family Planning Program in Nepal Department of Social Science, NIMS College, Lalitpur, Nepal. NJOG 2011;6(2):14–9.
14. Mishra V, Muslims and nonMuslim differentials in fertility and family planning in India. East west

centre working papers. Population and health series. No. 112, January 2004. Reproductive Health 2009; 6:3.

15. Mwaikambo L, Speizer IS, Schurmann A, Morgan G, Fikree F. What works in family planning interventions: A systematic review of the evidence. Stud Fam Plann. 2011 Jun;42(2): 67–82.

16. Najafi-Sharjabad F, Yahya SZS, Rahman HA, Hanafiah M, Manaf RA.Barriers of Modern Contraceptive Practices among Asian Women: A Mini Literature ReviewGlob J Health Sci 2013 Sep; 5(5):181–92.

17. Neelofur-Khan D. Adolescent pregnancy–unmet needs and undone deeds. A review of the literature and programmes issues in adolescent health and development. Geneva; 2007. (http://apps. who.int/iris/bitstre am/10665/43702/1/ 9789241595650_ eng.pdf).

18. PMCID: PMC2621397.

19. PMID: 19209272

20. Published online 2008 Oct.

21. Raheel H, Karim MS, Bharwani S, Saleem S. Knowledge, Attitudes and Practices of Contraception among Afghan Refugee Women in Pakistan: A Cross-Sectional Study. Published: November 2, 2012 https://doi.org/10.1371/ journal. pone.0048760

22. Riyami, Afifi M, Mabry RM. Women's Autonomy, Education and Employment in Oman and their Influence on Contraceptive Use. Reproductive Health Matters. 2004;12(23):144–54.

23. Saleem S, Bobak M. (2005). Women's autonomy, education and contraception use in Pakistan: A

national study. Reproductive Health, 2, 8. doi:10.1186/1742-4755-2-8.

24. Saxena S, Copas AJ, Mercer C, Johnson AM, Fenton K , Eren B , Nanchahal K , Macdowall W, Wellings K. Ethnic variations in sexual activity and contraceptive use: National cross-sectional survey. Contraception. Sept. 2006;74(3):224–33.

25. Senarath U, Gunawardena NS. Women's autonomy in decision making for health care in South Asia. Asia Pac J public Health 2009;21(2):137–43.

26. Sharma J, Dorairajan G, Chinnakali P. Knowledge and attitude towards contraceptive methods for spacing and decision making factors regarding its use in postpartum women. Int J Reprod Contracept Obstet Gynecol. 2015 Jun;4(3):750–4.

27. UN ICPD in Cairo 2013.

28. Ushma D. Upadhyay , Jessica D. Gipson, Withers M, Lewis S, Erica J. Ciaraldi, Fraser A, Huchko MJ, Prata N. Women's empowerment and fertility: A review of the literature. Social Science & Medicine 115,(2014):111e120

29. Westley E, Hertzen H, Faundes C. Expanding access to emergency contraception. International Journal of Gynecology and Obstetrics (2007) 97, 235–7.

30. Williamson LM, Wight D, Petticrew M, Hart GJ. Limits to modern contraceptive use among young women in developing countries: A systematic review of qualitative research. https://doi.org/ 10.1186/1742-4755-6-3© Williamson et al. licensee BioMed Central Ltd. 2009.

31. Wright KP, Johnson JV. Evaluation of extended and continuous use oral contraceptives 2008 Oct;4(5):905–11.

Rape in South Asia: Healing Unspoken Wounds

Mariam Iqbal, Asifa Naureen, Rubina Sohail

BACKGROUND

South Asia is a dynamic region which constitutes many countries which have quite a diverse culture, political framework and economic status. Many of these countries are struggling with political skirmishes and most are undergoing ever changing socioeconomic revolutions. In this rapidly transforming part of the world which struggles constantly with a heavy population explosion and limited resources, issues of human trafficking, undocumented migrations and ever growing poverty, etc. have led to a rapid increase in crime rates including rape. World Health Organization (WHO) describes sexual violence including rape, in the report on violence and health, as "physically forced or otherwise coerced penetration—even if slight —of the vulva or anus, using a penis, other body parts or an object." Koss et al. describes rape as a "severe form of sexual aggression and includes completed vagina, oral, or anal penetration through misuse of victim's intoxicated state, threat, or use of physical force." The South Asian region where most societies are predominantly patriarchal, and women's role being subservient economically and socially, rape is quite prevalent but the most unreported crime. Lack of education, political influences, feudal and tribal cultures, misuse of religious interpretations, customs and so called "traditions" are some of the many factors which lead to under-reporting of this horrid crime. Some other important factors like gender inequality and low socio-economic status and lack of empowerment of women add fuel to this exploitation of women.

BURDEN OF DISEASE—UNSPOKEN GRIEF

The assessment of burden of sexual violence in South Asia is a huge challenge as the data is scanty and fragmented and probably the most under reported crime. Most women hesitate to report sexual violence to police because either they are embarrassed, ashamed or fear being blamed, not believed or otherwise ill-treated. The percentage of women who contact medical services for help is also relatively small so most remain unreported. According to an estimate, 67–84% of cases of sexual violence go un-reported, being a socially sensitive issue, making it even more difficult to access exact burden of the problem. It has been hypo-thesized that virginity is culturally associated with not only honor of the woman but also the family which discourages the victim and family to report this crime and hence avoid being stigmatized.

Reported incidences in literature vary because of discrepancy in the definitions used by different studies, the diverse nature of the methodology and samples employed. Very few studies have compared results across different countries. Even the few official reports by UN and World Health Organization (WHO) surveys just show the tip of an iceberg.

In India, between 2009 and 2013, 8,342 rape cases were reported per year (23 women raped every day), 400,000 women and girls have been kidnapped over the last 10 years, most of whom were raped or sold for prostitution. In some rural areas, there have been rape cases reported by men of dominant castes of women belonging to lower castes like women and girls of Dalits (the lowest untouchable caste). These women and their families chose to remain quite about the incidences due to mistrust in police who would never support them and of course due to fear of being defamed. Women in villages have to go out in fields to pass stool which exposes women to being abducted and abused. In December 2012, the gang rape of a medical student Nirbhiya in a bus in New Delhi who died of internal injuries triggered demonstrations across India.

In remote villages of India, community's senior members or the heads of village committee would order rape of women as a means of punishment for wrong doings of the woman's family. Rapes have been reported as a tool of conflict during communal riots, in 2002, in Gujarat and then Muzaffarnagar riots in 2013. In Bangladesh, there were 757 reported cases of rape in 2016, among which 212 were gang rapes, and more than two-thirds of victims were sadly below the age of 18. However, the number of victims seeking legal or medical help is small due to fear of social stigma.

The Nepal Police reported a tremendous increase in the rape cases from 154 to 912, in 10 years from 2003–04 to 2013–14. Just like most South Asian countries rape is also a least reported crime due to social barriers as well as the limitation by law of reporting within 35 days of the crime

In Pakistan over 53,000 cases of violence against women were reported between 2011 and 2015: according to police statistics.[9] Punjab had the highest number of recorded cases in 2015, followed by Sindh and KP. Crimes targeting women, such as abduction, murder and rape are among the most common. In October 2016, the parliament passed anti-honor-killing and anti-rape bills, which extended sentences and prohibited victims' relatives from forgiving the criminals. HRCP (Human Rights Commission of Pakistan) report more than 250 incidents of rapes and gang rapes took place in the first 6 months of 2005 alone. Maximum number of victims was reported in the age group 10–19 years, 62.2%. Physical trauma was reported in 39% and genital trauma in 19% cases. The accused were identified as family friends (25%) and neighbors (23%). The recent incident of rape of a six-year-old child, Zainab on 4th Jan, 2018, in Pakistan stimulated a nation-wide protest which forced law enforcing agencies to not only arrest but also punish the abuser.

Sadly, enough most criminals enjoy impunity in this region and get away easily. A survey in Sri Lanka reported that over 95 percent of Sri Lankan men who committed faced no legal penalties. In Sri Lanka, India and most countries from the region, marital rape is not recognized as a crime. Lack of gender sensitivity, fear of being are some of the many factors which further discourage the rape victims and their families from pursuing legal action against their perpetrators. In India, only 3,860 of the 5,337 rape cases resulted in trials over a period of ten years. Offenders were either released due to lack of "proper" evidence or witnesses (reported by Indian National Crime Records Bureau). The failure of these countries to convict the abusers point to preponderance of gender inequalities and weak justice system in this region.

Afghanistan, being a war zone for many years, women suffered most under Taliban rule, as they were denied right to education, employment, health care, legal system. UNHCR quoted that 80% of Afghani women suffer due to atrocity of rape in refugee camps. In 2012, Afghanistan had 160 cases of rape, however, this is an underestimation as most cases are unreported and the actual numbers are much higher. The rate of rape in Maldives was estimated to be 1.4 cases per 100,000 populations while that of Bhutan was 7.7 cases per 100,000 populations in 2013.

What is the Issue?

Violence against women is not only a serious health concern but in fact is an urgent human rights issue. This extreme form of sexual aggression against women can lead to serious health consequences. These women suffer not only physical injuries but also are scarred emotionally. These victims are more prone to mental health issues like depression, anxiety and post-traumatic stress disorder and are more susceptible to committing suicide. They also have a higher risk of acquiring non-communicable diseases, including hypertensive disorders and cardiovascular disease.

These emotionally tormented women are also at an increased risk of sexual and reproductive health problems, including unwanted pregnancies, teenage pregnancies, unsafe abortions, adverse maternal and newborn health outcomes, sexually transmitted infections and HIV infection, and gynecological problems. Violence also has other long-term effects like emotional, social and behavioral problems which has a significant human and financial cost for victims as well as their families and in fact society as a whole. Rape survivors are vulnerable to many psychological disorders. Short-term consequences include shock, anger, irritability, intrusive memories, low self-esteem, self-blame, dissociation, low mood and depression, shame and guilt, fear, anxiety, bewilderment, and social withdrawal. People who are sexually assaulted are more likely to develop post-traumatic stress disorder (PTSD) than any other trauma and have symptoms like, emotional detachment, flashbacks, and sleeping problems. They also suffer from sexual and relationship difficulties later on. Psychological interventions for PTSD include

cognitive behavioral therapy (CBT) and eye-movement desensitization and reprocessing (EMDR).[15] Violence has reached its peak in many South Asian countries leading to a high prevalence of mental disorders among women which is more than men. In Bangladesh, male to female ratio for medical disorders was shown in a study to be 2:1 and that of suicide to be 3:1. A study from Nepal showed it to be 2.8:1. A meta-analysis of 13 studies in India showed a prevalence rate of 64.8 per 1000 in women. Sexual violence is a major cause of mental health illnesses and sometimes depression also sets in due to the negative social responses to the incident by others including family sometimes.

Teenage pregnancy is also common in this part of the world. This is a result of not only early marriages but also the non-availability of emergency contraception and abortion-related services. Women are made to continue the pregnancies even when resulting from rape. The root cause is sexual myths and cultural norms that prohibit young, unmarried women from seeking assistance for reproductive health services. Other consequences of this crime include illegal abortions and spread of sexually transmitted disease including HIV.

When these women come in contact with a health care professional, things are no better as the poor medical response capability of the health facilities for victims of rape is also a major concern in the region. The health issues to be dealt with in these cases are all sensitive and specialized care is needed to deal with issues like physical injury and disability, mental health problems, reproductive health and sexual health problems. Health care personnel delay recognition of violence due to lack of training in this specific area. They are reluctant to talk about it or counsel perhaps again because of lack of training and sometimes fear of facing legal proceedings as a witness. Limited resources at most facilities are also a barrier in providing efficient care. Although most countries are vigorously trying to develop and improve their health facilities and systems by training staff and improving resources, however, there is a long way to go.

Families of these victims suffer, children of abused women experience anxiety and behavior problems, loss of home, search for safe space and loss of wages and income. Communities and societies suffer at large as they not only have to bear the high cost of providing services but also of lost producti-vity and loss of victim's, i.e. women's partici-pation in public life. Women and girls who experience violence need support and services, however, they face social stigma, fear being blamed and feel ashamed due to lack of support from family as well as community at large.

Rape as a weapon for war—deep and painful lessons

Rape and other forms of sexual aggression have been reported in literature, to be used in South Asia as a form of political weapon during battles. Amnesty International reports women's bodies becoming part of the terrain of conflict. The report blames conflicts in Colombia, Iraq, Sudan, Chechnya, Nepal and Afghanistan. Use of rape as a combat tool is a strategic military strategy to control the opposite force and also in some cases for ethnic cleansing as seen in Bosnian women. Some 200,000 women were raped during the battle for Bangladeshi independence in 1971. According to Amnesty report the pro-government Janjaweed militias in Sudan's Darfur region used rape as a hatred tool to control and humiliate non-Arab groups.

In 1995, guidelines for prevention and response to sexual violence among refugee populations were released by the office of the United Nations High Commissioner. Similarly, the International Rescue Committee has developed a program to combat sexual violence in refugee communities. These programs use participatory methods to assess the incidence of sexual violence in refugee populations, community workers to identify and rehabilitate cases and help in finding and handing in perpetrator .

Handling the situation: Turning Scars into Smiles

There is an urgent need to bridge health inequalities in South Asian region, a region which struggles endlessly with issues like poverty, gender discrimination, war conflicts and an internally displaced population and refugees. There is a need to identify rape as a serious human right violation and lack of reproductive health crisis as an emergency issue, if we are to safeguard reproductive rights of the young girls and give them a chance to develop their human capabilities and access to education and a decent life.

The only way forward is to promote gender equality and address multiple security threats. It is sad how most countries legal systems, health systems and governments have failed to respond proportionate to the magnitude of the problem. The following strategies can be adopted to combat this growing menace make a difference in these women's lives.

Reliable reporting systems, database and collecting evidence

There is a serious need for a reliable reporting system in both the health and legal system so that the victims feel secure to report their misfortune and are ensured that their stories will not be left unheard and the culprits will be punished.

Role of health systems

Women who experience violence may not report to law enforcing ages for fear of being mistreated, however, do reach out to health facilities which become their first and perhaps the only point of contact with a professional. The care a patient initially receives influences her recovery from the trauma suffered due to rape. Some women suffering in silence do seek medical help at some point in their lives and they may not be open about it, so health care providers need skills and training to give support and level of compassionate care to these women that they deserve.

Health Care Responses

Timely and appropriate management of these post-assault medical issues is crucial. At times, the safety and forensic issues surrounding sexual assault can create clinician anxiety, resulting in delay in the appropriate assessment of mental health administration of medical care. A victim's overall and referral for emotional support should be considered.

In many countries, where sexual violence is reported the health sector has the duty to collect medical and legal evidence to corroborate the accounts of the victims or to help in identifying the perpetrator. Unfortunately, in many countries rape victims are not examined by gynaecologist and instead are assessed by police examiners who are not trained or experienced in conducting these examinations. A study from Pakistan revealed that only 21% of the victims were examined by a doctor and specimens were obtainedin only 14.9% of the cases. Thereare no standard protocols or guidelines to standardize the treatment or document injuries.

There is a need to have and follow standard protocols and guidelines which would translate into considerably improved quality of care and psychological support of affected women. This will also ensure proper documentation and collection of evidence. A 'survivor-centered approach' should be adopted when examining them which involves respecting woman's autonomy to choose treatment and even report the case. The woman's safety is most important and there should be no discrimination when being examined. The victims right to confidentiality should be the highest priority.

A comprehensive protocol for examination and treatment of an assault victim should be as follows:

Documenting a full description of the incident, listing all the accumulated evidence:

Some countries use the *"sexual assault evidence kit"* that carries instructions, appropriate containers for collecting evidence, relevant legal forms and documents for recording histories. Examination of a rape victim is a sensitive and stressful situation. Adequate reassurance to the victim and explanation of procedure needs to be done. Use of a video to explain the procedure before starting an examination would make it more comfortable for the victim.

Recording gynaecological and contraceptive history

- Documenting of full physical examination preferably using a diagrammatic documentation for ease of site of injuries/lacerations needs to be done.
- **Assessment of the risk of pregnancy, providing emergency contraception and, where legal, counseling on abortion**
- Levonorgestrel—use within 72 hours of UPSI or contraceptive failure. If liver enzyme-inducing drugs have been used by the woman, a double dose (3 mg) is recommended.

  Copper-bearing intrauterine device with antibiotic prophylaxis. It can be used within the first 5 days (120 hours) following first unprotected sexual intercourse or within 5 days from the earliest estimated date of ovulation. It is important that antibiotic prophylaxis is given in the circumstances of sexual assault.
- Ullipristal acetate (if available).

Testing for and treating sexually transmitted diseases antibiotic prophylaxis (for gonorrhoea and chlamydia) can be considered in certain circumstances:

- 500 mg ceftriaxoneintramuscularly
- 2 g metronidazole orally and 1 g azithromycin orally as a single immediate dose
- The situations when antibiotic prophylaxis can be considered may include a patient who requires an emergency intrauterine device fitting or is unable to attend or access

screening (e.g. a patient that is likely to miss appointments, the alleged suspect is known to have an infection or foreign travel where medical care is difficult to access)

- A routine screen should be organised for approximately 10–14 days after the assault. The screen would be site-specific depending on the nature of the assault.
- Hepatitis B vaccination
- It may have a protective effect if administered within 6 weeks of the assault.
- An accelerated schedule can be considered where the three vaccines are given within 1 month (at exposure, 1 week post-exposure and 3 weeks post-exposure).

Prophylaxis for HIV Infection

The risk of transmission of HIV during rape is a serious concern, especially in countries with a high prevalence of HIV infection. The risk of HIV infection after a single episode of unprotected intercourse with an infected partner is comparatively little (approximately 1–2 per 1000, from male to female). However, after rape due to tears in vaginal mucosa, the risk is increased. Many women who arrive at a healthy facility right after will not be in the state of mind to fully understand information about need for testing and risks of HIV. There is an issue of losing these patients in follow-up so suggesting antiretroviral therapy seems like a reasonable offer, even though effectiveness after rape is not well established. Most recommend HIV post-exposure prophylaxis after sexual exposure (PEPSE) should be given only if highly suspected.

Centers providing comprehensive care to victims of sexual assault

The first "One-Stop Crisis Centre" was established in 1993 in the accident and emergency department of Kuala Lumpur Hospital in Malaysia. It was initially made for victims of domestic violence but later extended to deal with rape victims. The centre comprises experts from the hospital, women's groups, the police, medical social workers, the legal advisors and the Islamic Religious Bureau and they handle more than 30 rape cases a month. Similarly, India has commenced "one-stop shop" crisis centers for sexual assault victims. This was as an aftermath of the Delhi incident of rape of the medical student mentioned above. Because of the shortage of doctors in many countries, specially trained nurses have been used in some places to assist victims of sexual assault. In Canada, for example, nurses, known as "sexual assault nurse examiners" are trained to care for rape victims. These nurses refer clients to a physician when medical intervention is needed.

Providing Counseling, Support—Psychiatrist, Psychosocial

The importance of counseling and support group initiatives in rehabilitation of these women cannot be emphasized enough. Brief cognitive behavioral therapy has shown to be a promising tool of healing, if given shortly after assault. Many of these women tend to blame themselves for the incident and need psychological support to help them recover from memories of these silent wounds. However, this requires training and resources. Mostly in these countries these services are provided by NGOs and women organizations. However, the number of women who have access to these therapies is small and especially not in rural or far flung areas a solution to overcome this barrier could be establishing free of charge helplines for these victims. These helpline numbers should be advertised extensively. The staff taking the calls should be trained to offer basic counseling and should be well aware how to refer women to specific centers and women shelters. This would also help women who cannot access facilities and don't want to face anyone and rather talk on the phone from the comfort of their home where they probably feel more secure. Most victims find counseling helpful in the process of recovering and moving on with their life.

Many such helplines and NGOs exist in some of the countries but are definitely few when compared to the magnitude of the problem. To name a few are Aurat Foundation, Shirkat Gah, War Against Rape, APWA, etc. in Pakistan; women's foundation, Saathi group, National Women's Commission, etc. in Nepal; Naari today, Bell Bajao, MAVA, in India; one stop crisis centre (OCC), VAW helpline network, in Bangladesh and SAWNET, Women in need (WIN) in Sri Lanka.

Recommendations

A lot of work is required to plan interventions to reduce this menace from society.

Training for Health Care Professionals

Issues concerning sexual violence are sensitive issues which should only be dealt by trained personnel. This training should be part of undergraduate for medical students and nursing and allied as well as postgraduate training and curricula. Specialized counselors should be trained. These trainings should enable these providers to detect and handle cases of sexual violence in a sensitive but efficient manner.

In the Philippines, the Task Force on Social Science and Reproductive Health, designed training modules for nursing and medical students for sexual assault victims. Similar manuals can be designed and implemented in native languages and distributed. Sexual assault kits can be designed according to contextual needs and distributed to all centers.

Legal Reforms

There is an absolute need for encouraging people to report incidents of sexual violence to the police and to improve the swiftness and sensitivity of the processing of cases by the courts. There is a need to establish sexual crime units, gender training for the police and court officials, women-only police stations and courts for rape offences. South Asia also faces the challenge of legislation that addresses rape.

The legal definition of rape, age of consent, laws vary across different countries. The decisions are influenced by judges inter-pretation rather than the law. Legal inter-ventions that can be adopted are:

- Broadening and standardizing the defini-tion of rape
- Reforming the rules to define duration of sentence and on admissibility of evidence;
- Eliminating the necessity for victims' descriptions to be verified

Laws which are not women friendly, like 'Zina Ordinance' and the 'Qunan-e-Shahdat' should be amended to ensure equal rights of women and equal importance to their testimony.

Primary Prevention

Providing services for silent survivors of crime is of utmost importance, however, there is also a need to emphasize role of primary pre-vention. Policy-makers, researchers, donors and nongovernmental organizations should therefore be encouraged to contribute in this vital area.

Awareness and Educational Programs

There is a need for life-skills and other edu-cational programs for sexual and reproductive health promotion. These should be culturally, religiously and contextually adapted. Unfortunately, tradition, customs and religion are used to justify this atrocity in this religion so it is very important to have religious leaders, community heads to do advocacy for the rape victims to encourage arrest of perpetrator and rehabilitation of these women.

Community Activism by Men

There have been men groups who work in close collaboration with women organizations to combat sexual violence against women. The few programs targeting perpetrators of sexual violence have generally been aimed at men convicted of assault. They are found mainly in the west and their utility in South Asia will have to be assessed as most men who are involved do not even think they did something wrong and infact blame the victim sadly enough.

Community Based Efforts—Prevention Campaign

Media has an important role in creating awareness and changing attitudes towards sexual violence through advertising on hoardings ("billboards" and in public transport, and on radio and television). Educational and awareness programs for communities, schools and refugee camps should be designed and culturally sensitive and participatory approach should be used to change mindsets and behaviour. The only way to combat underreporting and prevalence of this horrid crime is promoting gender equality. There is a need to acknowledge that underlying socioeconomic causes of violence, include poverty and lack of education which needs to be addressed by providing job opportunities for young people. Parents should also be counseled to improve child rearing, reduce the helplessness of women and promote and inculcate more gender-equitable concepts of masculinity in these vulnerable young minds. Discussions with adolescents about myths about rape, how to set boundaries for sexual activity, and differentiating between sex, and violence should be done.

There is a need for international organizations like WHO, and UNO to join hands with the governments of South Asian countries and assist in policy making, amending laws, training of healthcare professionals, police, judges and establishment of specialized centres to help these women appropriately.

Regaining Self-Confidence and Rehabilitation of these Silent Survivors

However, despite the stigma of rape, women in some parts of South Asia refused to be silenced. They struggle at a great personal cost to give women the identity they deserve. In India, for example, women protested naked against the alleged rape, torture and murder of a local woman, Thangjam Manorama, by paramilitary soldiers in the north-eastern Indian state of Manipur, in July 2004 which led to protests all over the country and government was forced to reduce the power of forces in the area. Mukhtaramai from Pakistan, survivor of a gang rape, was brave enough to report and fight for her case who later became a women activist.

CONCLUSION

Sexual violence is a common but serious public health problem affecting millions of people each year throughout the region. It is propelled by many factors like social, cultural and economic contexts but at the heart of sexual violence directed against women is gender inequality. Health professionals are the first line army to see these victims and hence have a vital role to play in supporting the rape victims—medically and psychologically—and collecting evidence to assist convicting the perpetrators. The training of staff and sensitization of government and civil society is a pre-requisite to reduce sexual assault in the region. Reforming strengthening the legal rights and reforms and promoting gender equality and women empowerment by improving their access to resources, employment, and secondary education will make them less vulnerable to mistreatment and violence. These measures remain crucial to prevention of violence against women in Asia. Let's join hands to eliminate this threat and making South Asia a safer region for our girls by providing better health care policies.

BIBLIOGRAPHY

1. Ansar Abbasi. Cases of violence against women increase, News International, January 6, 2017, https://www.thenews.com.pk/print/177182-Cases-of-violence-against-women-increase.

2. Apart LB. Lives Blown Apart: Crimes Against Women in Times of Conflict, London: Amnesty International Publications 2004.

3. Asia Foundation. The state of conflict and violence in Asia 2017[Internet]. [cited 2019 Feb 17]. https://asiafoundation.org/wp.../The_ State_of_ Conflict _and_Violence_in_ Asia-1.pdf

4. Foa EB, Hearst-Ikeda D, Perry KJ. Evaluation of a brief cognitive behavioral program for the prevention of chronic PTSD in recent assault victims. Journal of consulting and clinical psychology 1995;63(6):948.

5. Hagen K, Yohani S. The nature and psychosocial consequences of war rape for individuals and communities. International journal of psychological studies. 2010;2(2):14–25.

6. Kalra G, Bhugra D. Sexual violence against women: Understanding cross-cultural intersections. Indian journal of psychiatry. 2013; 55(3):244.

7. Koss MP, Abbey A, Campbell R, Cook S, Norris J, Testa M, Ullman S, West C, White J. Revising the SES: A collaborative process to improve assessment of sexual aggression and victimization. Psychology of Women Quarterly. 2007;31(4):357–70.

8. Krug EG, Mercy JA, Dahlberg LL, Zwi AB. The world report on violence and health. The lancet. 2002 Oct 5;360(9339):1083–8.

9. Manzoor I, Hashmi NR, Mukhtar F. Medico-legal aspects of alleged rape victims in Lahore. Journal of the College of Physicians and Surgeons Pakistan. 2010;20(12):785–90.

10. Maria Tanyag. Sexual and reproductive health is a security issue for Southeast Asia, Australian Journal of International Affairs, 2018;72:6,495–9, DOI: 10.1080/10357718.2018.1 534943

11. Niaz U, Hassan S. Culture and mental health of women in South-East Asia. World Psychiatry. 2006;5(2):118.

12. Odhikar, Annual Human Rights Report 2016, 30.

13. Parnis D, Mont JD. Examining the standardized application of rape kits: An exploratory study of post-sexual assault professional practices. Health Care for Women International 2002;23(8):846–53.

14. Rape is used as a weapon of war (June 9, 2011) http://www.bbc.co.uk/news/world-africa-13707445

15. Violence against women and HIV/AIDS: Setting the research agenda. Geneva, World Health Organization, 2001 (document WHO/FCH/GWH/01.08).

16. Winzer L, Krahé B, Guest P. The scale of sexual aggression in southeast Asia: A review. Trauma, Violence, & Abuse. 2017 Jan 1:1524838017725312.

17. World Health Organization. Global plan of action: health systems address violence against women and girls. World Health Organization; 2016.

18. Yuan NP, Koss MP, Stone M. The psychological consequences of sexual trauma. Retrieved Sept. 2006;27:2007.

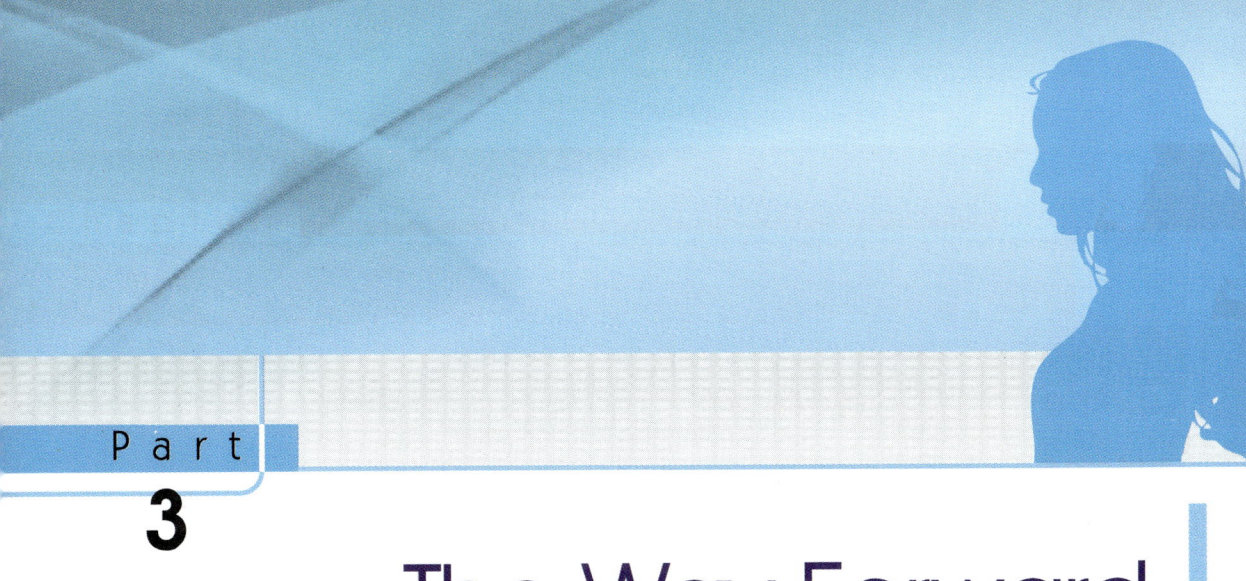

Part

3

The Way Forward

18

Integration of Human Rights in Physicians Practice

Rubina Sohail

INTRODUCTION AND BACKGROUND

Tremendous progress was made from the women's right perspective at the ICPD Conference in 1994 and Beijing Conference on Women in 1995 in bringing the agenda of women equality to the forefront. However, with millennium development goals (MDGs) and their deadline of September 2017, enough emphasis was not given on women's issues. Therefore, women's rights did not come out as strongly as was expected. The last decade saw a reduction in poverty mainly due to the efforts of two countries, China and India and there has been a global reduction in maternal mortality due to the growing number of skilled birth attendants, an increasing number of antenatal care visits and better EmOC. Despite this change, the decrease in morbidity and mortality has not been in proportion to the interventions done. In some countries, the MDG agenda did not get the attention that it deserved and in many countries, it was perceived as a donor driven agenda and not the need of the time. One of the lessons of MDGs was the fact that only numbers do not count, quality matters. Lack of women empowerment continued to be a reason for the lack of quality services for women and girls.

The SDG agenda has incorporated two important issues for women, firstly it has designated a goal to "gender equality, women's empowerment and women's rights" and secondly it proposes integration of gender equality in other key goals.

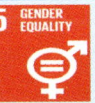 **SDG 5:** Achieve gender equality and empower all women and girls

Targets
- End all forms of discrimination against all women and girls everywhere
- Eliminate all forms of violence against all women and girls in the public and private spheres, including trafficking and sexual and other types of exploitation

Achieving gender equality by 2030 is a mammoth task and necessitates urgent action to eliminate the many root causes of discrimination that still curtail women's rights in private and public domains. For decades, women and girls have been discriminated against for food, education, health care, decision making, for employment and at workplace as well. This is compounded by long hours spent on household work, unsafe working environment and various forms of gender-based violence—emotional, physical and mental; all these have contributed to poor access and provision of health care services. Together, SDG 3 & 5 addresses the issues of gender equality, access to universal health and reproductive rights. Implementation of sexual and reproductive rights in clinical practice can help us achieve the objectives of SDG 3 & 5. The central principle of the *2030 Agenda for Sustainable Development* is to ensure that no one is left behind.

Target 5.6: Ensure Universal Access to Sexual and Reproductive Health and Reproductive Rights

Critical to SDG Goals 3 and 5 and Others

Target 5.6

Ensure universal access to sexual and reproductive health and reproductive rights as agreed in accordance with the program of action of ICPD and the Beijing platform for action and the outcome documents of their review conference.

Target 3.7

By 2030 ensure universal access to sexual and reproductive health care services, including for family planning, information and education, and the integration of reproductive health into national strategies and programs.

Target 5.2

Eliminate all forms of violence against all women and girls in the public and private spheres, including trafficking and sexual and other types of exploitation.

Target 5.3

Eliminate all harmful practices, such as child, early and forced marriage and female genital mutilation.

What are the rights?

A simplified list of The Universal Declaration of Human Rights adopted by the United Nations General Assembly on Dec 10, 1948

1. We all free and equal
2. I have right to freedom discrimination
3. I have the right to life
4. I have the right to freedom from slavery
5. I have the right to freedom from torture
6. I have the right to recognition even everywhere as a person before the law
7. I am entitled to equal protection before the law
8. I have right to legal assistance if my rights are being violated
9. I not be subjected to arbitrary arrest, detention or exile
10. I am entitled to a fair and public hearing
11. I am presumed innocent proven guilty
12. I have the right to privacy
13. I have the right to freedom of movement
14. I have the right to seek and enjoy in other countries asylum from persecution
15. I have the right to a Nationality
16. I have the right to marry and to found a family
17. I have the right to own private property
18. I have the right to freedom of thought and religion
19. I have the right to freedom of expression
20. I have the right to freedom of assembly
21. I have the right to participate in free and fair election
22. I have the right to social security
23. I have the right to work
24. I have the right to rest
25. I have the right to food and shelter
26. I have the right to education
27. I have the right to participate in cultural life and to the protection of author's rights
28. I have the right to social and international order
29. I have duties to the community
30. No one can take away my rights

Out of the long list of human rights, ten fundamental human rights contribute to optimal health care.

Health Care Rights

Health Care Rights
1. Life
2. Confidentiality
3. Right to decide on number and spacing of children
4. Health
5. Autonomy in decision making
6. Freedom from inhumane and degrading treatment
7. Privacy
8. Benefit from scientific progress
9. Information
10. Non-discrimination

Health is a fundamental human right. According to the constitution of World Health Organization (1948), "The enjoyment of the highest attainable standard of health is one of the fundamental rights of every human being without distinction of race, religion, and political belief, economic or social condition".

Dr Tedros Adhanom Ghebreyesus, WHO Director-General, on 10th December 2017, on human rights day said that "I call on all countries to respect and protect human rights in health—in their laws, their health policies and programs. We must all work together to combat inequalities and discriminatory practices so that everyone can enjoy the benefits of good health, no matter their age, sex, race, religion, health status, disability, sexual orientation, gender identity or migration status"

Importance of Integration of Rights

There is a strong association between reproductive health and rights, gender equality and the empowerment of women. The reproductive rights are fundamental to women's human rights and are the key to improving maternal health. Integrating the reproductive health rights into routine patient care by the physicians not only improves patient satisfaction, but also quality of health care leading to improvement in maternal health. Medical educationists have recommended that these rights and their integration to every day patient care should be a part of curriculum of nursing and medical students. During ICPD, it was proposed that curricula should promote gender equality and include life skills and sexual and reproductive health, in order to create awareness and build capacity of the schoolchildren to protect their own health.

How to Integrate Rights into Daily Practice

Integration of human rights into patients care is sadly lacking in medical teaching over the last many decades. The rights perspective and integration should be a part of curricula of doctors and nurses. In order to integrate the right into daily practice of physicians, sensitization and training is required. Physicians must be able to apply the principles of human rights to the daily practice of women's healthcare. In 2009, FIGO took up the responsibility of development and implementation of a curriculum of women's reproductive rights. This initiative was led by the FIGO committee on women's sexual and reproductive rights—Professors Diane Magrane and Lesley Regan. They developed competencies, teaching and learning tools which the physicians could easily introduce in their practice.

Integrated Competencies for Medical Practice

1. **Life: Everyone has the right to life.**
   - Discuss the impact of provision and denial of emergency healthcare services
   - Provide emergency life saving treatment independent of their own personal beliefs
   - Describe how health care systems can ensure or compromise the right to life.

2. **Health: Everyone has the right to the highest attainable standard of physical and mental health.**
   - Discuss the impact of availability, acceptability, accessibility and quality of care in health outcomes
   - Assess the quality of healthcare services for diverse populations in your community
   - Discuss how public health measures for screening of disease and injury prolong life expectancy

3. **Privacy: Everyone has the right to respect for privacy in the field of health care.**
   - Conduct the consultation, examination and treatment of the patient in a private space and in a manner that ensures privacy and respect
   - Recognize when there is a need for a third party or chaperone to be present
   - Maintain patient privacy in the presence of a chaperone or other individuals invited by the patient
   - Acknowledge and accommodate varying cultural attitudes towards modesty

4. **Confidentiality: Everyone has the right to confidentiality in relation to information on healthcare and health status.**
   - Maintain patient confidentiality and avoid unnecessary disclosure of information
   - Communicate to patients how confidentiality of all written and digital personal information are maintained
   - Discuss the potential harm and benefit of release of confidential information to third parties
   - Discuss how the interpretation of the laws on confidentiality affect the provision of healthcare for women
   - Discuss how decisions to protect or disclose confidential information are made

5. **Autonomy and decision-making: Everyone has the right to autonomous decision-making in matters concerning their health.**
   - Acknowledge and respect decisions that patients make about their own healthcare
   - Explore medical, social and cultural considerations affecting patient decision-making
   - Evaluate the capacity of an individual at any age to give consent
   - Ensure that the 'best interests' and evolving capacity of the child are considered in obtaining consent from children and their legal guardians

6. **Information: Everyone has the right to receive and impart information related to their health.**
   - Communicate risks/benefits/alternatives of accepting and declining therapies to patients
   - Offer full disclosure of test results and provide full information unless specifically requested otherwise by the patient
   - Use language in a manner that is culturally sensitive and understandable to the patient
   - Provide up to date information in understandable language to assist patients with informed decision-making

7. **Non-discrimination: No one shall be subject to discrimination on any grounds in the course of receiving healthcare. Discuss how principles of nondiscrimination result in improved health for everyone.**
   - Discuss the impact of societal and cultural roles and religious practices on healthcare
   - Discuss the extent to which women are ensured appropriate care in maternity services

   - Provide optimal healthcare services and establish mutually respectful relationships with men and women of all backgrounds and abilities

8. **Right to decide number and spacing of children: Everyone has the right to decide freely and responsibly on the number and spacing of children and to have access to the information, education and means to enable them to exercise these rights.**
   - Counsel patients about the risks, benefits, mechanisms of action and access to services for all methods of contraception
   - Provide information about the risks, benefits, mechanisms of action, and access to services for all methods of abortion, where it is legal
   - Discuss the effects of coercion or denial of contraceptive and abortion services upon the short- and long-term health of a woman and her family
   - Provide comprehensive preconception counseling
   - Discuss indications for referral for fertility problems

9. **Freedom from inhumane and degrading treatment: Everyone has the right to be free from torture or cruel, inhumane or degrading treatment or punishment in the field of healthcare:**
   - Identify and assist victims of physical, psychological and sexual violence and abuse, including domestic violence, trafficking, and political rape
   - Describe the effects of locally prevalent harmful practices such as female genital mutilation, early marriage, and polygamy
   - Discuss the harm resulting from involuntary sterilization and denial of medical treatment
   - Discuss how ethical standards for physician–patient relationships support standards of medical and surgical care

10. **Benefit from scientific progress: Everyone has the right to enjoy the benefits of scientific progress and its applications.**
    - Access and critically evaluate new information from a variety of sources
    - Inform patients of new evidence-based practices to maintain and restore health
    - Collaborate with patients to incorporate patients' health beliefs, community resources, and current medical therapies into effective healthcare plans

Source: GLOWM—Global Library for Women's Medicine—
See Appendix I for clinical application

Similarly, using the quality of care checklist, it can be determined whether the rights are protected or infringed upon by the providers and the health care system, during visit to a physician.

A Checklist for Quality Care

Life: Emergency health care is expected independent of personal beliefs
Health: The system presents no substantial barriers to available, acceptable, accessible, high quality health, including preventive screening for disease and injury
Privacy: Consultation, examination and treatment are conducted in a manner that ensures privacy, including times when chaperones and other invited individuals are present
Confidentiality: Conversation and medical records are maintained by procedures that ensure confidentiality and released to third parties only through appropriate legal procedures
Autonomy and decision-making: Decisions about healthcare are acknowledged and respected. When children are receiving care, their interests are protected in a manner that ensures their best interests and capacity for decision-making
Information: Understandable and up-to-date information about test results and risks/benefits/ alternatives of accepting and declining therapies are provided
Non-discrimination: Health care services that respect one's societal and cultural roles, religious practices, gender and abilities are provided
Right to decide number and spacing of children: When seeking counseling about pregnancy, fertility, contraception, or abortion, information about risks, benefits, mechanisms of action and access to services for all methods available are provided
Freedom from inhumane and degrading treatment: Seeking treatment for results of physical, psychological and sexual violence and abuse feels safe and without risk of involuntary treatment or denial of treatment from your healthcare provider
Benefit from scientific progress: Your healthcare provider helped you incorporate current scientific information, your own healthcare beliefs and knowledge of community resources into an acceptable healthcare plan

Source: GLOWM—Global Library for Women's Medicine

Case studies/scenarios have been developed for each competency and five questions are posed in all scenarios. These set of questions are applied to each scenario and in each case help in demonstrating the link between the rights and the health care outcome.

Five key Discussion Questions
1. What are the medical problems and health issues in this case?
2. What are the threats to human rights posed by the scenario?
3. How does this health care system support or infringe upon human rights?
4. What local practices and regulations affect the practitioner's ability to deliver human rights based patient care?
5. How could this healthcare encounter be improved to respect human rights and ensure quality health care?

CONCLUSION AND RECOMMENDATIONS

- A human rights approach to health is critical to address growing global health inequalities.
- WHO promotes the idea of people-centered care, which is actually the incorporation of human rights in clinical practice.
- Schools should promote gender equality and include life skills and sexual and reproductive health.
- Rights perspective should be added to the nursing, midwifery and medical curriculum
- Physicians must be able to apply the principles of human rights to the daily practice of women's health care.
- Teaching and training of physicians should be carried out, using the FIGO toolkit to build the capacity of physicians.
- Integrated competencies should be reviewed and ascertained.
- Use of checklist should be encouraged.
- GLOWM is a good source of information and has scenarios dealing with each of the rights, all of which could be used for teaching purposes.

APPENDIX I

Scenarios

Clinical Scenario # 01

Mrs. S.J., an 18-year-old mother of two, walks 7 kilometers to her local clinic in rural Africa to be evaluated for vaginal bleeding. Her last menstrual period was 14 weeks ago, and she has felt the familiar signs of nausea and breast tenderness of early pregnancy. The previous evening, she inserted some tablets into her vagina to induce an abortion. The friend who gave her the tablets told her they would make it seem like she was having a period, so her family would never know about the pregnancy.

The nurse at the clinic performs a vaginal examination and finds what appear to be retained products of conception lying within an open cervical os. The nurse also finds three white tablets in the vagina. The nurse records Mrs. S.J.'s history and physical examination in a handwritten note. She hands Mrs. S.J. an envelope with the note and a plastic specimen container with the three tablets, and then calls for an ambulance to transfer her to the district hospital.

After approximately 3 hours, the ambulance arrives to take Mrs. S.J. to the district hospital 300 kilometers away. Upon the patient's arrival, the doctor reviews the nurse's notes, examines the container of tablets, and asks her "Why did you murder your baby?" He conducts a cursory examination and adds a note to her records: "Criminal abortion, suspected use of misoprostol." Despite her profuse vaginal bleeding and rapid pulse, the doctor calls for an ambulance to take her to another hospital, which is 2 hours away. Mrs. S.J. continues to bleed throughout the long journey by ambulance and is pronounced dead on arrival at the provincial hospital.

Questions for discussion: Scenario # 01

1. What are the medical issues in this case?
2. What is the appropriate treatment for an incomplete abortion with active bleeding at this gestational age?
3. What are the health risks of delayed treatment of continued heavy bleeding after an incomplete abortion?
4. Using the Integrating Human Rights and Health Checklist, identify the human rights that were infringed in this case.
5. How did the responses of each of the health care providers respect or threaten the patient's right to life?
6. How should a health care provider reconcile his or her beliefs with the health care needs of the patient?
7. How did the policies and practices of this health care system support or infringe the patient's right to life?
8. What measures and policies need to be in place to avoid such situations recurring?
9. What policies in your health care system ensure quality care in situations like this?

Clinical Scenario # 02

Mrs. Z.B., a 35-year-old mother of four children (all under the age of 10 years), requests advice on effective methods of contraception. Her 11-month-old son was conceived while she was taking oral contraceptive pills. Although she took the pills regularly, on one occasion she was unable to obtain a new pack until almost a week after she was scheduled to begin them and during that period she became pregnant. She thinks that an intrauterine contraceptive device (IUCD) might be better for her. Both oral contraceptive pills and IUCDs are available at this clinic. Mrs. Z.B.'s last routine examination was 19 months ago, at the time of her first pregnancy consultation. She has no health complaints and no contraindications for either method of contraception.

The clinic doctor sees her at the end of a very busy day that has included two emergency procedures, 35 additional patients, and no lunch break. The doctor has a personal appointment immediately following clinic and Mrs. Z.B. is her last patient for the day. She reviews Mrs. Z.B.'s record and chooses not to conduct a physical examination. Dismissing Mrs. Z.B.'s questions about the IUCD, she tells Mrs. Z.B. that the pill is her best option. She quickly writes a prescription for oral contraceptives and leaves the clinic without advising Mrs. Z.B. on follow-up.

One year later, Mrs. Z.B. returns to the clinic, pregnant again.

During the course of her examination she is found to have a lesion on her cervix. A biopsy reveals cervical cancer.

Questions for discussion: Scenario # 02

1. What are the medical issues in this case?
2. What are the health risks and benefits of oral contraceptives, IUCDs, and pregnancy?
3. What routine screening is recommended at the time of counseling for contraception?
4. Using the Integrating Human Rights and Health Checklist, identify the human rights that were infringed in this case.
5. In what ways did the physician provide or deny optimal health care to Mrs. Z.B.?
6. What laws and policies in your country/ state/province address the issue of neglecting to provide proper care to patients?
7. What changes in policies and practices in this clinic would better ensure that all patients receive the highest standard of care possible?

Clinical Scenario # 03

Mrs. R.L. is a medical student at the teaching hospital in the capital city of a developing country. She has heard that women in the area generally know that when they attend the hospital's gynecology outpatient clinic, they will be interviewed and examined by student doctors and nurses along with the teaching consultant. Mrs. R.L. is one of six students assigned to work with Professor M.S., who has a reputation as an excellent teacher and clinician. Today Mrs. R.L. joins three other medical students and two nursing students to learn to perform vaginal speculum examinations.

Professor M.S. and a female nurse see patients in a clinic room that has no curtains or partitions. During the consultation, the women must remove their clothes in full view of the students. The consultant does not ask the women if they are agreeable to the students being present at the consultation and does not seek the patients' permission to teach the students how to place a vaginal speculum.

C.P. is a 32-year-old patient who is being seen in the clinic for heavy bleeding and a lower abdominal mass. She is embarrassed and distressed by the large number of people in the room and by the fact that she is menstruating. She asks Mrs. R.L. whether it is absolutely necessary for them to remain while she undresses. When Mrs. R.L. relays this query to Professor M.S., he retorts, "She knows she has come to a teaching hospital. I cannot have all the students leaving the room every time I ask a woman to undress and lie on the examination table, and then reenter to watch my examination. We do not have enough time to offer women that degree of privacy in this clinic "and manage to get through 30 patients in the same morning. Tell the patient to undress or to come back another time."

Questions for discussion: Scenario # 03

1. What are the medical issues in this case?
2. What is the differential diagnosis for the patient's symptoms?
3. Using the Integrating Human Rights and Health Checklist, identify the human rights that were infringed in this case.

4. How might privacy policies and practices of this clinic have an impact on the health of women in the community?

5. How might this clinic's procedures be redesigned to accommodate patient privacy and the need to train medical students?

6. What policies and practices regarding privacy are in place at your outpatient clinic?

Clinical Scenario # 04

Mrs. J.M., a 35-year-old professional woman, attends her first pregnancy visit at 8 weeks' gestation. As per the clinic's routine, she is offered an HIV antibody test. She accepts after stating that she does not want her partner to find out that she has taken the test, whatever the result may be.

When her doctor telephones to inform her that her HIV test is negative, she reminds him of her request that her partner is not to be informed about the test. The doctor reassures her that it is standard practice to record test information only in her medical record, which is confidential.

At her next visit, Mrs. J.M.'s partner accompanies her for the ultrasound scan to date the pregnancy. After a particularly long wait, Mrs. J.M. goes to the bathroom. Before she returns, the nurse calls her to see the doctor; in Mrs. J.M.'s absence, the nurse hands her antenatal record to her partner, saying, "Please go in to see the doctor as soon as she comes back." Glancing through her antenatal notes, Mrs. J.M.'s partner discovers that she has undergone an HIV test. He is happy that Mrs. J.M. is HIV negative but concerned that she needed to take the test and that she did so secretly. Earlier in their relationship, they had undergone HIV testing together, and they had both been found negative.

Questions for discussion: Scenario # 04

1. What are the risks and benefits of HIV screening in pregnant women?

2. Using the Integrating Human Rights and Health Checklist, identify the human rights that were infringed in this case.

3. What are the potential consequences to the patient of this loss of confidentiality?

4. How could the clinic staff have better protected the patient's record?

5. What are the laws/policies/regulations regarding medical confidentiality in your country/region?

6. How would you have counseled the woman about the sharing of results before she undertook the HIV test?

7. What actions would the doctor need to take if the woman's HIV test result had been positive?

Clinical Scenario # 05

Mrs. O.P., an unmarried 15-year-old high school student, finds herself pregnant by her 17-year-old boyfriend of several months. She estimates she is 10 weeks pregnant and visits a doctor to ask for an abortion.

Mrs. O.P.'s parents have made it very clear that they would no longer allow her to live at home and would withdraw all financial support were she to become pregnant before marriage. Mrs. O.P. has always aspired to attend college and graduate school. Her family knows about her relationship with the young man but they are unaware of its sexual nature. In her country, the law requires parental consent in all health care services for minors under the age of 16 years. It also provides for abortion for any woman upon request, up to 12 weeks of pregnancy. However, the doctor refuses to perform an abortion for Mrs. O.P. unless one of her parents provides consent for the procedure.

Questions for discussion: Scenario # 05

1. What are the medical issues in this case?

2. What are the health risks and benefits of a termination procedure at 10 weeks' gestation?

3. How do these risks change if the procedure is delayed for a further 4–6 weeks?

4. What are the health risks if this girl undergoes an unsafe abortion?

5. What are the likely health and social outcomes of a pregnancy for this 15-year-old?

6. Using the Integrated Human Rights and Health Checklist, identify the human rights that were infringed in this case.

7. How does the law in your country/state/province recognize the principles of evolving capacity or best interest of the child as it applies to medical care?

8. How do your responses to the above questions guide your support of O.P.'s decision-making authority free from parental consent?

Clinical Scenario # 06

At the time of consultation for a pelvic mass, the family of Mrs. S.Y. asks the gynecological surgeon to withhold the diagnosis from Mrs. S.Y. if she proves to have cancer. Mrs. S.Y. is a 46-year-old woman from a very traditional family, as is her surgeon. Their families share a long-held belief that if a patient is diagnosed with a terminal illness, the doctor should inform the family members but not the patient herself, as a kindness to the patient. The surgeon listens to S.Y.'s family's request and responds, "Let's wait and see how the surgery goes first."

Surgery reveals that Mrs. S.Y. has stage II epithelial ovarian cancer. The surgeon informs her family of the diagnosis and of the need for further treatment. The family repeats their request to withhold the information from Mrs. S.Y. Thus, the doctor informs Mrs. S.Y. that the surgery has gone well but that further treatment will be required to prevent recurrence of the mass. Mrs. S.Y. asks no further questions. Her doctor prescribes oral chemotherapy, which he refers to as "medication" and which her family calls "health supplements."

Soon, severe medication-related nausea and vomiting limits S.Y.'s ability to conduct her daily duties for several days following each administration. Mrs. S.Y. refuses to continue taking the drugs. In response to incessant pressure from family members to "take her health supplements," she moves to another small town, where she dies of cancer within 8 months.

Questions for discussion: Scenario # 06

1. What are the medical issues in this case?

2. What is the appropriate treatment for stage II ovarian cancer?

3. What are the health consequences of the interruption of postoperative chemotherapy for stage II ovarian cancer?

4. Using the Integrating Human Rights and Health Checklist, identify the human rights that were infringed in this case.

5. What are the health consequences of failing to fully inform the patient of her condition and treatment?

6. What hospital policies and laws in your state/province/country protect patients' rights to health information?

7. How would you respond to the strong cultural pressures to comply with the family's wishes and meet the ethical obligation to support the patient's right to information about her diagnosis, prognosis, and treatment?

8. What measures need to be put in place to avoid similar situations occurring in the future?

Clinical Scenario # 07

At 36 weeks into her second pregnancy, Mrs. A.R. is still undecided about where to deliver. A.R.'s midwife at the primary health center strongly encourages her to take up residence at a local hospital maternity waiting home where she delivered her first child. That delivery was complicated by a severe postpartum hemorrhage.

Mrs. A.R. is reluctant to make the 50 kilometer journey to the maternity home because of her previous experience with the hospital's religious policies.

The hospital is faith based but receives 20% of its annual funding from the state in return for providing public services. Hospital policy requires that all residents of the maternity home attend Sunday church services in the hospital's chapel, where only the religion of the hospital founders is recognized. Mrs. A.R. does not practice that religion and finds the services disturbing. During her last pregnancy, she requested to be excused from Sunday services and was accused of being ungrateful for the free lodging and meals provided to her during her stay. Her pregnancy care was excellent but she felt humiliated by the experience.

This time she does not go to the maternity waiting home. At 38 weeks, Mrs. A.R. goes into labor and within 3 hours she delivers a healthy daughter at the primary health center. She again bleeds profusely when the placenta is delivered. The clinic midwife gives her an injection of oxytocin and applies compression while waiting for the ambulance to arrive to take her to the hospital. Still bleeding, Mrs. A.R. is transferred to the same district hospital where her first child was born. Upon arrival, the doctors pronounce her dead of exsanguination. The pastors give her body the blessings of the church and release it to her family.

Questions for discussion: Scenario # 07

1. What are the medical issues of this case?
2. What are the possible complications during the delivery of a woman who has a history of postpartum hemorrhage?
3. What is the appropriate antepartum management of a patient with previous postpartum hemorrhage?
4. What is the appropriate management of acute postpartum hemorrhage?

5. Using the Integrating Human Rights and Health Checklist, identify the human rights that were infringed in this case.
6. How did the policies for religious observation at the maternity home cause discrimination against A.R.? What were the health consequences of that discrimination?
7. What laws and/or policies of your state or country protect against discrimination in health care settings?
8. How might the system of maternity care offered by this district hospital become more inclusive and welcoming for women and continue to respect the wishes of the religious organization that finances the project?

Clinical Scenario # 08

Doctor D. and Mr. M., the administrator of the hospital where Dr. D. practices, meet to discuss a letter of complaint from a patient who had an abortion in the outpatient surgical clinic 3 months previously. The letter states that the patient was forced to undergo a painful vacuum aspiration of a 10-week pregnancy without anesthesia and that Dr. D. ignored her screams of pain and requests for pain relief.

Dr. D. suspects that Mr. M. shares her belief that far too many women are having abortions. She assumes that he will support her opinion that providing pain relief only encourages these women to have more abortions. Although Dr. D. professes that she supports legal and safe abortion, she believes that the current laws make it too easy for women to terminate their pregnancies. Dr. D. considers that a little pain during the procedure discourages women from having unprotected sex.

Mr. M. expresses his disbelief that Dr. D. would purposely withhold pain relief for women undergoing operative surgical procedures. Dr. D. replies, "Only those having abortions, Mr. M. You have to be cruel in order to be kind." She continues, "There is only a little cramping if they lie still on the table. But if they move, they pay the price."

Horrified, Mr. M responds, "Do you mean to say that this woman is not the only one? How many times have you performed this procedure without anesthesia? This former patient of yours claims she has recurrent nightmares and is no longer able to function at work as a result of your cruelty and lack of professionalism. How do you expect the hospital to respond to this complaint?"

Questions for discussion: Scenario # 08

1. What are the medical issues in this case?
2. What measures can be taken to assess and provide pain relief during outpatient surgical procedures?
3. What are the risks and benefits of providing or not providing pain relief for a patient having a vacuum aspiration of the uterus?
4. Using the Integrated Human Rights and Health Checklist, identify the human rights that were infringed in this case.
5. What standards of practice in hospitals and outpatient surgery clinics ensure a patient's right to be free from degrading and inhuman treatment?
6. How should the hospital administrator respond to the patient's letter of complaint?

Clinical Scenario # 9

Mrs. R.S., a 22-year-old woman, is admitted to the emergency department at 13:00 for evaluation of assault. She reports taking the bus home after a long day of work at the supermarket and then attending evening classes at the local community college. About three blocks from the bus stop, a man with a knife in his hand appeared from the shadows of a vacant parking lot. He pushed her into the bushes, raped her, and ran off. She gathered her clothing and ran the remaining five blocks home, where her mother was anxiously awaiting her arrival. Her mother drove her to the local hospital emergency department and now sits in the waiting room during the examination.

A nurse cleans multiple abrasions on Mrs. R.S.'s thighs and knees and takes blood samples for HIV testing. The doctor sutures and bandages a small wound on her forehead, then performs a pelvic examination; he sends swabs to be cultured for sexually transmitted infections (STIs) and collects a few blades of grass for forensic documentation.

When she is discharged, Mrs. R.S. asks for emergency contraception and voices concerns about STIs, including HIV. She is given an injection of penicillin and told that she must wait for the HIV results before the doctor will consider prescribing antiretroviral drugs. The doctor explains, "These drugs are much too expensive to be used for anyone who does not already have HIV infection. You must wait until your test results are available. Furthermore, I will *not* prescribe emergency contraception. I have never performed an abortion and I do not intend to begin with you!" Exhausted and distressed, Mrs. R.S. leaves the hospital with her mother.

Questions for discussion: Scenario # 9

1. What are the medical issues in this case?
2. What are the health risks and standards of care for a woman who suffers sexual violence from an unknown aggressor?
3. What therapies are available to reduce the risks of pregnancy, STIs, including HIV? What is the mechanism of action of each of these therapies?
4. What are the consequences of denying access to these therapies?
5. Using the Integrated Human Rights and Health Checklist, identify the human rights that were infringed in this case.
6. How did the practices of this emergency department support or infringe upon the patient's right to benefit from scientific progress to prevent sequelae of sexual assault?

7. What changes in policies and practices of this department would improve care and protection of the rights of patients who are being examined for sexual assault?

BIBLIOGRAPHY

1. Amnesty International. Prescription for Change: Health Professionals and the Exposure of Human Rights Violations. International Secretariat; 1996.
2. Bueno de Mesquita J, Kismödi E. Maternal mortality and human rights: landmark decision by United Nations human rights body. Bulletin of the World Health Organization. 2012 ;90(2):79-A.
3. Farmer P. Pathologies of power: Health, human rights, and the new war on the poor. North American Dialogue. 2003;6(1):1–4.
4. Geiger HJ, Cook-Deegan RM. The role of physicians in conflicts and humanitarian crises: Case studies from the field missions of Physicians for Human Rights, 1988 to 1993. JAMA. 1993;270(5): 616–20.
5. Global Library of Women's Medicine. Integrating Human 286 Rights and Women's Health | GLOWM https://www.glowm.com/Integrating_womens_rights
6. Hannibal K, Lawrence RS. The health professional as human rights promoter: ten years of Physicians for Human Rights (USA). Health and human rights. 1996:110–27.
7. Human Rights Council. Eleventh Session. Resolution 11/8. Preventable maternal mortality and morbidity and human rights. United Nations. A/HRC/RES/11/8. 17 June 2009. http://ap. ohchr.org/Documents/ E/HRC/resolutions/ A_HRC_RES_11_8.pdf. Accessed 27 Dec 2016.
8. Human Rights Council. Fifteenth session. Resolution 15/17. Preventable maternal mortality and morbidity and human rights: follow-up to council resolution 11/8. United Nations General Assembly. A/HRC/RES/15/17. 7 October 2010. https://documents-ddsny.un.org/doc/ UNDOC/GEN/G10/167/35/PDF/G1016735. pdf. Accessed 27 Dec 2016.
9. Iacopino V. Istanbul Protocol Model Medical Curriculum. Physicians for Human Rights. 2013. Web site.
10. MacNaughton G, Forman L. The value of mainstreaming human rights into Health Impact Assessment. International journal of environmental research and public health. 2014;11(10): 10076–90.
11. Mann JM, Gostin L, Gruskin S, Brennan T, Lazzarini Z, Fineberg HV. Health and human rights. Health and human rights. 1994:6–23.
12. Mann JM. Health and human rights. Protecting human rights is essential for promoting health. BMJ. 1996;312:924–5.
13. Mohanty A, Gurpur S, Beerannavar CR. Rethinking Inclusive Development: A Human Rights Critique of South Asia. Procedia-Social and Behavioral Sciences. 2014;157:128–36.
14. Muhunthan K, Arulkumaran S. Medical Ethics and Human Rights in Reproductive Health. Nepal Journal of Obstetrics and Gynaecology. 2014; 9(1):5–7.
15. OECD/WB (2013) 'Integrating Human Rights into Development: Donor Approaches, Experiences, and Challenges', 2nd edition, World Bank; Organisation for Economic Cooperation and Development, Washington, DC.
16. Piron LH, O'Neil T. Integrating Human Rights into Development. A synthesis of donor approaches and experiences. 2005 Sep.
17. Reproductive Health and Rights: Key to Achieving the Millennium Development Goals; 27 October 2004.
18. Shaw D, Cook RJ. Applying human rights to improve access to reproductive health services. International Journal of Gynecology & Obstetrics. 2012;119(S1).
19. Sirkin S, Iacopino V, Grodin M, Danieli Y. The role of health professionals in protecting and promoting human rights: A paradigm for professional responsibility. The Universal Declaration of Human Rights: Fifty years and beyond. 1999: 357–66.
20. World Health Organization. WHO global strategy on people-centred and integrated health services: Interim report. World Health Organization; 2015.

19

Respectful Maternity Care

Hemantha Senanayake, Mohammed Rishard
Probodhana Ranaweera, Chandana Jayasundara

Sri Lanka is a lower middle-income country, whose healthcare system has been held out as a model for other developing countries. Its maternal mortality rate is the lowest in South Asia: According to the last estimates, the reported maternal mortality ratio (MMR) is relatively low (33.7/100 000). 99% from a predominantly rural-based economy to one that is urban oriented around manufacturing and services. Major progress has been made in maternal healthcare in past decades. However, no significant improvement in the MMR has been observed in the last 10 years. The leading causes of MMR have shifted from direct to indirect causes making respiratory and heart disease complicating pregnancy contributing mainly to MMR. Similarly, deaths from morbidly adherent placenta related complications are also rising reflecting the year-on-year of births occur with skilled attendance in a hospital setting, with a total of 85% delivering in a facility that has the services of a specialist obstetrician. Since the end of the civil war in 2009, the economy has grown on average at 6.2% per year, transiting increase in cesarean section rates, which has now reached 37%. Almost 80% of the deaths occurred in hospitals where specialized facilities are available thus suggesting possible gaps in the quality of care provided. Inappropriate practices are suggested also by other indicators, such as the rising rate of caesarean section (CS), peaking above 50% in selected facilities. The estimated rate of induction of labor in Sri Lanka is currently among the highest in Asia (35.5%), and the rate of inductions without medical indication is reported to be 27.8%. These observations suggest possible gaps in quality of care provided. There is a need for a shift from provision of care merely to reduce maternal mortality to one that addresses patient centered care provision that empowers the woman to obtain evidence-based quality care, which suits her needs. Although the level of care in general ensures safe delivery, issues in quality have much room for improvement.

SITUATION REGARDING RESPECTFUL CARE IN SRI LANKA

Most women in Sri Lanka will deliver in hospitals that have strong fundamentals that ensure safe delivery. There has been strong emphasis on safety that has borne results. Labor is conducted in labor wards where beds are usually separated by fabric curtains. Less than a handful of state sector hospitals will allow the facility of a labor companion and most Sri Lankan women will go through labor unaccompanied. A similar situation exists in visits to antenatal clinics, where the women will be seen by a doctor or other healthcare worker unaccompanied.

In the private sector however, allowing a labor companion is the norm and some hospitals will even allow a male partner to be present during cesarean section.

In 2018, the Ministry of Health issued circular encouraging healthcare facilities to allow a female labor companion. This has been observed more in the exception by providers, rather than in the affirmative.

The Problems with Abuse and Disrespect During Childbirth

Childbirth is a deeply emotional experience for women. These experiences could have potentially major short and long effects on a woman's well-being and relationships. While for some, birth will be a joyful, fulfilling experience, others will have experiences that result in post-traumatic stress disorder. The approach taken by the care providers will be a major determinant of these outcomes. For example, a care provider's prejudices regarding pain relief in labor could result in a woman having to endure a long labor without analgesia.

Modern obstetrics has tended to lay emphasis on making labor safe for mother and baby. From delivering at home supported by women from their social and family networks, women are being encouraged to deliver in hospital, to make childbirth safer. Undoubtedly, this has led to a reduction in maternal mortality due to childbirth related complications. However, this approach led to a situation where undermine the emotional aspects of labor, which is crucial for a woman's positive birth experience. Some countries are actively encouraging this shift to birth in hospital, offering incentives to mothers and to those who are accompanying them to hospital. In settings with high rates of home deliveries resulting in high maternal mortality rates due to suboptimal care, this would be an approach that is reasonable. However, in trying to achieve this objective, emotional aspects of labor, which are crucial for a woman's birth experience, have become sidelined.

Labor is unique from the care provider's perspective, in that women will remain totally dependent on their care providers during the process of giving birth.

Issues of gender inequality and provider prejudices could come into play during its course. In many geographic settings, women's lives are not valued and their well-being and quality of care received will receive low priority. Health systems may be institutionalizing and normalizing some of these anomalies. Authors have expressed concern regarding childbirth becoming 'dehumanized' across high, middle and low income countries. In general, it is the women of who are from lower socioeconomic strata who bear the brunt of this dehumanization, while women who are more empowered will enjoy a different birthing experience. There is great inequity in the care received by pregnant women even within countries.

As would be discussed later in this chapter, health care systems and leaders may be institutionalizing these anomalies.

Abuse and disrespect during birth could have major consequences for healthcare systems, particularly in settings where attempts are being increase hospital delivery rates. Women may opt not to deliver in a facility, based on previous experience of poor quality care, abuse or disrespect during childbirth.

Recent years have seen a great research interest in abuse and disrespect during childbirth, with 18 papers on the subject being published in the year 2018, from all over the world, including Sri Lanka. These describe disrespect and abuse ranging from physical to psychological violence. As mentioned earlier in this chapter, in the context of women being helpless disempowered and totally dependent on their care providers during labor, such eventualities are possible.

What is respectful maternity care?

As a means of addressing abuse and dis- respect, the concept of respectful maternity care (RMC) is being introduced. RMC is more than a mere absence of abuse and disrespect, but until recently, there has been no consensus regarding what constitutes it. Shakibazadeh et al., conducted a systematic review of 67 publications from 32 countries on RMC and came up with a qualitative synthesis of evidence to refine what this concept should include. They identified twelve domains in RMC, which are essentially third-order themes derived from a more detailed second order. The twelve domains are reproduced below. These were synthesized based on information provided by mothers and care providers.

Table 19.1: Twelve domains of respectful maternity care derived from the qualitative findings

Being free from harm and mistreatment
Maintaining privacy and confidentiality
Preserving women's dignity
Prospective provision of information and seeking informed consent
Ensuring continuous access to family and community support
Enhancing quality of physical environment and resources
Providing equitable maternity care
Engaging with effective communication
Respecting women's choices that strengthens their capabilities to given birth
Availability of competent and motivated human resources
Provision of efficient and effective care
Continuity of care

Source: Shakibazadeh et al.

These domains have a resemblance to the ten universal rights of women's healthcare identified by the FIGO (International Federation of Obstetrical & Gynecological Societies). The domains are interrelated, in the sense that if one is taken care of, others will automatically be taken care of. RMC also features prominently in the recent publication of the World Health Organization regarding Recommendations for a Positive Childbirth Experience, which emphases many of the domains.

RMC goes way beyond the mere absence of violence, mistreatment and abuse. For example, in the first domain, which refers to freedom from harm and mistreatment includes not using a loud voice and a professional approach. In the domain on maintaining privacy and confidentiality, women and care providers alike stated that awareness regarding this aspect was poor. Women appreciated ensuring privacy during examinations and procedures and limiting the number of personnel present in the labor ward as important. In the domain of preserving the woman's dignity, they appreciated feeling welcomed into the labor ward, kind attitudes, time spent with the woman, being calm, tactful, warm, smiling and caring. Being treated as 'persons' and avoidance of non-consented care were also considered important by women. Regarding prospective provision of information and seeking informed consent, women considered that taking consent prior to vaginal examinations as important. This underscores the fact that while care providers may consider such intimate examinations as 'routine' and an essential part of good care, that these procedures must not be taken for granted. These examinations and interventions must be considered major invasions of a woman's privacy and personal space. There is much that contributes to abuse and disrespect in labor that could be considered as being done in the name of good care, but the importance of participation of the woman in decision-making and consenting process cannot be overemphasized.

Person Centered Maternity Care (PCMC)—An Expansion of RMC

Person-centered maternity care (PCMC) is an overarching concept that that could supplement RMC. It is defined as "maternity care that is respectful of and responsive to individual women and their families' preferences, needs, and values".

The WHO recommendations for a positive childbirth experience emphasize RMC, effective communication, and companionship during labor and childbirth as key dimensions of PCMC that should be provided to every woman throughout labor and birth.

PCMC takes quality of care beyond merely ensuring safety of childbirth. Recent interim data from a baseline assessment of a quality improvement project in a tertiary care hospital in Sri Lanka shows that "person centered care"(PCMC) given in maternity wards falls short of satisfactory levels (Unpublished data, Rishard M).

PCMC was assessed with a questionnaire developed by Afulani, which was validated in India, using 30 items on three key domains: dignity and respect, communication and autonomy, supportive care. Each item has a four-point response scale, from 0 ("no, never") to 3 ("yes, all the time").

One hundred and twenty women who had a vaginal delivery participated in this study. The Afulani (PCMC) tool mean score was 41.7 (range 14–82, in a possible range between 0 and 90). For the dignity and respect domain, the mean score was 12.7 (range 5–21, versus a possible range 0–21). For communication and autonomy the mean score was 9.4 (range 2–23, versus a possible range 0–27). For supportive-care the mean score was 19.7 (range from 6–39, versus a possible range 0–42). This data, indicates that despite safety of childbirth being at a high level.

Can the Presence of a Labor Companion Address Issues of Disrespect and Abuse?

In many parts of the world including Sri Lanka, women will endure labor alone, being confined to a labor room. During the whole duration of labor, the only human contact women will have will be with care providers. In many settings in the developing world,

labor wards are out of bounds for persons from the mother's family or social circle. Historically, mothers have been supported during labor by other women from their social and family circle. With childbirth moving from home to hospital, the process has been made more sterile and devoid of social dimensions.

Shakibazadeh et al., found that some healthcare workers and most women considered continuous contact with the family as a basic human right. Its denial would constitute also an infringement of the principles of equity and woman or family-centered care. In settings where the norm is for mothers not to be allowed to have a companion during labor, others who are more privileged would be able to access this facility in private hospitals. In some societies, however, this facility will be denied to mothers in both the private and state sectors, based on social norms. Nevertheless, in most settings, denial of the facility of a labor companion (LC) would represent a violation of the principle of equity in healthcare.

It could be argued that the presence of a LC would be a safeguard against abuse and mistreatment during labor. It would convert a woman from being someone who is utterly helpless and totally dependent on care providers to one who is empowered.

Would the presence of a LC have benefits that go beyond mere companionship and empowerment? In fact, there has been much data regarding the effect of this intervention. It has been the subject of two Cochrane Reviews. These showed that the presence of a LC will increase the chances of a woman having a spontaneous vaginal birth and a shorter labor while lessening the requirement of labor analgesia, requirement of an operative delivery, chances of the woman reporting negative feelings regarding the childbirth experience and birth of a baby with low Apgar scores. Studies have shown also an improvement in breastfeeding after a mother has had an LC. In a review of interventions during labor, the American Journal of Obstetrics & Gynecology described a LC as one of the most effective interventions in labor. In some countries, the facility of a 'doula', a helper who provides nonmedical and informational support to laboring women. We found that the positive effects of a LC will still be preserved irrespective of whether the companion had training or not. While the WHO and other guidelines dealing with improving childbirth experience recommends allowing a companion of choice, in many developing countries, the infrastructure of labor wards will not be able to provide adequate privacy for a male partner to be present. However, other laboring women would probably find the presence of female companions acceptable even when the facilities to provide privacy are rudimentary. Our own experiences, in labor wards that allow little room between beds that are separated by fabric curtains, support this view.

The presence of a LC would result in improved empowerment of laboring women. This would compel the care providers to approach the woman in a more respectful way. This would then result in better communication, often cited as a shortcoming in healthcare settings in the developing world. Improvements in many other aspects of RMC would follow when a companion is present. Therefore, we could consider the presence of a LC as central to effectively executing respectful care.

It would be pertinent to inquire as to why despite evidence regarding benefits of allowing a LC, the practice is not followed in developing countries. In a study among Sri Lankan obstetricians, it was found that the knowledge of the obstetrician regarding the benefits of having a companion was a crucial factor in their decision to allow LCs in the labor wards as a policy. A higher workload, unwillingness of other staff and having to share the labor ward with another colleague were other factors that were associated with not allowing a LC.

How can RMC be Promoted?

Health care systems and providers in maternity care must begin to consider the client's experience of care. These aspects are hardly ever considered in developing countries. It is possible that improvements client satisfaction would result in improved outcomes as well. This could be true of all domains of RMC, with the allowing of a LC being probably the best example of improved outcomes resulting from improvement of client satisfaction.

Tools are available to assess client satisfaction in maternity care, which can be adapted to local settings for service evaluation. Gathering information regarding women's perspectives in institutions should be a driving force for administrators and clinicians to improve quality of care.

It is probable that healthcare workers of all categories have little knowledge of what RMC is and that it could improve outcomes. It is imperative that to improve this situation conducting in-service training and including these aspects in training must be done. Awareness must be created that obstetric interventions represent major invasions of a woman's privacy and that she has a right to autonomy, to privacy and to be involved in decision making regarding her health.

One of the problems that promotes disrespect and abuse in healthcare systems is the lack of awareness among care providers of the rights of the consumer, who in this case is the patient or mother. Creation of awareness is the only solution to this and curricula in schools could be a starting point.

As communication and use of good language is an important aspect in RMC, proficiency of minority languages should be made mandatory. In developed countries, certified interpreters are available but the norm in less privileged settings is that communication with them will happen via relatives or other staff whose prejudices may color the interpretations. Women from minorities with imitations communication with health care providers must be considered to be vulnerable to suboptimal outcomes. This problem is also reported from the developed world where minority groups are a risk group for maternal death.

A language guide should be introduced to help healthcare workers to communicate with clients in a culture-sensitive way and to instill a culture of using respectful words in communicating with pregnant women. Patient's satisfaction scores and feedback from clients should be used as a "key performance index" among all categories of health care workers.

Health care systems in developing countries must strive to break down barriers between health workers and clients by regular meetings and dialogues would help to minimize the paternalistic care and improve the RMC. In some respects, this may be very simple—as part of RMC as described by Shakibazadeh et al., women appreciated being welcomed into the labor ward. Health care professionals develop a professional identity in their training and sometimes this may go against effective communication. Many aspects of disrespect may arise from desensitization that arises from considering day-to-day activities as 'routine' rather than one that is a sentinel event for the client and her family.

Similarly, it would become important to re-examine day-to-day practices of care provision. In Sri Lanka and probably in many parts of the developing world, women will attend antenatal clinics in public hospital by themselves. However, if they were accompanied, the care would automatically become more respectful. This would even make the interaction of a better quality, since there would be more opportunities for clarifying doubts regarding instructions that are given.

Finally, a key aspect of promoting RMC is improving awareness among care providers. The importance of addressing this aspect by embedding these aspects in curricula cannot be overemphasized.

CONCLUSION

With medicalization of birth, many aspects of RMC have become sidelined. Globally, there is concern regarding dehumanization of birth. It is important for healthcare workers and systems to be sensitive to the fact that they may be helping to institutionalize such practices. These may be due to desensitization of care providers to the emotional aspects of day-to-day maternity care. Allowing a labor companion from the woman's social circle will go a long way towards addressing issues of disrespect and abuse. RMC also has the potential to improve physical outcomes of birth.

BIBLIOGRAPHY

1. Afulani PA, Diamond-Smith N, Golub G, Sudhinaraset M. Development of a tool to measure person-centered maternity care in developing settings: Validation in a rural and urban Kenyan population. Reprod Health. 2017;14:118.
2. Afulani PA, Phillips B, Aborigo R, Moyer CA. Person-centred maternity care in low-income and middleincome countries: analysis of data from Kenya, Ghana, and India. Lancet Glob Health 2019; 7: e96–109.
3. Berghella V, Baxter JK, Chauhan SP. Evidence-based labor and delivery management. Am J Obstet Gynecol. 2008 Nov;199(5):445–54. doi: 10.1016/j.ajog.2008.06.093.
4. Bohren MA, Hofmeyr G, Sakala C, Fukuzawa RK, Cuthbert A. Continuous support for women during childbirth. Cochrane Database of Systematic Reviews 2017, Issue 7. Art. No.: CD003766. DOI: 10.1002/14651858.CD003766. pub6
5. Bohren MA, Hunter EC, Munthe-Kaas HM et al. Facilitators and barriers to facility-based delivery in low-and middle-income countries: A qualitative evidence synthesis. Reprod Health. 2014 Sep19; 11(1):71. doi: 10.1186/1742-4755-11-71

6. Family Health Bureau Ministry of Health and Indigenous Medicine. Analyses of Maternal deaths 2015. 2014 http://fhb.health.gov.lk/web/index.ph p?option=com_phocadownload&vie w=category&id=40:maternal-childmorbidity-mortalitysurveillance& Itemid=150&lang=en# (Accessed 25 Jan 2019).

7. Family Health Bureau Ministry of Health and Indigenous Medicine. Analyses of Maternal deaths 2015. 2014 http://fhb.health.gov.lk/w eb/index.php?option=com_phocado wnload&view =category&id=40:mater nal-child-morbidity-mortalitysurveillance& Itemid=150&lang=en# (Accessed 25 Mar 2018).

8. Family Health Bureau. Health statistics. http://fhb.health.gov.lk/web/index.php?option=com_statistics&view=islan dwideallresult&Itemid =134&lang=en accessed 02 Feb 2019

9. Goonewardene M, Kumara DMA, Arachchi DRJ, et al. The rising trend in caesarean section rates: should we and can we reduce it? Sri Lanka Journal of Obstetrics and Gynaecology 2012;34:11–18. doi:10.4038/sljog.v34i1.4816

10. Hodnett ED, Gates D, Hofmeyr GJ, Sakala C. Continuous support for women during childbirth. Cochrane Database Syst Rev. 2013;7:CD003766

11. Hodnett ED, Gates D, Hofmeyr GJ, Sakala C. Continuous support for women during childbirth. Cochrane Database Syst Rev. 2013;7:CD003766

12. Martin CR, Martin CH, Redshaw M. The Birth Satisfaction Scale-Revised Indicator (BSS-RI). BMC Pregnancy and Childbirth. 2017; 17:277.

13. Maternal Death Surveillance and Response (MDSR) - outcomes of 2014. http://fhb.health.gov.lk/web/ind ex.php?option=com_phoca download&view=category&id=40:maternal child-morbidity-mortalitysurveillance& Itemid =150&lang=en#(Accessed 25 Mar 2018)

14. Perera D, Lund R, Swahnberg K et al. 'When helpers hurt': women's and midwives' stories of obstetric violence in state health institutions, Colombo district, Sri Lanka. BMC Pregnancy Childbirth. 2018 Jun 7;18(1):211. doi: 10.1186/s12884-018-1869-z.

15. Senanayake H, Goonewardene M, Ranatunga A, et al., Achieving Millennium Development Goals 4 and 5 in Sri Lanka. BJOG. 2011;118(Suppl 2): 78–87.

16. Senanayake H, Wijesinghe RD, Nayar K. Is the policy of allowing a female labor companion feasible in developing countries? Results from a cross sectional study among Sri Lankan practitioners. BMC Pregnancy Childbirth. 2017; 17(1):392. doi: 10.1186/s12884- 017-1578-z)

17. Senanayake HM, Somawardana U, Samarasinghe M. The effect of a female labor companion and the effect of educating her regarding support during labor on perinatal and labor outcomes. Sri Lanka Journal of Obstetrics and Gynaecology. 2014;35 (4):112–5.

18. Shakibazadeh E, Namadian M, Bohren MA, et al. Respectful care during childbirth in health facilities globally: a qualitative evidence synthesis. BJOG 2018;125:932–42.

19. The World Bank. Sri Lanka overview. http://www.worldbank.org/en/country/srilanka/overview (Accessed 02 Feb 2019).

20. Unicef Sri Lanka. Statistics. https://www.unicef.org/info bycountry/sri_lanka_statistics. html#1 22 (Accessed 23 Mar 2018).

21. Vogel JP, Souza JP, Gülmezoglu AM et al. Patterns and Outcomes of Induction of Labour in Africa and Asia: a secondary analysis of the WHO Global Survey on Maternal and Neonatal Health. PLoSOne 2013;8:e65612. doi:10.1371/journal.pone.0065612

22. World Health Organization. WHO recommendations: intrapartum care for a positive childbirth experience. WHO. 2018; [cited 2018 Feb 28]. Available from: http://www.who.int/reproductive-health/publications/intrapartum-careguidelines/en/

Looking for Solutions?
The Way Forward

Rubina Sohail, Mariam Iqbal, Asifa Naureen

The South Asian region, accounts for around one-fourth of the world's population, two-thirds poor people, and around half of the illiterate adult population. It is one of the most fast growing, poor regions of the world where there is rampant illiteracy and malnourishment and lacks gender sensitivity making it one of the most deprived regions of the world. Women constitute 48.45 % of the population of south Asia (2016).

The issues in South Asia have a huge impact on the world. The region needs education, prosperity, security and an urgent need to address problems related to women and adolescents. The women related issues and violation of their sexual and reproductive rights need to be addressed on a war footing. No single step can bring about a change. It needs a multidisciplinary integrated approach over a number of years. Only then can we witness a substantial change in women's health and rights. Over the last two decades, work has been done in South Asia to reduce maternal and neonatal mortality with focus on three delays, skilled birth attendant, improved antenatal care, and there has been a reasonable improvement in these parameters. However, the cross cutting issue of sexual and reproductive rights has not been addressed appropriately in South Asia.

Time is ripe for South Asia to change its mindset, and an aggressive campaign needs to be initiated for improving sexual and reproductive rights, leading to improvement in women's health. Developmental partners and WHO have put their weight behind the issue but lasting change will need a firm government commitment, concrete steps in place for behavior change, transformation in society attitudes towards women, self-awareness in women and most importantly change in attitudes of the health care provider to become the catalysts of change themselves. Not only can the health care providers identify women in distress, but can also provide in patient care, integrate human rights in daily practice and implement rights in true sense of the word.

This chapter aims at highlighting the measures that can be taken to safeguard the physical, mental, social and psychological well-being of the women. This is only possible, if we the physicians, are able to play our roles in safeguarding the interest of women in terms of sexual and reproductive rights.

South Asia Facts

Current population –South Asia	1,906,520,522 (Thursday, March 7, 2019: Latest United Nations estimates)
Proportion of total world population	24.81%
Population density in South Asia	299 per km² (774 people per mi²)
Total land area	6,400,127 km² (2,471,102 sq. miles)
Urban population	35.9 % (687,617,321 people in 2019)

One of the cardinal reasons for these women related issues is the pervasive gender inequality which is a global issue but rampant in South Asia. Over the years, women in South Asia have suffered silently from gender based discrimination. Unfortunately, communities, religious leaders, families and the governments, have not done enough in this regard.

SOLUTIONS—GENERAL MEASURES

Environment at home The social and cultural norms of Asian societies are very difficult to modify. Therefore, changing their mindset is one of the most challenging steps. A stringent behavior change campaign is the need of the hour. Media can be an important tool for this behavioral change. Right from the birth of a girl, nurturing her at home, providing a conducive environment, giving her the same food variety, equal opportunities for education are important steps that need to be taken. The elders should have a positive conversation with emphasis on health, safe sexuality and respect for women with these vulnerable growing up teenagers. Discussions with adolescents about myths about rape, how to set boundaries for sexual activity, and differentiating between sex, and violence should be done. Parents need to nurture a more gender balanced environment and prevent stereotyping of gender roles.

- **Awareness at community level:** An environment with gender equality and respect for women rights has to be promoted through awareness, training of young boys and girls and adolescents and community support. Notions of masculinity that frame sexual aggression as a strong or *admirable quality for men needs to be discouraged and derided.*

The involvement of elders or influential persons in community to create awareness can be a useful tool. In Asian societies religious leaders, community heads, politicians and elders of a community really influence minds of people around them. They can play a vital role in creating an environment of respect for women. Public figures, charismatic personalities and popular media stars should act as role models and help in creating awareness against violence.

- **Education:** Girls should get equal opportunities for education as boys. In schools focus on ensuring that the girls develop confidence in their abilities, teaching them self-defence, life-skills and other educational programs for sexual and reproductive health promotion, like HIV prevention and gender issues go a long way. Sexual education should be part of school and college curriculum and made a part of teaching and assessment. Teachers, mentors and parents need to teach young children and adolescents, especially boys about consent, and what to do if someone does not give consent. Children in school should be taught concept of good and bad touching using age appropriate material and language and enhance their ability and confidence to take control over their own bodies.

- **Media:** The power of media can never be underestimated in bringing about societal change, Media can play an important role in reducing the culture of rape and violence through advertising on hoardings ("billboards") and in public transport, and on radio and television. Media needs to stop objectifying females. Media that dehumanizes women by treating them as sex objects contributes to rape and violence culture.

Social media in this region has also attracted a large audience and can be an effective modality to create awareness. Educational and awareness programs for communities, schools and refugee camps should be designed and culturally sensitive and participatory approach should be used to change mindsets and behavior.

- **Women empowerment and job opportunities:** Unfortunately, Pakistan has the lowest variables of empowerment with estimated education of only around 2.4 years, economic participation of only twenty-three percent (in 2007). Bangladesh and Afghanistan have similar statistics, which is no surprise as cultural similarities within the region include men being the head of the family who takes all the decisions, where women merely follow; polygamy is allowed for men and women are either denied inheritance or are given half. These biases are mostly cultural norms and some use religion to justify them. South Asia is also way behind other regions in political empowerment, which is judged by the number of women in parliament and percentage of women in legislature. The sky rocketing crime rate against women, especially rape and other forms of gender violence also points to poor state of empowerment in the region, hence, it is evident how women are marginalized in South Asian society.

The only way forward in this regard is to empower the girls and women so they can stand up for their rights and protect themselves. Empowerment can only be achieved when girls have an improved access to quality education, financial independence and when they are given a voice in society, all three of which are interrelated as quality education will translate into better job opportunities and an automatic financial independence and standing in society. Women's economic contribution can only be ensured if they are provided with a favorable and safe working environment, women friendly, respectful work places and better labour laws. Right to inheritance and property rights are essential for continued progress in women's empowerment.

SOLUTIONS—SPECIFIC MEASURES

- **Political Will:** A strong political will and government commitment is necessary to promote and protect women's rights and to eliminate discrimination against women.
- **Laws and Implementation:** There is a need to translate recommendations into national laws and policies and to ensure implementation of these laws. All countries in South Asia have laws against domestic violence, but fail to translate these laws into practices. Nearly all laws exclude unmarried intimate partner's violence. There is limited awareness among women about laws pertaining to violence, which hinders women's legal protection. As an example in Pakistan, there is a strong legal framework exists. However, there is limited awareness amongst the general public. These include the Punjab Protection of Women against Violence Act (2016), Domestic Violence (prevention and protection) Act (2013), Acid Control and Acid Crime Prevention Act (2010), and the Protection Against Harassment of Women at the Workplace Act (2010).

Laws which are not women friendly, like 'Zina Ordinance' and the 'Qunan-e-Shahdat' should be amended ensure equal rights of women and equal importance to their testimony.

- **Preventing child marriages:** To avoid child marriages, increasing the age of marriage from 18–21 years of age is recommended and should come up as a legislative change.
- **Multisectoral response:** There is need to implement a multisectoral response to urgently address gender-based violence against women and girls across this diverse region. A collaborative and synchronized response is needed in every country, so that a concrete guidance is available, building on existing standards and applies to the health,

social services, police, and justice sectors, as well as to overall governance and coordination. There is need for survivor centered approach and care, with involvement of social workers. A coordinated approach is followed with strengthening the capacity of police, health and justice department workers. This includes providing integrated health and counseling services, legal aid, and economic opportunities. Framework should be implemented that promotes the integration of women's rights into all government sectors.

- Women friendly police stations: There is a need to create a safe and reliable environment at police stations to maximize reporting as women fear "slut-shaming" and victim-blaming. A way forward could be women friendly police stations where women feel safe. There is an urgent need for encouraging people to report incidents of sexual violence to the police and to improve the swiftness and sensitivity of the processing of cases by the courts.

- One stop crisis centers: *Centers providing comprehensive care to victims of sexual assault.* There is a need for specialized centers to provide specialized multidisciplinary care. One such solution could be ''One-Stop Crisis Centre''. The first of this kind of centre was established in 1993 in the accident and emergency department of Kuala Lumpur Hospital in Malaysia. The centre comprises experts from the hospital, women's groups, the police, medical social workers, the legal advisors and the Islamic Religious Bureau. Similarly India, Bangladesh, Pakistan have one stop crisis centers. However, the number may still not be optimal. In India it happened as an aftermath of the Delhi incident of rape of the medical student.

- *Providing Counseling, Support: Psychiatrist, psychosocial* support groups consisting of social workers, physicians, lawyer, police officers, community, women and

adolescents. The importance of counseling and support group initiatives in rehabilitation, cannot be emphasized enough.

Brief cognitive behavioral therapy has shown to be a promising tool of healing, if given in a short period of time. Mostly in South Asian countries these services are provided by NGOs and women organizations. However, the number of women who have access to these therapies is small and especially not in rural or far flung areas. A solution to overcome this barrier could be establishing free of charge helplines. This would also help women who cannot access facilities and do not want to face anyone and rather talk on the phone from the comfort of their home where they probably feel more secure. Many such helplines and NGOs exist in some of the countries but are definitely a few when compared to the magnitude of the problem.

- **Role of health care systems:** Training of health care professionals is an essential solution as issues concerning sexual violence are sensitive issues which should only be dealt by trained personnel. Health care providers should be able to detect early signs of violence and the steps that they need to proceed further with the issue. They need skills to give support and level of compassionate care to these women. Training should be a part of undergraduate and postgraduate curricula of doctors, nurse and affiliated personnel. Specialized counselors should be trained. These trainings should enable these providers to detect and handle cases of sexual violence in a sensitive but efficient manner.

- **Health care responses:** Health care providers should be trained to integrate sexual and reproductive rights in daily practice. Timely and appropriate management of violence and assault victims is essential. At times, the safety and forensic issues surrounding sexual assault can create clinician anxiety, resulting in delay in the administration of appropriate medical care. A 'survivor-centred approach' should be adopted when examining them which involves respecting woman's autonomy to choose treatment and even report the case. The woman's safety is most important and there should be no discrimination when being examined. The health professionals dealing with this vulnerable group should be non-judgmental and empathetic. The victims right to confidentiality should be the highest priority. There is a need to have and follow standard protocols and guidelines which would translate into considerably improved quality of care and psychological support of affected women.

Examination of a rape victim is a sensitive and stressful situation. Adequate reassurance to the victim and explanation of procedure. Documentation of full physical examination preferably using a diagrammatic documentation for ease of site of injuries/lacerations needs to be done. Some countries use the *"sexual assault evidence kit"* that carries instructions, appropriate containers for collecting evidence, relevant legal forms and documents for recording histories.

Assessment of the risk of pregnancy should be done and emergency contraception should be provided. Testing and treating sexually transmitted diseases and give hepatitis B and HIV prophylaxis is important.

Women in crisis need special attention and it is the physician's job to safeguard women patients sexual and reproductive rights. Ideally she should be examined in a private place where conversation cannot be overheard or interrupted and language and cultural norms of the women need to be subscribed to, by the health care personnel.

- **International collaborations:** International treaties are important as they set standards for national legislation and provide a lever for local groups to campaign for legal reforms.

Many international organizations like WHO has designed strategies to bring reforms in countries in the region. UNHCR also helped in especially reducing rape being used as a war weapon. All NGOs, international organizations, government and nongovernmental organizations, should prioritize reproductive health as one of the key health services included in the planning, coordination, funding, implementation, and monitoring and evaluation of activities for their projects.

CONCLUSION

All efforts need to be made to make the world safe and equitable for the women of South Asia region.

TEN STEPS TO IMPROVE—SUMMARY

1. Empowerment of women
2. Training of healthcare professionals, police and lawyers
3. Reforms in current law to make it women friendly
4. Better reporting facilities with adequate collection of data
5. Women-only police stations
6. Awareness campaigns
7. Community involvement
8. Active role of government
9. Adequate counseling and rehabilitation of victims
10. Collaboration with NGOs and international organization

ASKING ABOUT VIOLENCE

Here are some statements you can make to raise the subject of violence before you ask direct questions:

- "Many women experience problems with their husband or someone else they live with."

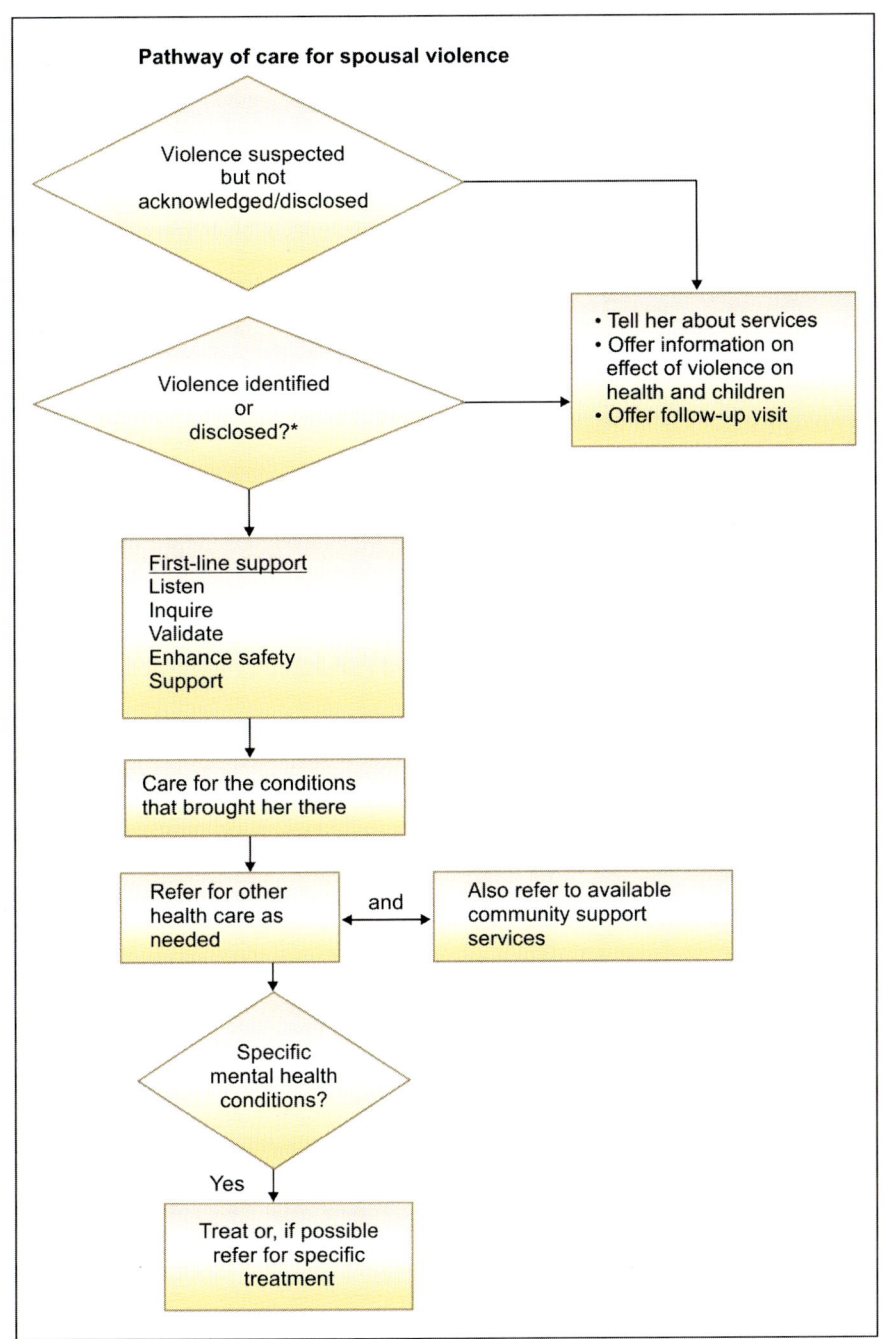

Pathway of care for spousal violence

Violence suspected but not acknowledged/disclosed

- Tell her about services
- Offer information on effect of violence on health and children
- Offer follow-up visit

Violence identified or disclosed?*

First-line support
Listen
Inquire
Validate
Enhance safety
Support

Care for the conditions that brought her there

Refer for other health care as needed — **and** — Also refer to available community support services

Specific mental health conditions?

Yes

Treat or, if possible refer for specific treatment

*Some women may need emergency care for injuries. Follow standard emergency procedures.

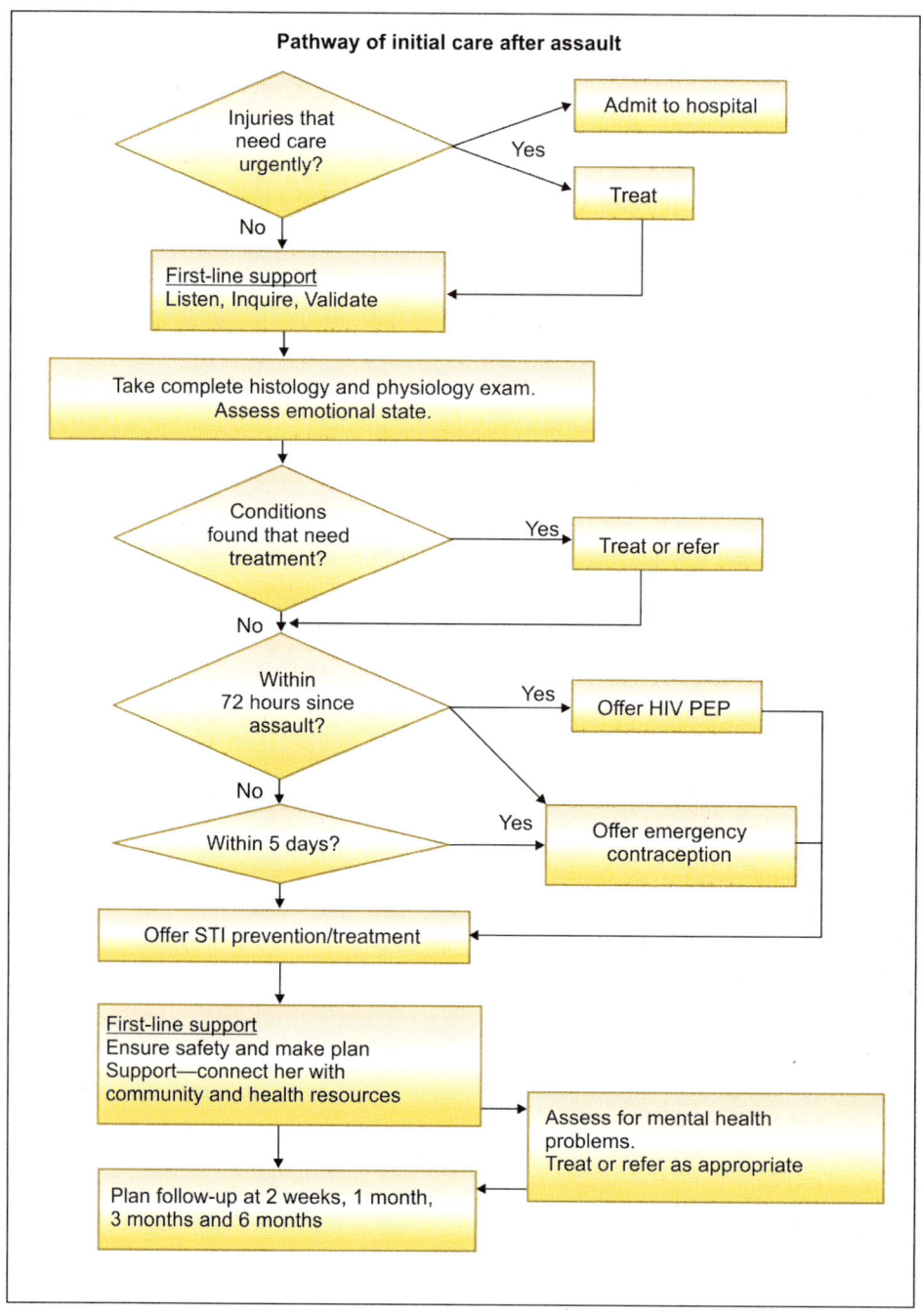

Pathway of initial care after assault

- "I have seen women with problems like yours who have been experiencing trouble at home."

Here are some simple and direct questions that you can start with that show you want to hear about her problems. Depending on her answers, continue to ask questions and listen to her story. If she answers "yes" to any of these questions, offer her first-line support.

"Are you afraid of your husband?"

"Has your husband or someone else at home ever threatened to hurt you or physically harm you in some way? If so, when has it happened?' "Does your husband or someone at home bully you or insult you? "Does your husband try to control you, for example, not letting you have money or go out of the house?' "Has your husband forced you into sex or forced you to have any sexual contact you did not want?" "Has your husband threatened to beat and kill you?"

First-line support involves 5 simple tasks. It responds to both emotional and practical needs at the same time. The letters in the word "LIVES" can remind you of these 5 tasks that protect survivors's lives:

Listen	Listen to the woman closely, with empathy, and without judging.
Inquire about need and concerns	Assess and respond to her various needs and concerns—emotional, physical, social and practical (e.g. childcare)
Validate	Show her that you understand and believe her. Assure her that she is not to blame.
Enhance safety	Discuss a plan to protect herself from further harm if violence occurs again
Support	Support her by helping her connect to information, services and social support.

BIBLIOGRAPHY

1. Apart LB. Lives Blown Apart: Crimes Against Women in Times of Conflict, London: Amnesty International Publications 2004.
2. Barbara Rodriguez, Sofia Shakil, Adrian Morel. Four Things to Know About Gender-Based Violence in Asia. March 14, 2018.
3. Chaudhuri S. Women's empowerment in South Asia and Southeast Asia: A comparative analysis.
4. Factsheet August 30, 2018 Factsheet: Update on Addressing Gender-Based Violence in Development Projects
5. Foa EB, Hearst-Ikeda D, Perry KJ. Evaluation of a brief cognitive behavioral program for the prevention of chronic PTSD in recent assault victims. Journal of consulting and clinical psychology. 1995;63(6):948.
6. Foubert JD, Newberry JT, Tatum J. Behavior differences seven months later: Effects of a rape prevention program. NASPA Journal. 2007;44(4): 728–49.
7. Hagen K, Yohani S. The nature and psychosocial consequences of war rape for individuals and communities. International journal of psychological studies. 2010;2(2):14–25.
8. http://www.unwomen.org/en/whatwe-do/ending-violence-againstwomen/facts-and-figures
9. Nelasco S. A Study on Women Empowerment in South-Asian Countries: A Contemporary Analysis. In Book of Proceedings 2012 Sep 4 (p. 20).
10. Sharma I. Violence against women: Where are the solutions? Indian journal of psychiatry. 2015; 57(2):131.
11. The United Nations Office on Drugs and Crime (UNODC) by the Wednesday, June 28, 2017 [Press Release]
12. UNICEF (2017). A Familiar Face: Violence in the lives of children and adolescents, p. 73, 82.
13. United Nations Office on Drugs and Crime (2018). Global Study on Homicide 2018, p. 10.
14. UNODC (2016). Global Report on Trafficking in Persons 2016, p. 7, 28.
15. WHO Clinical Hand Book for Health Care for survivors of Gender Based Violence in Pakistan.
16. WHO global plan of action on health systems response to violence against women and girls.

17. Winzer L, Krahé B, Guest P. The scale of sexual aggression in southeast Asia: A review. Trauma, Violence, & Abuse. 2017 Jan 1:1524838017725312

18. World Bank Group (2018). Women, Business and the Law 2018, database

19. World Health Organization, Department of Reproductive Health and Research, London School of Hygiene and Tropical Medicine, South African Medical Research Council (2013). Global and regional estimates of violence against women: prevalence and health effects of intimate partner violence and non-partner sexual violence, p. 2. For individual country information, see The World's Women 2015, Trends and Statistics, Chapter 6, Violence against Women, United Nations Department of Economic and Social Affairs, 2015 and UN Women Global Database on Violence against Women.

Index